Carol W

Restorative Care:
Fundamentals for Certified Nursing Assistants

Barbara Acello, MS, RN

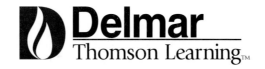

Africa • Australia • Canada • Denmark • Japan • Mexico • New Zealand • Phillipines
Puerto Rico • Singapore • Spain • United Kingdom • United States

NOTICE TO THE READER

Delmar Staff

Business Unit Director: William Brottmiller
Developmental Editor: Marjorie A. Bruce
Executive Marketing Manager: Dawn Gerrain
Channel Manager: Nicole L. Benson

Project Editor: Stacey Prus
Production Coordinator: John Mickelbank
Art/Design Coordinator: Mary Colleen Liburdi
Cover Design: TDB Publishing Service

COPYRIGHT © 2000
Delmar is a division of Thomson Learning. The Thomson Learning logo is a registered trademark used herein under license.

Printed in the United States of America
2 3 4 5 6 7 8 9 10 XXX 05 04 03 02 01 00

For more information contact Delmar, 3 Columbia Circle, PO Box 15015, Albany, NY 12212-0515; or find us on the World Wide Web at http://www.delmar.com

International Division List

Asia
Thomson Learning
60 Albert Street, #15-01
Albert Complex
Singapore 189969
Tel: 65 336 6411
Fax: 65 336 7411

Japan
Thomson Learning
Palaceside Building 5F
1-1-1 Hitotsubashi, Chiyoda-ku
Tokyo 100 0003 Japan
Tel: 813 5218 6544
Fax: 813 5218 6551

Australia/New Zealand
Nelson/Thomson Learning
102 Dodds Street
South Melbourne, Victoria 3205
Australia
Tel: 61 39 685 4111
Fax: 61 39 685 4199

UK/Europe/Middle East
Thomson Learning
Berkshire House
168-173 High Holborn
London
WC1V 7AA United Kingdom
Tel: 44 171 497 1422
Fax: 44 171 497 1426

Thomas Nelson & Sons LTD
Nelson House
Mayfield Road
Walton-on-Thames
KT 12 5PL United Kingdom
Tel: 44 1932 2522111
Fax: 44 1932 246574

Latin America
Thomson Learning
Seneca, 53
Colonia Polanco
11560 Mexico D.F. Mexico
Tel: 525-281-2906
Fax: 525-281-2656

South Africa
Thomson Learning
Zonnebloem Building
Constantia Square
P.O. Box 2459
Halfway House, 1685
South Africa
Tel: 27 11 805 4819
Fax: 27 11 805 3648

Canada
Nelson/Thomson Learning
1120 Birchmount Road
Scarborough, Ontario
Canada M1K 5G4
Tel: 416-752-9100
Fax: 416-752-8102

Spain
Thomas Learning
Calle Magallanes, 25
28015-MADRID
ESPANA
Tel: 34 91 446 33 50
Fax: 34 91 445 62 18

International Headquarters
Thomas Learning
International Division
290 Harbor Drive, 2nd Floor
Stamford, CT 06902-7477
Tel: 203-969-8700
Fax: 203-969-8751

Library of Congress Cataloging-in-Publication Data
Acello, Barbara.
    Restorative care: Fundamentals for certified nursing assistants / Barbara
Acello.
       p. cm.
    Includes bibliographical references and index.
    ISBN 0–8273–8141–7
    1. Rehabilitation nursing. 2. Nurse's aides. I. Title.
    [DNLM: 1. Rehabilitation Nursing—methods. 2. Nurses' Aides.
3. Long-Term Care. WY 150.5 A173r 1999]
RT120.R4A25 1999
610.73'6—dc21
DNLM/DLC   99–17380
for Library of Congress: CIP

Contents

Foreword

It is not unusual to hear the phrase, "It takes a very special person to be a nursing assistant." This is so true, but it takes more than good intentions to truly do the right thing for residents. Sometimes what we think is the best course of action can, over time, bring harm to a person's overall health and well being. For example, it may seem kind to "wait" on a person in a nursing facility as if they were in a hotel, handing them things outside their immediate reach to save them from getting out of a chair, making their bed, dusting their room, bringing them a pan of warm water with which to wash so they will not have to get up and go to the sink. These are all things we may do for a hospital patient who has just had a procedure that makes it impossible for him or her to get out of bed, but to complete a task for anyone who can do any part of that task for themselves is actually unkind. Restorative nursing is kind.

A long-term care facility is the home of its residents. They *reside* there; they are not *patients*. What would they be doing if they lived in their own home? They may have different degrees of independence, so we must experiment to help them discover what they can and cannot do, then allow them to maintain their self-esteem and dignity by encouraging them to do those things for themselves for as long as possible. If they are capable of doing at least part of their bath, allow them however much time it takes to do that part. You finish the rest. This is restorative nursing.

Getting every bed made and everyone's bath completed by 9 AM should not be the priority of the morning. Yes, schedules must be followed or there would be total chaos, but not to the detriment of a human being's self-esteem and his or her need to feel they still have a purpose in life—a reason for living. Allowing the resident to make the bed is restorative nursing. It may not be as neatly made as if a staff member had done it, and it may take longer, but the resident is showing a degree of independence for which he or she feels worthwhile. Considering the residents' self-esteem and independence is restorative nursing.

Let us not forget that the resident's room is the only home the resident has, and we should respect their home. Never enter their room without knocking first, whether you think they can hear you or not. Knocking is a sign of respect. Respecting residents' rights is restorative nursing.

Never begin to do something for a person unless you have first told them what you are about to do. Informing the resident of your actions may help prevent fear. This is simple common courtesy. This is restorative nursing.

Use common sense and always think a situation through to the end results—to what the long-term outcome will be. This is restorative nursing.

You will be required to follow guidelines wherever you work, but you can suggest ideas that might benefit the people in your facility. All care plans should be based on Restorative Nursing Concepts, and all caregivers are invited to offer input. Be creative. Suggest ideas to help residents feel they are able to help themselves and others in some way. Always remember to thank the residents and praise all their efforts. This is restorative nursing.

Allowing and encouraging people to do as much as possible for themselves provides exercise. This keeps the muscles toned and enhances the blood circulation carrying vital nutrients and oxygen to all parts of the body, including the brain. Range of motion movement keeps their joints mobile. In just the last several years we have made huge strides in understanding the corrective measures of restoring range of motion. It is vital that nursing assistants are taught that contractures are 100% preventable and contractures resulting from immobility are correctable—at least to varying degrees. The time frame is hard to determine but we know that astounding improvements can be achieved in a relatively short time. This is restorative nursing.

The effect on staff and other residents is astounding when they see a man walk on straight legs who once spent all of his time in a wheelchair because he had been allowed to develop knee contractures. Unless a contracture is totally rock hard (very few are, but may appear that way because of neurological conditions as a result of brain injury commonly seen after a stroke, closed head injury, or from birth) the angle of that joint has the potential to be increased. However, it takes more than just range of motion exercises. The area must be massaged, slowly stretched *just to the point of resistance,* then a dynamic type of orthotic device must be placed on the joint at that degree. Because the dynamic device is flexible, it allows the patient to pull the joint inward in flexion, then the device pulls the joint back to extension, allowing the patient to do their own range of motion exercise and stretching. Once the desired extension is achieved, the resident must remain on a maintenance program to prevent the re-injury of the muscles and tendons reshortening. This is restorative nursing.

Everyone who works a night shift in any type of medical or nursing facility must remember that even though it is your time to work, for everyone who lives there, it is time to sleep. It is all too common for a nursing home to be as brightly lit at midnight as it is at noon, and the 11–7 staff is just as loud as those during the day. If ice is passed at 4 AM, you can hear the noise from anywhere in the facility. Nursing staff need to understand sleep patterns. If a resident does not have long enough sleep cycles, it can lead to disorientation that might not be recognized as a correctable condition caused by the environment of the nursing home. It often results in an inappropriate diagnosis and medication that may sedate or be otherwise harmful for the person. Understanding rest and sleep cycles, and promoting regular sleep is restorative nursing.

Never make anyone wait to go to the bathroom. Not only is this inhumane and humiliating for the person, but it can also damage the body's way of telling them that they need to empty their bowel or bladder. Elimination procedures are an important part of restorative nursing.

Human touch should be one of the most important and easiest things we do for residents. Just knowing another human being cares and is near can make a world of difference. Can you imagine never being hugged or touched? Just being at eye-level with someone and laying your hand on theirs when you are talking to them can mean a lot. This is restorative nursing.

Most of the elderly have reached a mature relationship with a higher power, and religion is very important to them. Whether you are a religious person or not, you must respect their beliefs. There may be a time when they are upset and lonely and their need is not for medicine, but just to have someone with whom to pray or who will take the time to sit down and patiently listen to whatever they need to say. Listening is restorative nursing.

People are moved to a nursing facility because they have lost something. Perhaps it is a loss of independence after an accident or because of physical or mental decline; perhaps it is the loss of a spouse or primary caregiver. When they move to a nursing facility, we put them in a room with a total stranger with whom they may or may not be compatible. They must eat the food we serve them after someone else has decided whether they can eat the foods they like and have always eaten—food that makes them feel secure. They must eat when we tell them to, no matter when they were used to eating. They are told when they will get up (or we make so much noise that we awaken them) and when they will go to bed. They are told when they will be bathed. Respecting residents' rights to make choices and control their own routines is restorative nursing.

People cannot lie in bed or a reclined geri-chair too much and be healthy. It adversely affects every organ and system of the body, including the skin—increasing the potential for bedsores. Adequate fluid intake is vital for the entire body, not just the kidneys and bowels. Confusion can result from not having enough fluids in the body, therefore creating an electrolyte imbalance. Preventing pressure sores and dehydration are restorative nursing.

Repositioning is important, not just to prevent bedsores, but also for comfort. Can you sit in a car for three hours without becoming uncomfortable? Imagine someone who cannot change their position because of their arthritic joints. They are forced to sit or lie hour after hour with no one thinking to even take their hands to allow the person to pull on them, slightly shifting their weight and bringing some relief. Repositioning residents and making them comfortable is restorative nursing.

When you go home at the end of a shift after working as a caregiver, confident that you have done your best to meet the needs of those in your charge, and that you have made a difference in someone's life, you will know that all of your hard work is well worthwhile. This is restorative nursing.

The most important lesson you can ever learn is to protect people's dignity, and that without quality of care, there is no quality of life! This is what restorative nursing care is all about! You are taking a gigantic step into advancing your career, and improving the quality of life of the residents you care for. Godspeed in your work. This book will help you to attain your personal and professional goals. Using the information herein will improve the quality of care you deliver. Spread the word to others! Restorative nursing care is considerate, compassionate care that truly benefits the residents. You will receive a great deal of satisfaction in seeing changes in your residents. You will be gratified knowing that you made a difference in the lives of many residents in your facility. The restorative nursing assistant is an advanced care provider. This book provides you with sensitive, holistic information that will open doors in your career. You may sometimes feel frustrated, but be persistent in your studies and in your work. The rewards will far outweigh the negatives. Immense personal satisfaction is a benefit of providing restorative nursing!

Karen Bonn, RN
Restorative Medical, Inc.
Brandenburg, Kentucky

Preface

▰▰ INTRODUCTION

For years, health care providers have trained nursing assistants to work as rehabilitation or restorative aides. Medicare reimbursements to facilities began changing in 1998. The change in reimbursement is being phased in gradually, until all Medicare certified nursing facilities are being reimbursed under the new program called PPS (prospective payment system). This change in reimbursement has significantly affected long-term care facility care and increased the demand for trained, qualified restorative nursing assistants. It has caused some facilities to expand restorative nursing assistants' responsibilities.

Evolution of Restorative Nursing

Restorative nursing has evolved and developed into a specialty area over the past 25 years. This is particularly true in the long-term care setting, in which facilities follow the requirements of the Omnibus Budget Reconciliation Act (OBRA) of 1987. The OBRA '87 laws place a major emphasis on restorative care. Theoretically, all nursing care should be restorative in nature. Restorative care is the nuts and bolts of nursing. It is just plain, good nursing care! A major emphasis of restorative nursing is resident independence and positive self-esteem. Interestingly, these are also two of the founding principles of the OBRA laws.

As we approach the twenty-first century, the role of the restorative nursing assistant is increasing in importance in the long-term care industry. Before the OBRA '87 laws, we used the medical model of care, in which we looked only at the resident's medical condition. Long-term care has evolved so that we now look at the resident as a whole. This change has been very beneficial to residents, but it has increased the restorative assistant's responsibilities. Assisting licensed nurses and therapists, encouraging residents, making observations, trying various approaches, and reporting the effectiveness of these approaches is an integral part of the restorative nursing assistant's job. The long-term care industry has changed immensely.

Restorative nursing care involves seeing the resident as a whole person with many strengths and weaknesses. These strengths and weaknesses must be considered when developing and implementing programs to meet the needs of each resident. Weaknesses must be considered because they affect the whole person. Strengths can be developed or maximized to compensate for weaknesses. The emphasis of care is on the resident's ability, and not his or her disability. Programs designed to maintain the resident's current level of function, preventing declines, are also restorative in nature. Providers of restorative care believe in this type of nursing and know that it works. They spread their philosophy to their coworkers. Long-term care facilities that provide active restorative programs have higher percentages of residents who return to their own homes. Resident and staff attitudes are positive about the outcome of restorative nursing care.

▰▰ WHY THIS BOOK WAS WRITTEN

This book was written to meet a need identified by long-term care facilities. For the most part, restorative nursing assistant training has been given as one-to-one instruction from a licensed therapist or nurse, or on-the-job training. There are a limited number of formal training programs. Learning and reference material for the restorative nursing assistant is scarce. Often, references are photocopies of material from nursing and therapy textbooks, or materials written for other health care providers.

The United States is a diverse country. The laws governing nursing assistant education and practice vary in each state. Likewise, the role of the nursing assistant and restorative nursing assistant varies widely from one long-term care facility to the next. Since there is no requirement for formal training or certification of the restorative nursing assistant, we have tried to take a middle of the road approach in this book. We have provided brief information on subjects in which the restorative nursing assistant normally has little exposure. We have placed more emphasis on subjects that the restorative nursing assistant will deal with frequently. Overall, the emphasis of the text is on holistic resident care.

▰▰ PREREQUISITES

This book was developed to meet the needs of the nursing assistant who practices as a restorative or rehabilitative nursing assistant. The book is designed for experienced nursing assistants who have completed the basic nursing assistant program and passed the state certification test. Restorative training is, essentially, an advanced, specialized level of training. Completing a restorative nursing assistant class and delivering restorative care is something to be proud of! We have used the term restorative, because it reflects the emphasis on nursing practice, instead of rehabilitative, which emphasizes therapy. Nevertheless, some nursing assistants fill a dual role, working in both disciplines. We have tried to address dual responsibilities, whenever applicable, in the text.

We assume that the restorative nursing assistant is familiar with the basic concepts of being a nursing assistant. Very little basic information is provided here. The purpose of this text is to supply new information about restorative nursing. It is designed to assist the student in becoming a strong restorative clinician. This is an advanced text that prepares highly qualified assistants to deliver restorative care!

Selecting the Content

Writing a text for restorative nursing assistants has been a challenging task. We are treading in uncharted waters. This is largely because there are no certification or training requirements for this important caregiver. Qualifications and training vary from one facility to another. The material in the book was selected by assessing facility needs in various states. However, the scope and depth of practice vary widely. In some states, certain tasks cannot be performed by unlicensed caregivers. All of the procedures in this book are being used by restorative nursing assistants in the United States. Your instructor will adjust the material to the meet the needs of your facility and your state. In some states, all of the material will be applicable. In others, only part of the material will apply.

We recognize that terminology varies in different health care settings, and regionally throughout the United States. The terms "patient," "resident," and "client" refer to the recipient of health care. These terms are somewhat interchangeable. The terms "rehabilitation" and "restoration" are sometimes used interchangeably as well. As you will soon discover, "rehabilitation" and "restoration" are not synonymous. They refer to two distinctly different types of care. For purposes of this text, we will use the word resident when referring to the recipient of care, since most restorative care is delivered in the long-term care setting. However, the content and procedures in this text are also applicable to other health care settings. Masculine and feminine pronouns are used interchangeably.

Responsibilities of the Restorative Nursing Assistant

The restorative nursing assistant's responsibilities cross over many different health care settings. The procedures described in this book apply to restorative care in any health care setting. Restorative nursing is part of routine care in facilities providing long-term care and subacute care setting. Restorative nursing principles also apply to care given in hospitals, in clients' homes, adult day care, and other outpatient settings. Knowledge of basic nursing assistant practice and procedures is essential. The assistant must also be familiar with some procedures delivered by physical, occupational, speech, and respiratory therapy. He or she may assist the restorative nurse with some procedures, as well. The restorative nursing assistant is a valuable health care provider. He or she is a "jack of all trades," whose contribution to the residents' overall well-being is enormous. The author and publisher commend and respect this caregiver, and recognize the valuable contribution that he or she makes to the interdisciplinary health care team.

▓ FUNDAMENTAL CONCEPTS AND CONTENT PRESENTED

▓ The text begins with an explanation of the OBRA requirements for rehabilitative and restorative care, describing declines in condition, and the dangers of immobility. Compliance with the intent and requirements of the OBRA '87 guidelines is emphasized throughout.

▓ It progresses to an explanation of the nursing process in restorative care, including the MDS 2.0 and the importance of care planning. We have included current information on the 1998 changes to the minimum data set and reimbursement. Basic human needs, aging changes, developmental tasks, and resident comfort are reviewed.

▓ Important survey alerts are highlighted in text boxes throughout the book. The symbol ⓢⒶ in red signifies a "Survey Alert". The symbol is placed at the beginning of content crucial to meeting care standards as defined by regulatory agencies. The failure to meet these standards commonly results in deficiencies noted during surveys. The symbol is repeated in black ⓢⒶ to indicate the end of the specific content. The symbols appear in the body of the text and in selected tables and guidelines. At times, the entire table or guideline may be marked as the Survey Alert; at other times, only a portion of the table or guideline is marked. Remember that each alert covers an area of performance that is rated by surveyors.

▓ Infection control responsibilities, including the 1996 CDC recommendations are discussed in detail, including the restorative nursing assistant's responsibilities for maintaining a clean, safe environment.

- The text describes the principles of restoration and rehabilitation, and caring for residents with many conditions seen in residents of long-term care facilities. Emphasis is placed on musculoskeletal, neurological, and integumentary system disorders because a large part of the restorative nursing assistant's time is spent assisting residents with problems related to these conditions.

- Ergonomics is a subject that has become popular in the health care industry over the past few years. The text introduces this subject and provides basic information about workplace design, ergonomics programs, and general principles.

- Personal safety is emphasized, and information describing ergonomics, and preventing personal injury are included.

- Several chapters are devoted to resident exercise and mobility, including use of assistive devices.

- A section is devoted to matching the wheelchair size to the resident. This important information is not included in most nursing assistant textbooks, and has a major effect on resident independence and safety.

- Mealtime is an important part of the residents' day. Besides the pleasures derived from eating, the ability to self-feed affects the resident's self-esteem. One chapter details restorative eating programs, and the assistant's responsibilities for restorative dining and feeding.

- Information on assisting residents with activities of daily living is integrated throughout the text.

- Many long-term care facility residents are incontinent. One chapter details the assistant's responsibilities in meeting the needs of residents with bowel and bladder incontinence.

- Meeting the special needs of residents with respiratory disorders and behavior management is summarized.

- A chapter describing restorative documentation completes the text.

- The appendices provide many useful items, including employment information, forms, useful reference information, communication tools, federal guidelines for restorative care, a summary of the Americans with Disabilities Act, and a review of basic nursing assistant procedures that are useful for the restorative nursing assistant.

- The information in the text provides a comprehensive explanation of the restorative nursing assistants' responsibilities in the long-term care facility, and will be useful to assistants working in other settings as well.

SUPPORT MATERIALS

Delmar is committed to providing the instructor with a package of teaching and supportive materials to help students master the principles of restorative nursing care. Using these materials in combination will enable the instructor to assist students to become strong clinicians, with advanced knowledge in restorative nursing care.

End of Chapter Review Material

Each chapter provides an end of chapter review called "Key Points in Chapter" for student study. This section contains a summary of the key information and nursing principles from the chapter. A clinical applications section concludes each chapter. The clinical applications are critical thinking questions. Many situations in this section are based on real facility situations. This section will help students combine basic nursing assistant principles with the restorative nursing information in the text. Using the critical thinking questions will help students use good judgment in applying the principles of restorative nursing care.

Instructor's Manual

For instructors of formal restorative nursing assistant programs, a companion instructor's manual provides teaching tools to use in helping the assistant master the material. The instructor's manual contains numerous resources that will be useful to both the student and the instructor. Some of these provide the instructor with additional information and resources. Some may be used as classroom handouts to enhance student learning. Example restorative nursing forms from facilities across the United States are included. Seeing the forms others use provides an overview of what works well in other facilities. Use these to develop your own forms, capture additional reimbursement, or duplicate them and use for students to practice documentation in class, if desired. A crossword puzzle is provided for each chapter. Crossword puzzles are fun alternative teaching tools that help students master vocabulary words and proper spelling of medical terms. The manual also contains a quiz for each chapter. The puzzles and quizzes may be duplicated and used as homework, for extra practice, or for classroom testing. The manual also contains a comprehensive final examination for use upon course completion. One section contains patterns for restorative equipment that can be made in the facility.

Computerized Test Bank

We have developed a computerized test bank to provide the instructor with a simple means of developing additional testing materials. Using the test bank enables the instructor to combine information from multiple chapters into one quiz or test. The instructor has the flexibility of selecting questions in various formats from the test bank, or to write his or her own questions. The quizzes from the instructor's manual may be used for review or homework. The instructor can develop additional quizzes or testing materials using the test bank, or vice versa. Using the test bank gives the instructor a great deal of flexibility in helping students master the material. It also enables the instructor to develop make up quizzes for students who miss class on testing day. Quizzes and tests are difficult to write, and using the test bank makes this task virtually painless for the instructor.

▣ PUTTING IT ALL TOGETHER

The text begins with an explanation of the OBRA legislation, assessment, and care planning requirements. It progresses by introducing the principles of restorative nursing, and describes restorative care of residents with self-care deficits affecting each body system. Combining the textbook material with the quizzes from the test bank or instructor's manual helps students master the principles of restorative nursing care. Reviewing and discussing the clinical applications with students in class is useful in guiding students to develop critical thinking skills that are essential on the nursing units.

▣ ABOUT THE AUTHOR

Barbara Acello, MS, RN is an independent consultant in Denton, Texas. She has 30 years experience in health care delivery, management, consultation, and education in the public and private sectors. Mrs. Acello is a graduate of a diploma RN program, with a Bachelor's degree in health care administration and a master's degree in education. She has completed additional courses in restorative nursing, and has diverse experience in restorative nursing care in multiple states. Mrs. Acello has implemented and supervise many restorative nursing programs in long-term care facilities. She participated in the development of the Texas Curriculum for Nurse Aides and is committed to helping nursing assistants enhance their image and level of professionalism.

Mrs. Acello is a member of the Texas Nurses Association, Association of Nurses in AIDS Care, and Iowa Emergency Medical Services Association. She has written numerous books and journal articles for nurses, nursing assistants, and other health care professionals.

▣ ACKNOWLEDGEMENTS

The author wishes to thank Dawn Gerrain, the acquisitions editor, and the staff at Delmar Publishers for their dedication to providing high quality textbooks. I especially appreciate your wisdom, foresight, and commitment to meet the needs of this specialized group of restorative nursing assistants. Marge Bruce, the developmental editor, has nurtured me through this project, and has spent many hours working to ensure that this is the best product possible. She always goes beyond the call of duty for me, making my job much easier. I can not imagine writing a Delmar book without her. I sincerely appreciate her support, encouragement, and assistance. Brooke Graves provided the copy editing. The copy editor is responsible for making the book grammatically correct when my language is less than polished. I am always delighted when she lends her very special talents to my books.

A special thanks to Briggs Corporation, in Des Moines, Iowa. I am always pleased to feature the Briggs forms, signs, and products in my books. Briggs has been a leading health care supplier for more than 50 years. The company offers total solutions that include regulatory guidance, industry knowledge, and more than 9000 products in the areas of documentation, charting supplies, activity and recreational products, medical supplies, education and training, and professional resources and rehabilitation products.

A special note of thanks to Pat Carroll, M.S., R.N., who assisted me with the respiratory therapy information. Pat is committed to quality health care education, and I am honored to have such a valued colleague and friend.

Sharon Laney, OTR/L was a major source of information and assistance. She has spent many hours assisting with this book, and has been a valuable source of occupational therapy information. I sincerely appreciate her contributions.

Karen Bonn, RN, provided a great deal of information and enlightened me about contracture management. Ms. Bonn is an outstanding resident advocate and restorative nurse, and I sincerely appreciate her assistance. Mr. Jim Klimek has inspired me about the true value of restorative care. My husband, Francis Acello, and daughter, Laura Fowler, were invaluable in helping me put the finishing touches on the draft manuscript, and assisted with the art manuscript. As usual, Dennis Clarkson, CNA, was a blessing during the photo shoot. I am proud to feature him in my textbooks. He is a true example of a professional nursing assistant. Kristi Kirschnek, R.N., and the staff at Aristocrat West/West Park Health Care Facilities, Cleveland Ohio, generously shared forms and job descriptions used in their facility. Skip Baker of Skip Baker Photography, and Pat Cassidy of the Journal of Nurse Assistants assisted me in pulling the photos and art together. The staff and residents of Good Samaritan Nursing Center in Denton, Texas, and East Galbraith Healthcare Community in Cincinnati, Ohio graciously allowed us to take photographs in their facilities. Mr. Duncan Kinder wrote the summary of the American's with Disabilities Act, and allowed me to copy it from his outstanding web page. I appreciate his dedication in providing and maintaining a comprehensive web page for sharing this important information with others.

Last, but by no means least, a note of thanks to other contributors to the art manuscript:

Acme United Corporation
Restorative Medical, Inc.
Sammons-Preston
Medline Industries, Inc.
Hudson RCI

A team of peer reviewers dedicated many hours to reviewing this manuscript and providing helpful comments throughout the text development. Your input was invaluable, and I sincerely appreciate your cooperation and dedication:

Alison P. Bell, RN, C, BSN: Eastern Maine Technical College, Bangor, ME

Karen L. Bonn, RN, ROF: Restorative Medical, Inc., Brandenburg, KY

Susan Brooks: Community College of Southern Nevada, Las Vegas, NV

Carole Broxson, RN, PhD: Sinclair Community College, Dayton, OH

Saitofi Anne Deem: Fontana High School, Fontana, CA

Genevieve Gipson, RN, MEd: Career Nurse Assistants' Programs, Inc., Norton, OH

Kristi Kirschnick, RN: Secretary, The Florence Project, Ohio coordinator, North Ridgeville, OH

Stephen Tardy, RN, ICSO, DSD, ASBA: Mount San Jacinto College, Menifee, CA

Mary Therriault: Our Lady of Mercy Life Center, Albany, NY

Judith H. Thom, RN, MA: Learey Technical Center, Tampa, FL

FEEDBACK

We hope you find this package of training materials useful in helping students master the principles of restorative nursing care. We endeavor to provide you with distinctive, useful training materials that have been peer reviewed by experienced restorative nurses and nursing assistant instructors from a variety of educational settings in multiple states. Quality health care lies in a combination of proper training and personal motivation. We are delighted that you have selected us to assist you in your mission! Please feel free to contact me personally through Delmar or via e-mail at bacello@aol.com if you have questions, comments, or suggestions.

Barbara Acello, MS, RN

Abbreviations and Acronyms

AAROM	active assisted range of motion
ABC	antecedent/behavior/consequences
ADA	Americans with Disabilities Act
ADLs	activities of daily living
AIDS	acquired immune deficiency syndrome
AROM	active range of motion
CDC	Centers for Disease Control and Prevention
CNA	certified nursing assistant
COPD	chronic obstructive pulmonary disease
CVA	cerebrovascular accident
EPA	Environmental Protection Agency
FWB	full weight bearing
HCFA	Health Care Financing Administration
HD	Huntington's disease
HEPA	high-efficiency particulate air
HMO	health maintenance organization
IADLs	instrumental activities of daily living
LPN	licensed practical nurse
LVN	licensed vocational nurse
MDS 2.0	Minimum Data Set 2.0
MRSA	methicillin-resistant *Staphylococcus aureus*
MS	multiple sclerosis
NIOSH	National Institute for Occupational Safety and Health
NPUAP	National Pressure Ulcer Advisory Panel
NREM	nonrapid eye movement
NWB	nonweight bearing
OA	osteoarthritis
OBRA	Omnibus Budget Reconciliation Act of 1987
ORIF	open reduction internal fixation
OSHA	Occupational Safety and Health Administration (or Act)
PCP	*Pneumocystis carinii* pneumonia
PD	Parkinson's disease
PMEs	pelvic muscle exercises
POMR	problem-oriented medical records
PPE	personal protective equipment
PPO	preferred provider organization
PROM	passive range of motion
PUSH	Pressure Ulcer Scale for Healing
PWB	partial weight bearing
RA	rheumatoid arthritis
RAI	Resident Assessment Instrument
RAPs	resident assessment protocols
REM	rapid eye movement
RN	registered nurse
RNA	restorative nursing assistant
SDC	staff development director
SOAP	Subjective/Objective/Assessment/Plan
SOMR	source-oriented medical records
TTWB	toe-touch weight bearing
VA	Veterans Administration
WBAT	weight bearing as tolerated

Introduction to Restorative Nursing

Introduction to Rehabilitation and Restorative Nursing Care

After reading this chapter, you should be able to:

Spell and define key terms.

List five purposes of the OBRA legislation.

Describe the purpose of restorative care.

List some positive effects of restorative care on residents.

List the role and responsibilities of the restorative nursing assistant.

Explain how facilities are reimbursed for rehabilitation and restorative care.

Explain why a basic understanding of reimbursement is important for the restorative nursing assistant.

Define declines.

Explain the emotional impact of declines.

State the purpose of rehabilitation and restorative nursing care.

Explain why safety is a major consideration in restorative care.

List five factors to consider when evaluating residents' safety.

Describe one negative effect of immobility on each body system.

THE OBRA '87 LEGISLATION

OBRA '87 is an abbreviation for the Omnibus Budget Reconciliation Act. Each year, there is OBRA legislation. The OBRA legislation of 1987 was designed to improve the quality of life, care, health, and safety for residents in long-term care facilities. OBRA '87 mandated major changes in the long-term care industry. It actually changed the way facilities provide care. Before OBRA '87, the emphasis of care was on meeting residents' physical needs. ⑤Ⓐ The OBRA '87 laws require facilities to look at residents as complex individuals with many needs. Needs can be physical, mental, social, or spiritual. Other needs, such as financial needs, may also be considered. The OBRA '87 legislation focuses on:

▦ Prevention of deterioration, or functional **declines** in condition. This is done by identifying **risk factors.** The facility takes steps to prevent problems from developing. Risk factors are conditions that can cause the resident's health to worsen.

▦ Assisting residents to be as independent as possible **(Figure 1–1).**

▦ Meeting residents' psychosocial needs.

▦ Improving residents' quality of care.

▦ Improving the quality of life, as perceived by the residents.

▦ Eliminating restraints whenever possible.

▦ Providing a home-like environment.

▦ Requiring nursing assistants to complete a training program and be entered into the state registry to work in long-term care facilities.⑤Ⓐ

RESTORATIVE NURSING CARE AND REHABILITATION IN THE LONG-TERM CARE FACILITY

⑤Ⓐ Rehabilitation and restorative care **(Figure 1-2)** are based on belief in the dignity and worth of each resident. Each resident is a unique individual. Both services are designed to assist the resident to

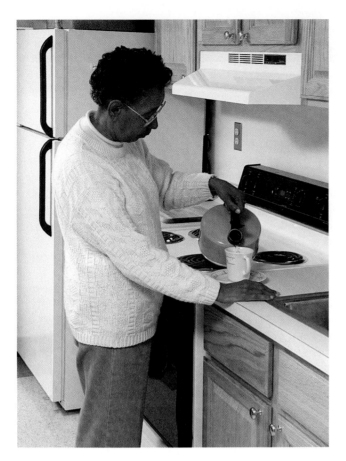

Figure 1–1 This alert, independent resident uses good safety judgment, and fixes herself coffee between meals.

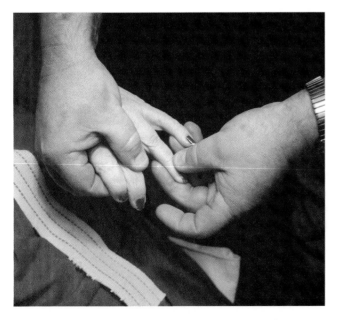

Figure 1–2 The restorative nursing assistant performs passive range-of-motion exercises on a resident with arthritic deformities of her hands.

attain and maintain the highest level of function possible. The maximum level is viewed in light of the resident's individual needs.⊛ **Restorative nursing care** is given by nursing staff. The caregiver may be licensed or unlicensed. **Rehabilitation** is skilled care given by licensed therapy staff and their assistants.

⊛ The resident's physical condition affects self-esteem and quality of life. Restorative nursing care is given 24 hours a day, 7 days a week.⊛ Restorative care is good nursing care. It can be given in any setting. To be successful, all staff must be aware of the restorative program. The care given is in keeping with the restorative goals and approaches established by the interdisciplinary team. Keys to success of the restorative nursing program are:

▪ **Consistency**

▪ **Continuity of care**

▪ Good communication

▪ Using the care plan

Consistency and continuity of care mean that all staff care for the resident in the same manner. Examples of restorative nursing programs are listed in **Table 1–1.**

In contrast, rehabilitation is provided by licensed therapists **(Figure 1–3, p. 5).** The goal of rehabilitation is the same as restorative care, but the skill level of the caregiver is higher. The care is more complex and specialized. Rehabilitation services are given from 1 to 4 hours a day in the long-term care facility. Residents participate in most rehabilitation programs 5 days a week. In some facilities, rehabilitation is available 6 or 7 days a week. For example, a resident with a fractured hip receives gait training for 1 hour, twice a day, 6 days a week.

Some facilities use the terms *rehabilitation* and *restoration* interchangeably. However, rehabilitation is really a higher level of care. It is always provided by licensed personnel. The terms *restoration* and *restorative care* are interchangeable. The restorative approach provides continuity of care. This is because many staff members are working on the same goals and using the same approaches to the residents' problems. This type of care benefits the residents. Most progress quickly when restorative care is given.

▪ THE RESTORATIVE NURSING ASSISTANT

Many long-term care facilities employ **restorative nursing assistants (RNAs).** This position was created out of need. The government agencies that regulate long-term care do not require this position. Facilities know that assistants functioning at an advanced level are needed to work in rehabilitation and restorative care and these facilities recognize

Table 1–1 Examples of Restorative Nursing Programs

Program	Purpose/Benefits
Positioning	Proper positioning is important for residents in bed, chair, or wheelchair. Proper positioning increases function, prevents contractures, and maintains skin integrity. Adaptive equipment and other props, such as pillows and foam wedges, may be used to maintain body alignment.
Restorative Dining	Restorative dining techniques assist residents to become as independent as possible with eating. Dining programs promote dignity. Proper feeding techniques reduce the risk of choking. For some residents, adaptive dining equipment may be used to improve self-feeding skills and promote independence.
Reality Orientation, Cognitive Enhancement, and Mental Stimulation	These programs provide a supportive environment. Dignity and acceptance are important. The programs help to maximize residents' abilities, promote self-esteem, and provide normal day-to-day activities that stimulate mental awareness.
Validation	Validation promotes dignity and self-control by helping residents resolve life tasks, release emotions, and validate their feelings.
Relaxation	Relaxation programs use music or other special techniques to relieve stress and pain, and promote feelings of self-worth and well-being.
Active and Passive Range of Motion	Active and passive range of motion maintain or increase joint range of motion, preserve function and mobility, and prevent contractures, pain, and deformities. Good joint motion promotes a healthy appearance, comfort, body alignment, and overall health.
Ambulation	Ambulation programs may require the use of assistive devices. Ambulation helps improve overall health and well-being. All systems benefit. Circulation, digestion, elimination, muscle strength, emotional satisfaction, and socialization are improved. Restorative ambulation programs focus on safety and consistency.
Wheelchair Mobility	These programs increase or maintain the residents' ability for independent movement and assure proper, safe, and comfortable positioning and body alignment when in a wheelchair.
Bowel and Bladder Retraining or Maintenance	There are several types of bowel and bladder programs to assist residents in becoming continent and as independent as possible. Some programs minimize episodes of incontinence through scheduled intervention. Bowel and bladder programs promote self-esteem and dignity, and maintain skin integrity.
Bathing, Dressing, and Grooming Programs	Personal hygiene and grooming programs help residents maintain or improve self-care abilities. Special techniques or adaptive devices may be used to promote independence and dignity.
Communication Programs	Several types of communication programs are provided that use assistive devices, computers, or communication boards to assist residents to communicate independently.

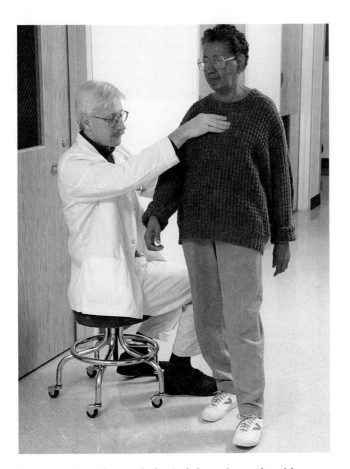

Figure 1–3 A licensed physical therapist works with residents on gait training.

the importance of the position. They understand the benefits of restorative care to the residents. Some facilities employ only one RNA. Others employ several.

Because the RNA position is not mandatory, there is no formal training requirement. Many facilities train nursing assistants to work in this position. Some progressive businesses and schools offer programs to prepare the RNA. Therefore, the training and preparation for this position vary widely.

The qualifications and responsibilities of the RNA also vary widely. Each facility establishes a job description, listing job requirements. Many factors are considered when developing the RNA duties. A sample job description is found in Appendix A. The RNA is often promoted from within the facility. He or she is usually an experienced nursing assistant who sets a good example for others and has a record of providing excellent resident care. He or she has good attendance and is dependable. In most facilities, the RNA is a state-tested or certified nursing assistant. He or she typically has at least 6 months to 1 year's experience as a nursing assistant.

Some facilities also employ restorative nurses. This person is usually a registered nurse who has education and training in restorative nursing care.

The nurse oversees the restorative program. If your facility employs a restorative nurse, he or she will probably be your supervisor. In some facilities, the director of nursing or someone in the therapy department supervises the restorative assistants. The supervisor varies with the facility. Report changes in resident condition to your supervisor or the designated person in your facility.

Likewise, the restorative assistant's responsibilities vary greatly from one facility to the next. In some facilities, this individual works in the therapy department. In some, he or she works in nursing. In others, the assistant has responsibilities in both departments. This book is designed to prepare you to work in both departments, but the emphasis is on nursing. ⓈⒶ Your responsibilities may be determined by your state rules and regulations. Some states allow assistants to perform certain procedures, such as sterile technique. Other states do not permit assistants to perform these same procedures. Your job description will be designed by your facility to encompass the things that you can legally do.ⓈⒶ

Your supervisor will assign you to certain residents and tasks each day. ⓈⒶ If you have questions, or do not know how to perform a procedure, ask your supervisor. You will find that some of the things you do each day were learned in your nursing assistant class. Do not perform procedures that you are not trained and qualified to do. If you are not sure whether you may legally perform a procedure, consult your supervisor.ⓈⒶ The information in your job description will guide you in your responsibilities.

The restorative nursing assistant is an advanced care provider. He or she has received additional training in rehabilitation and restorative care. Becoming an RNA is something to be proud of, and is a step up the career ladder!

▓▓ FINANCING HEALTH CARE

Health care is expensive for both the consumer and the facility. The facility must make enough money to pay wages and expenses. The resident must pay for health care services. Health care is paid for in many different ways. Some individuals pay for care out of their personal bank accounts. Many pay a premium to insurance companies, which in turn pay the facility for providing care. Many individuals depend on state and federal government programs to pay for their care.

Medicaid

Medicaid is a health care program funded by the state and federal governments. It pays for health care for individuals with a low income. Medicaid may also be called Title XIX. A person must be eligible and qualify to receive these benefits.

Medicare

Medicare is a federally funded health care program. It pays for some care for individuals who are elderly or disabled. The Health Care Financing Administration (HCFA) administers the program. Medicare pays for certain services in the hospital, long-term care facility, and home health care setting. Facilities must be approved to participate in the Medicare program. Some facilities do not accept payment from the Medicare and Medicaid programs.

Health Maintenance Organizations

A **health maintenance organization (HMO)** is a group of health care providers and hospitals. The HMO may be funded by Medicare, Medicaid, or the patient's private money. Members are given a list of health care providers and facilities where they may go to receive care. The HMO pays the health care provider a set fee each month for each member. This fee is **all-inclusive:** it covers all care the individual receives. No additional payments are made for extra services or supplies. Facilities participating in HMO programs must be very cost-efficient.

Preferred Provider Organizations

Preferred provider organizations (PPOs) also pay for health care. The PPO provides a list of its health care providers and facilities to members. The member can go anywhere for care. However, going to providers who are not on the PPO list will result in a higher cost to the member.

Other Methods of Financing Health Care

Other sources may also pay for health care. Charitable and community agencies may fund care in some situations. The Veterans Administration (VA) cares for veterans in government hospitals. To qualify, the illness must be related to military service. Occasionally, the VA also pays for care in long-term care facilities.

▉ PAYING FOR REHABILITATION AND RESTORATIVE CARE

Payment for long-term care is very limited. This presents a serious dilemma. The population is aging. The demand for long-term care services is increasing. The criteria for payment are rigid and many individuals do not qualify. Many do not have enough money to pay for care. For this reason, the Medicare and Medicaid programs pay for most long-term care.

The Medicare Program

Medicare pays for long-term care in different ways. **Medicare Part A** pays the hospital or long-term care facility a set rate for its services. The rate includes room, board, and all care and supplies. Medicare Part A payment for long-term care is not automatic. Many people do not understand this. Coverage is very limited. The resident must meet certain criteria for Medicare Part A to pay for the care. Most residents do not qualify for Medicare benefits.

Residents whose payment source is Medicare Part A reside in a specific area of the facility, commonly called the **skilled unit.** While in this unit, Medicare pays the long-term care facility one fee for all services the resident receives. The amount of payment is determined by information the facility submits to the state. The state, in turn, transmits the information to the HCFA. The rate is based on the amount and type of care the resident needs and receives. Rehabilitation services are included in the Part A fee. Residents receiving therapy under Part A need skilled services to restore and maintain function. Safety is a major consideration.

To be eligible for payment under Part A, the resident must need complex care. The skills and judgment of a licensed health care professional are needed every day. This sounds simple. However, most long-term care services are not considered skilled, according to the Medicare criteria. To be eligible for coverage for therapy, the resident must need the skills and judgment of a licensed therapist at least 5 days a week. A physician's order is necessary for skilled therapy.

Medicare Part B is an additional service. If a Medicare beneficiary wants to use Part B, he or she must pay a premium each month. Some individuals are unwilling or unable to pay the premium. These persons do not have Part B Medicare coverage. Part B pays for some diagnostic tests, splints, braces, prosthetics, and therapy evaluations and services. Payment for rehabilitation under Medicare Part B is very limited.

Medicaid Reimbursement

The Medicaid program pays for health care for persons who cannot afford health insurance and do not qualify for Medicare payment. Payment is administered by the state. Each state sets its own criteria for eligibility. The state also decides what services will be provided, and how much reimbursement will be made for care. Because of this, payment is different in each state. Part of the state Medicaid money comes from the federal government.

All long-term care facilities are required to provide restorative care. In some states, Medicaid will pay the facility for restorative services. In some states, there is no extra reimbursement. Some states approve therapy services under the Medicaid program; others do not. Payment for therapy by Medicaid must be pre-approved. Your supervisor will describe how payment is made in your state. He or she will teach you how this affects your documentation and responsibilities.

Other Forms of Payment

Insurance companies, HMOs and PPOs also pay for rehabilitation and restorative services. They require very precise documentation. Very few residents have private long-term care insurance. This limits HMO, PPO, and insurance payment in long-term care.

Documentation

Documentation of restorative care and the resident's response is very important. (SA) Records must support the resident's need for care. Documentation must show the resident's response to care and progress. (SA) If the documentation is absent or insufficient, payment will be denied. The facility loses a great deal of money if an agency denies payment. In some situations, governmental agencies will also deny payment. The important thing to remember is that documentation must be accurate and complete. Documentation is described in detail in Chapter 19.

▦ DECLINES IN CONDITION

(SA) A **decline** is a deterioration in condition. It is not permitted, according to OBRA '87, unless it is medically unavoidable. Saying that a decline was caused by normal aging or a chronic illness may not be acceptable. Licensed facility staff assess the resident on admission and make a record of this assessment. The facility must maintain or improve the resident's condition compared with how he or she was at the time of admission. For example, if the resident could walk at the time of admission, the facility must maintain this ability. If the resident cannot walk, the facility must do everything possi-

ble to restore **mobility** (the ability to move about). If walking is not possible, mobility is provided by an assistive device or wheelchair. If the skin was clear on admission, the facility must prevent pressure sores and injuries. If pressure sores were present on admission, the facility must take steps to heal them. These are simple examples that apply to the musculoskeletal and integumentary systems. Declines can occur in all areas of the resident's life. Restorative care is highly individualized **(Figure 1–4).** Restoring the resident to his or her former status may not be possible. Nevertheless, restorative care is still very beneficial. (SA)

Reasons for Decline

Declines in function occur for many reasons. Conditions such as stroke, falls, fractures, or an illness such as pneumonia cause weakness and loss of function. Other conditions that increase the risk of declines are:

- cognitive impairment
- inability to ambulate
- unresponsive condition
- poor skin integrity
- poor nutritional intake
- inadequate fluid intake
- chronic pain
- deformities
- spasticity
- edema
- generalized weakness
- restraints
- multiple medications
- certain medical conditions
- terminal diagnosis

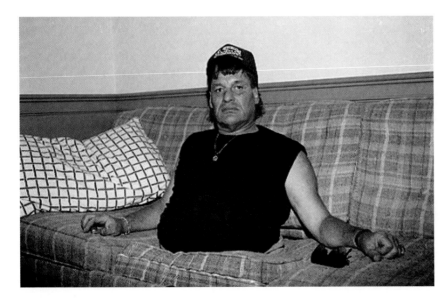

Figure 1–4 This young resident has a below-the-waist amputation. His restorative care is designed to assist him to return home and live independently in the community.

EMOTIONAL IMPACT OF DECLINES

Long-term care facilities must promote independence. Restorative care helps residents function at their highest level. Their individual situations are considered. Being partially independent is better than being dependent on others. Residents who are completely immobile can still exercise control by verbally directing their care **(Figure 1–5).** Restorative care has many physical benefits. It is also important to help residents feel good about themselves. Being independent promotes a healthy self-esteem.

Sometimes the staff will do things for the residents that they could do themselves, just because doing so is faster. This violates the intention of the OBRA '87 laws. Surveyors will write deficiencies for this. If the resident does not use the self-care skills, he or she will lose the ability to do them. Sometimes the staff does not know what the resident can and cannot do. This is particularly true with confused residents. Staff members assume that the resident cannot be independent because of the confusion. In fact, these residents can do many things. Encourage them to be as independent as possible. Studies have shown that prompting and encouraging most cognitively impaired residents to perform simple tasks takes only 1 to 2 minutes longer than it would for staff to complete the task.

Many residents have low self-esteem because they cannot care for themselves. When providing restorative care, give only the assistance necessary. Set up the needed materials. Give simple instructions. Allow adequate time to complete the task. Encourage the resident. If he or she cannot complete a task, offer to finish it. Provide positive feedback about the part of the task that the resident completed. Avoid making residents feel they have

failed. Stressing the resident's ability and not the disability is very important. This type of care takes patience and determination. However, it pays off in improved resident self-esteem and satisfaction. Over time, restorative programs makes the staff's work easier as well. Everyone benefits!

Sympathy and Empathy

Sympathy means feeling sorry for residents and accepting their feelings as your own. **Empathy** is understanding how the resident feels. It means connecting with and supporting a resident when he or she works through difficult times. Feeling sorry for residents will not help. Try to understand residents' feelings of frustration and take action to help them. Listening and providing support will help. Successful restorative care depends on this action. Your attitude is important to the success of the restorative program. It affects the residents' motivation. You must believe in what you are doing and in the benefits to the residents **(Figure 1–6).**

The Grieving Process

You learned about the grieving process in your nursing assistant program in the death and dying unit. The steps in the grieving process are listed in **Table 1–2.** People grieve because of other types of losses as well. For example:

- Loss of spouse
- Loss of health
- Loss of ability to leave the facility
- Loss of ability to make decisions
- Loss of control over the environment

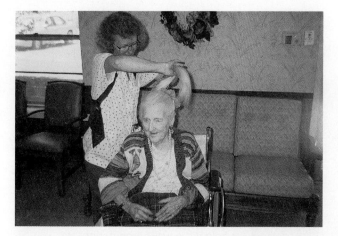

Figure 1–5 This alert resident has limited range of motion because of arthritis. She takes pride in her appearance, and directs the nursing assistant in styling her hair.

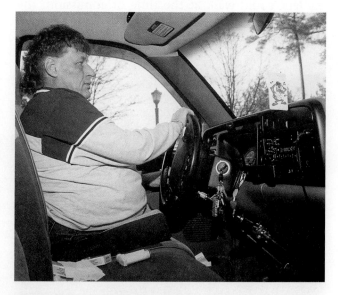

Figure 1–6 The resident in Figure 1–4 received active rehabilitation and restorative care. He has returned home and drives his truck about the community.

Table 1-2 The Grieving Process

Stage of the Grieving Process	Resident Reaction	How the Nursing Assistant Can Help
Denial	May exhibit false hope, tell untrue stories, refuse to participate in care, not follow directions, and in general deny that a problem exists.	Paraphrase the resident's statements. Avoid confirming or denying the fact that the resident is dying.
Anger	Anger with self, family, doctor, and God. Often is angry with caregivers for no apparent reason.	Try to understand why the resident is angry. Listen and provide support. Meet reasonable requests and demands quickly.
Bargaining	Bargains with God or higher power for favors. May ask for more time to live or restored physical ability. Usually promises something in return.	Meet the resident's requests, if possible. Listen carefully and provide support. Avoid giving the resident false hope.
Depression	Feeling regret, apathy, decreased concentration, insomnia, fatigue, crying, poor appetite, lack of interest in people and environment.	Avoid dismissing the resident's fear and pain. Do not try to cheer the resident by saying that things could be worse. Show that you care. Listen and provide support.
Acceptance	Feels empty and peaceful, has less emotional pain. Understands that he or she must accept the situation.	Avoid assuming that the resident is not afraid of death, although he or she has accepted it. Show that you care. Listen and provide support.

Residents who suffer physical losses go through the grieving process. For example, a person has a stroke and loses the ability to move one side of the body. This resident will grieve for the loss of function. This is a normal reaction. You must understand grieving and recognize stages of grief if you are going to help the residents. Your understanding will help you move the resident through the process. Once the resident has accepted the diagnosis, living with decreased physical ability is easier. Restorative care helps the resident pick up the pieces. It enables the resident to make the best use of whatever ability remains. Look at this as a positive step, with physical and emotional benefits.

▀▀ SAFETY CONCERNS

Safety is a primary concern when there is a loss of function. If a resident's condition changes, evaluate his or her awareness. If the level of consciousness and mental status have changed, report to your supervisor. Changes in consciousness and mental status may indicate serious problems. Other important observations that should be reported are:

▬ Whether the resident is aware of the change

▬ Whether the resident asks for assistance when needed

▬ The resident's desire to remain independent despite the increased safety risk

▬ Whether the resident denies that there has been a change

▬ Any falls that you know of

▬ Changes in vision

▬ Changes in bowel and bladder control

▬ The resident's ability to ambulate

▬ Problems with standing, balance, or coordination

If you observe any of these changes, notify your supervisor immediately. A licensed health care professional will assess the resident. He or she makes other team members aware of the changes. They will reevaluate the care plan and write new approaches, if necessary. The restorative program will be designed with the changes in mind. The overall goal is keeping the resident safe.

If the resident has been on bed rest for a long time, he or she must gradually increase activity. Inactivity and bed rest cause changes in blood pressure and balance. Your supervisor will develop a schedule to gradually increase the length of time that the resident will be up.

▆▆ THE DANGERS OF IMMOBILITY

Many years ago, sick people stayed in bed for long periods of time. Now we know that early activity is best. It positively affects the resident both physically and emotionally. Rest is important to the treatment of many illnesses. However, too much rest and too little activity often worsens the condition. Bed rest is a medically prescribed treatment. Bed rest, inactivity, and immobility adversely affect every body system. A summary of the major complications of immobility appears in **Table 1–3.**

Table 1–3   Complications of Immobility

System	Complication
Respiratory	Fluid and secretions collect in the lungs. The resident has more difficulty expanding the lungs, increasing the risk of pneumonia and other lung infections.
Circulatory	Blood clots caused by pooling of blood and pressure on the legs. Edema may be caused by lack of movement. The heart must work harder to pump blood through the body. Changes in the blood vessels may cause dizziness and fainting when the resident is placed in the upright position.
Integumentary	Pressure ulcers may develop in a short time from lack of oxygen to the tissues. Pressure ulcers may worsen quickly and be difficult or impossible to reverse.
Muscular	Weakness and atrophy from lack of use. Contractures develop because of the resident's position. Contractures may be painful and are difficult or impossible to reverse.
Skeletal	Calcium drains from the bones when they are inactive. This may contribute to fractures, non-healing, osteoporosis, and other complications.
Genitourinary	The extra calcium in the system from the bones promotes the development of kidney stones. Retention of urine is common, and is often caused by the resident's position in bed. Overflow of a full bladder leads to incontinence. The resident is at high risk of urinary tract infection.
Gastrointestinal	Indigestion and heartburn may result if the resident is not positioned properly for meals. Loss of appetite may occur from lack of activity, illness, and boredom. Constipation and fecal impaction result from immobility.
Nervous	Weakness and limited mobility. Insomnia may result from sleeping too much during the day, then being unable to sleep at night.
Mental changes	Irritability, boredom, lethargy, and depression result from the resident's frustration and feelings of helplessness.

KEY POINTS IN CHAPTER

The OBRA '87 legislation emphasizes preventing declines, promoting independence, meeting psychosocial needs, and improving quality of care and quality of life.

The resident's physical condition affects self-esteem and quality of life.

Restorative care is designed to maintain or improve the resident's overall condition.

Consistent care is a key to a successful restorative program.

Rehabilitation and restorative care may be financed by Medicare, Medicaid, insurance, and other private sources of funding. Funding for long-term care is limited.

Accurate documentation is necessary to be reimbursed for rehabilitation and restoration.

The OBRA '87 legislation states that the resident's condition should not decline, unless the decline is medically unavoidable.

Functional declines have a negative effect on the resident's self-esteem.

Safety is a primary concern when a resident has a loss of functional ability.

Bed rest has a negative effect on all body systems.

CLINICAL APPLICATIONS

1. Mr. Hernandez is a 77-year-old resident who has had a stroke. He has a potential for skin breakdown because of immobility. He is up in a wheelchair most of the day. He becomes irritable if you suggest that he return to bed. He becomes upset if you reposition him in the wheelchair. Mr. Hernandez has a poor appetite. His intake and output are measured. His fluid intake is approximately 550 cc each day on the 7 AM to 3 PM shift. He has lost weight. What measures can the restorative nursing assistant take to assist Mr. Hernandez?

2. Mrs. Lange has multiple medical problems. She was hospitalized 2 weeks ago for pneumonia. She recently returned to the facility. Before going to the hospital, Mrs. Lange was active and independent. She is now lethargic, on bed rest, and very weak. What kind of restorative programs do you think this resident will benefit from?

3. Mr. Chung is mentally confused. He keeps his hands in very tight fists. The occupational therapist has assessed him. She states that he has full range of motion in both wrists and fingers. Is there potential risk for a problem? If so, what? Will this resident benefit from a restorative program? If a program is ordered, what observations will you make about the resident? What will you report?

CHAPTER 2

The Nursing Process in Restorative Nursing Care

OBJECTIVES

After reading this chapter, you should be able to:

Spell and define key terms.

Identify the members of the interdisciplinary team and describe the responsibilities of each.

State the purpose of the nursing process.

Describe the four steps of the nursing process.

State the purpose of the RAI and explain why it is important.

Identify and define the MDS, triggers and RAPS.

Describe how the care plan is developed from the MDS.

State the purpose of the care plan.

Explain why the care plan is important and how it is used.

Define holistic care and explain why this type of care is important.

Describe how restorative programs are developed and explain why restorative care is important.

Define risk factors and explain what must be done if a risk factor is identified.

RESIDENT'S CONDITION ON ADMISSION TO A LONG-TERM CARE FACILITY

Hospital patients are discharged as soon as they become medically stable. Because today's patients are discharged so quickly, they often need more time to complete their recovery. Many go to the long-term care facility, skilled nursing unit, or sub-acute care center, or receive care in their homes. Residents entering the facility from the hospital may be very ill. Many require skilled nursing and therapy services to recover. Common conditions are fractures, cerebrovascular accidents, and medical illnesses. Some residents become weak and unstable because of medical problems. They will receive therapy to restore them to their former state of independence. If this is not possible, care is designed to help them become as independent as possible.

THE INTERDISCIPLINARY APPROACH TO RESTORATIVE CARE

Ⓢ The OBRA '87 legislation is designed to assist us in working as a team. No single discipline has all the answers. It takes everyone working together to meet the needs of each resident.Ⓢ

Members of the Interdisciplinary Team

The resident is the most important member of the interdisciplinary team. He or she must be the center of attention **(Figure 2–1).** The resident should be involved in planning his or her own care. The family's attitudes, interests, and desires are also considered. They affect the resident's response to care. The family should know what is being done for the resident, unless the oriented resident objects. Whenever possible, families are encouraged to participate in care planning. They may also assist with the restorative program. Other team members and their responsibilities are listed in **Table 2–1.**

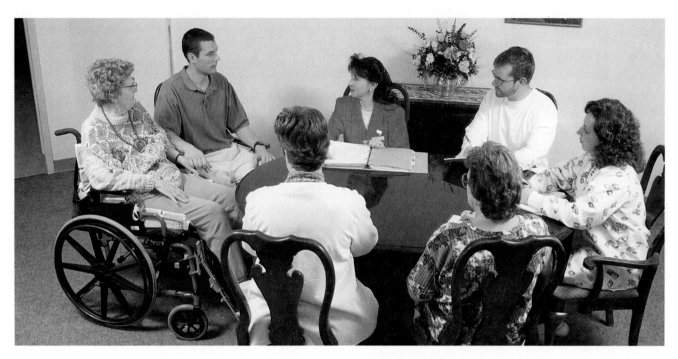

Figure 2–1   This resident is the most important member of the interdisciplinary team and is actively involved in planning her own care.

Table 2–1	Interdisciplinary Team Members and Responsibilities
Team Member	**Responsibility**
Physician	Directs medical care. Many restorative services and treatments require a physician's orders. Others may be ordered by a licensed health care professional.
Rehabilitation team	Composed of licensed therapists, licensed and certified therapy assistants, and restorative nursing assistants. This team evaluates and treats residents, designs rehabilitation and restorative programs, teaches and trains facility staff and family members, and serves as consultants when needed.
Physical therapist	Prevents physical disability; uses physical methods to evaluate and treat pain, disease, and injury. Responsible for teaching ambulation and transfers.
Occupational therapist	Evaluates and treats residents for self-care, work, and activities of daily living (ADLs). This therapist is concerned with increased function and prevention of deformity. He or she modifies tasks and the environment to help the resident become independent.
Staff development director	Orients and teaches the restorative philosophy to all personnel. He or she teaches new staff members the skills and techniques of basic restorative care. The SDC may teach the basic nursing assistant training program. He or she monitors staff performance, periodically reviews employees' skills, and provides education on new techniques and information.

(continues)

Table 2–1   Interdisciplinary Team Members and Responsibilities, *continued*

Dietary personnel	Provide proper diets and ensure that individual dietary needs are addressed; order groceries, cook, prepare meals, and wash dishes.
Dietitian	Plans the menus; develops special diets to address residents' medical problems and needs.
Social worker	Helps residents adjust from living in the community to life in the facility. He or she helps residents and families with problems affecting the resident's response to care. Some social workers design behavior management programs and do psychosocial counseling. The social worker coordinates the services of other individuals and agencies. He or she is responsible for discharge planning, which begins on the day of admission. As the resident progresses, the social worker will arrange for the resident to make the transition to a lesser care setting or return to his or her own home.
Speech therapist	Uses special techniques and skills to help residents with communication and swallowing disorders.
Licensed and certified therapy assistants	Individuals with several years of education in their specialty. They can do many of the things licensed therapists do, but assistants cannot assess.
Respiratory therapist	Works with residents who have problems with oxygenation, and performs breathing treatments.
Licensed nurses (RN, LPN/LVN)	Assess the residents. Communicate residents' needs and progress to the physician; responsible for taking physicians' orders and seeing that the medical plan of care and orders for restorative services are followed.
Restorative nurse	RN with special training in rehabilitation and restoration; he or she oversees the restorative care program and acts as a liaison with therapies. The nurse develops restorative programs, assesses the residents' response to care, and trains and supervises restorative nursing assistants.
Restorative nursing assistant	Meets residents' needs on many levels. He or she is responsible for performing tasks for residents in restorative mobility, ADL, and other programs. Reinforces the teaching that the therapist and restorative nurse have done. May also have responsibilities for assisting in the rehabilitation department.
Nursing assistants	OBRA '87 requires facilities to deliver restorative care 24 hours a day, 7 days a week. Assistants use the restorative approaches each time the resident performs the ADL skill.
Activities director	Provides useful and purposeful activities to help residents maintain their lifestyles. Activities empower residents and promote healthy self-esteem.
Other team members	At times, other departments will be involved with the restorative program. For example, maintenance and housekeeping may make environmental adaptations in residents' rooms. Facilities should modify the environment whenever possible to promote independence. Representatives of outside agencies working with the resident, or the clergy, may also participate in care conferences from time to time. Some facilities have a pastoral care department to meet residents' spiritual needs.

▨ THE NURSING PROCESS

Upon admission to a long-term care facility, a resident is assessed by members of the interdisciplinary team. The team develops a plan of care based on the assessment. The care plan is revised periodically to reflect improvements or declines in the resident's condition. The resident's progress toward care plan goals is evaluated. If he or she is progressing, the goals are continued. If the resident is not progressing, the team will attempt to learn why. They will revise the plan of care accordingly. This is called the **nursing process.** The term *nursing process* does not truly describe the process because many disciplines participate in the assessment and care planning. However, the process is coordinated by a registered nurse. It follows a pattern used by all nurses in care plan development. The four steps of the nursing process are listed in **Table 2–2.**

Table 2–2 The Nursing Process in Restorative Care

Nursing Process Step	Description and Action
Assessment	A complete evaluation of the resident's condition. It answers questions about what is happening with the resident. The nursing assistant participates in the assessment by gathering information such as vital signs, height, and weight, and submitting the findings to the licensed nurse. He or she contributes observations, information, and knowledge about the resident's condition, care, likes and dislikes, and personal preferences, such as the type of bath and time of day preferred for bathing. Assessment is an ongoing process and continues throughout the course of the resident's stay.
Planning	The second step in the nursing process. It answers questions about what is possible for the resident. The course of action is determined based on the resident assessment. The nurse makes decisions about the resident's initial care based on the information gathered. Medical problems, high-risk conditions, functional ability, and other factors are considered. Next, an initial plan of care is developed. The plan describes problems, goals, and approaches to use when caring for the resident. The initial care plan contains basic nursing information to provide guidance in resident care until a more thorough assessment is completed. When the interdisciplinary team meets for the first time, the care plan is expanded and revised. The revised plan reflects a more comprehensive assessment and interdisciplinary team approach. Thereafter, the plan is revised whenever there is a deterioration, improvement, change, or acute illness. Licensed professionals can make minor changes to the care plan at any time necessary.
Implementation	The third step in the nursing process involves putting the care plan into action. It answers questions about how care will be given and things will be done. Staff follow the plan when caring for the resident. When all staff are familiar with and follow the care plan, the resident benefits and the staff is well organized.
Evaluation	The fourth step in the nursing process. It answers the question, "How do we know if anything has changed?" Evaluation is ongoing throughout the resident's stay. It involves critically reviewing care plan goals and approaches to see if they are working. If they are not, the plan is modified until it is effective for the resident.

▬▬ THE RESIDENT ASSESSMENT INSTRUMENT

(SA) All care begins with an assessment. The facility must help all residents function at the highest level possible. This level is determined by considering the resident's situation. To do this, facilities use a written tool developed by the government. This tool is called the **Resident Assessment Instrument (RAI).** The purpose of the RAI is to improve quality of care and quality of life. It helps staff assess the resident. The RAI identifies problems, needs, and risks. It provides the foundation for the care plan. The government also uses the tool to set payment to the facility. As you can see, this is a very important document. It must be completed within specific timeframes. Completing the RAI requires a high degree of accuracy.(SA) The RAI helps team members to:

▪ Use the nursing process

▪ Develop a care plan that maintains or improves the resident's condition

▪ Identify risk factors and develop approaches to prevent declines

▪ Identify the need for restorative programs

▪ Consider the whole person

▪ Focus on resident strengths

▪ See how strengths and needs in one area can affect the whole person

▪ Improve communication among departments

▪ Appreciate the roles, responsibilities, and contributions of other departments in resident care

▪ Work as a team rather than providing discipline-specific care

▪ Assist residents to achieve their maximum potential, improving their quality of life

▪ Ensure that the facility is paid for providing services the residents need and receive

The Minimum Data Set

The RAI consists of three parts. The first part is a comprehensive assessment called the **Minimum Data Set 2.0 (MDS 2.0), Figure 2–2.** It is one of many assessments that the facility uses to evaluate the resident and plan care. Using the MDS 2.0 causes facility personnel to look at many facts. All of these influence the resident's care and well-being. The other parts of the RAI are triggers and RAPs.

Triggers

When the team completes the MDS 2.0, some conditions activate **triggers.** Conditions that activate a trigger usually need a care plan intervention. A condition will trigger for one of three reasons:

▪ The resident has an actual condition with the potential for complications, including declines in condition

▪ The resident has a **risk factor,** or condition that could cause his or her health to worsen

▪ The resident is a candidate for a restorative program

RAPs

Triggers are like bridges. They lead personnel to the third component of the RAI, the **resident assessment protocols (RAPs).** The RAPs are lists of information and guidelines. They link the MDS 2.0 with care plan goals. The RAPS are problem-oriented. They guide staff in problem identification, care planning, and treatment decisions.

Timeframes for RAI Completion

The OBRA '87 requirements state that the MDS 2.0, triggers, and RAPS must be completed within 14 days of admission. An additional 7 days are allowed from the date of completion to develop a care plan. Most facilities take the entire 21 days for this process. Because the care plan is not required until day 21, the nursing process is used to develop the interim care plan. This plan directs the resident's care for the first three weeks. Using the 21-day timeframe gives staff adequate time to assess the resident. During this time, they will begin to develop a workable, realistic care plan. The interim care plan guides staff until the MDS 2.0 is completed and the interdisciplinary care plan developed.

The Medicare program requires an MDS 2.0 on day 5, day 14, day 30, day 60, and day 90. Residents on Medicare have complex needs. They require at least daily services from licensed personnel. Their condition and care may change quickly. The care plans usually change with every MDS 2.0.

A summary of the MDS 2.0 and care plan schedule appears in **Table 2–3.**

Quarterly Review. A short version of the MDS 2.0 is completed for all residents quarterly. The care plan is revised if necessary. The care plan is reviewed and revised each time the MDS 2.0 is done. Some facilities complete triggers and RAPs during the quarterly review. These are not required, but may be helpful.

Reassessments. A complete, new MDS 2.0 is completed annually. It is also done if the resident has a significant change in condition that is major or is likely to be permanent. A significant change may indicate a decline or improvement. Changes

SECTION G. PHYSICAL FUNCTIONING AND STRUCTURAL PROBLEMS

1. (A) ADL SELF-PERFORMANCE—*(Code for resident's PERFORMANCE OVER ALL SHIFTS during last 7 days—Not including setup)*

   0. INDEPENDENT—No help or oversight—OR—Help/oversight provided only 1 or 2 times during last 7 days
   1. SUPERVISION—Oversight, encouragement or cueing provided 3 or more times during last 7 days—OR—Supervision (3 or more times) plus physical assistance provided only 1 or 2 times during last 7 days
   2. LIMITED ASSISTANCE—Resident highly involved in activity; received physical help in guided maneuvering of limbs or other nonweight bearing assistance 3 or more times—OR—More help provided only 1 or 2 times during last 7 days
   3. EXTENSIVE ASSISTANCE—While resident performed part of activity, over last 7-day period, help of following type(s) provided 3 or more times:
      —Weight-bearing support
      —Full staff performance during part (but not all) of last 7 days
   4. TOTAL DEPENDENCE—Full staff performance of activity during entire 7 days
   8. ACTIVITY DID NOT OCCUR during entire 7 days

   (B) ADL SUPPORT PROVIDED—*(Code for MOST SUPPORT PROVIDED OVER ALL SHIFTS during last 7 days; code regardless of resident's self-performance classification)*
   0. No setup or physical help from staff
   1. Setup help only
   2. One person physical assist
   3. Two+ persons physical assist
   8. ADL activity itself did not occur during entire 7 days

			SELF-PERF (A)	SUPPORT (B)
a.	BED MOBILITY	How resident moves to and from lying position, turns side to side, and positions body while in bed A = 1 = 5A; A = 2, 3, or 4 = 5A, 16; A = 8 = 16		
b.	TRANSFER	How resident moves between surfaces—to/from: bed, chair, wheelchair, standing position (EXCLUDE to/from bath/toilet) A = 1, 2, 3, or 4 = 5A		
c.	WALK IN ROOM	How resident walks between locations in his/her room A = 1, 2, 3, or 4 = 5A		
d.	WALK IN CORRIDOR	How resident walks in corridor on unit A = 1, 2, 3, or 4 = 5A		
e.	LOCOMO-TION ON UNIT	How resident moves between locations in his/her room and adjacent corridor on same floor. If in wheelchair, self-sufficiency once in chair A = 1, 2, 3, or 4 = 5A		
f.	LOCOMO-TION OFF UNIT	How resident moves to and returns from off unit locations (e.g., areas set aside for dining, activities, or treatments). If facility has only one floor, how resident moves to and from distant areas on the floor. If in wheelchair, self-sufficiency once in chair A = 1, 2, 3, or 4 = 5A		
g.	DRESSING	How resident puts on, fastens, and takes off all items of street clothing, including donning/removing prosthesis A = 1, 2, 3, or 4 = 5A		
h.	EATING	How resident eats and drinks (regardless of skill). Includes intake of nourishment by other means (e.g., tube feeding, total parenteral nutrition) A = 1, 2, 3, or 4 = 5A		
i.	TOILET USE	How resident uses the toilet room (or commode, bedpan, urinal); transfers on/off toilet, cleanses, changes pad, manages ostomy or catheter, adjusts clothes A = 1, 2, 3, or 4 = 5A		
j.	PERSONAL HYGIENE	How resident maintains personal hygiene, including combing hair, brushing teeth, shaving, applying makeup, washing/drying face, hands, and perineum (EXCLUDE baths and showers) A = 1, 2, 3, or 4 = 5A		

2. BATHING — How resident takes full-body bath/shower, sponge bath, and transfers in/out of tub/shower (EXCLUDE washing of back and hair). **Code for most dependent** in self-performance and support. A = 1, 2, 3 or 4 = 5A

   (A) BATHING SELF-PERFORMANCE codes appear below.
   0. Independent—No help provided
   1. Supervision—Oversight help only
   2. Physical help limited to transfer only
   3. Physical help in part of bathing activity
   4. Total dependence
   8. Activity itself did not occur during entire 7 days
   (Bathing support codes are as defined in Item 1, code B above)

(A)	(B)

3. TEST FOR BALANCE (See training manual) — *(Code for ability during test in the last 7 days)*
   0. Maintained position as required in test
   1. Unsteady, but able to rebalance self without physical support
   2. Partial physical support during test; or stands (sits) but does not follow directions for test
   3. Not able to attempt test without physical help

   a. Balance while standing
   b. Balance while sitting—position, trunk control 1, 2, or 3 = 17*

4. FUNCTIONAL LIMITATION IN RANGE OF MOTION (see training manual) — *(Code for limitations during last 7 days that interfered with daily functions or placed resident at risk of injury)*

   (A) RANGE OF MOTION
   0. No limitation
   1. Limitation on one side
   2. Limitation on both sides

   (B) VOLUNTARY MOVEMENT
   0. No loss
   1. Partial loss
   2. Full loss

		(A)	(B)
a.	Neck		
b.	Arm—Including shoulder or elbow		
c.	Hand—Including wrist or fingers		
d.	Leg—Including hip or knee		
e.	Foot—Including ankle or toes		
f.	Other limitation or loss		

5. MODES OF LOCOMOTION — *(Check all that apply during last 7 days)*
Cane/walker/crutch	a.	Wheelchair primary mode of locomotion	d.
Wheeled self	b.		
Other person wheeled	c.	NONE OF ABOVE	e.

6. MODES OF TRANSFER — *(Check all that apply during last 7 days)*
Bedfast all or most of time 16	a.	Lifted mechanically	d.
Bed rails used for bed mobility or transfer	b.	Transfer aid (e.g., slide board, trapeze, cane, walker, brace)	e.
Lifted manually	c.	NONE OF ABOVE	f.

7. TASK SEGMENTATION — Some or all of ADL activities were broken into subtasks during last 7 days so that resident could perform them
   0. No   1. Yes

8. ADL FUNCTIONAL REHABILITATION POTENTIAL
Resident believes he/she is capable of increased independence in at least some ADLs 5A	a.
Direct care staff believe resident is capable of increased independence in at least some ADLs 5A	b.
Resident able to perform tasks/activity but is very slow	c.
Difference in ADL Self-Performance or ADL Support, comparing mornings to evenings	d.
NONE OF ABOVE	e.

9. CHANGE IN ADL FUNCTION — Resident's ADL self-performance status has changed as compared to status of 90 days ago (or since last assessment if less than 90 days)
   0. No change   1. Improved   2. Deteriorated

Figure 2–2 The full MDS is completed upon admission, annually, and any time there is a significant change in condition. An abbreviated version is completed quarterly. (Courtesy of the Health Care Finance Administration. Reprinted with permission of Briggs Corporation, Des Moines, IA 50306 [800] 247-2343.)

can be either physical, mental, or psychosocial. The government has defined *significant change* as a major change in the resident's status that:

- *Is not* **self-limiting;** this means that the condition will not resolve itself without intervention
- Affects more than one area of the resident's health
- Requires interdisciplinary review or revision of the care plan

Some conditions are not permanent but still have a major impact on the resident. Because the change is important, a comprehensive reassessment is required, although the change is not permanent. For example, a resident falls and fractures a hip. This condition affects ambulation, toileting, elimination, and activities. In general, a reassessment is necessary if the resident has declines in ADLs. A new MDS 2.0 is necessary if the resident has declines or improvements in two or more ADLs.

Electronic Transmission of the RAI

The RAI has been used since the early 1990s. The government changed the rules for using the RAI several times, most recently in 1998. Facilities must complete the RAI using a computer. The data is electronically transmitted to each state. The state transmits the information to the federal government. Medicaid and Medicare payments to the facility are based upon the residents' condition and needs as

SA Table 2–3

Minimum Data Set Assessment and Care Plan	Type of Assessment and Time Frame
Resident on Medicare	Complete, comprehensive MDS 2.0 　　day 5—with RAPs on day 5 or 14 　　day 14—with RAPs on day 5 or 14 　　day 30—RAPs not required unless significant change 　　day 60—RAPs not required unless significant change 　　day 90—RAPs not required unless significant change Complete, comprehensive care plan initially, then review and revise as appropriate.
Resident not on Medicare	Complete, comprehensive MDS 2.0 with RAPs by day 14 of admission. Review care plan and revise as needed.
All residents	Quarterly review, within 3 months of original MDS 2.0. The quarterly review is a shorter version of the comprehensive MDS 2.0. RAPS are useful, but not required. Review care plan and revise as needed.
All residents	Complete, *comprehensive MDS 2.0 with RAPs by day 14, and whenever a significant change in condition occurs.* Review care plan and revise as needed. A new care plan may be necessary.
All residents	Complete, comprehensive MDS 2.0 with RAPs annually. Review care plan and revise as needed. A new care plan may be necessary. SA

identified on the RAI. The information is also used to track patterns of declines in the facility. Many declines in a facility can trigger a survey. Surveyors will arrive unannounced to investigate the cause.

As you can see, the RAI is a very important document. Using it correctly benefits the resident. It ensures that declines will be avoided whenever possible.

CARE PLANNING

Staff members from many departments participate in the assessment. The RAI is the minimum assessment required. It is not the only assessment. Facilities can complete as many assessments as necessary to plan the resident's care. Many assess bowel and bladder, therapy, and nutritional status. After the RAI and other assessments are complete, staff from each department meet for a conference. This is also called a *care plan meeting*. During the meeting, team members plan the resident's care for the next 90 days. The assessments provide the basis for the care

plan **(Figure 2–3)**. However, additional information about the resident may be included. Additional information comes from:

- Physician's orders, including medications, treatments, special equipment, and procedures
- The physician's history and physical examination
- Laboratory reports
- Consultant notes
- Therapy evaluations
- Information in the nurses' notes
- Special needs
- Information provided by the resident and family
- Information provided by nursing assistants and restorative nursing assistants

The resident and family members of the resident's choice are invited to participate in the care conference.

MARYSVILLE CARE CENTER	CARE PLAN	09/07/XX
		FORM # 280L

PROBLEM	SHORT TERM GOAL	APPROACH
(1) FLUID VOLUME DEFICIT RELATED TO DECREASED FLUID INTAKE. ONSET TARGET RESOLVE 09/06/XX 12/05/XX / /	(1) REHYDRATE/ESTABLISH FLUID BALANCE. BEGIN TARGET RESOLVE 09/06/XX 12/05/XX / /	(1) RECORD INTAKE AND OUTPUT EVERY SHIFT. DISC: NSG (2) CHECK & RECORD B.P. AS ORDERED. DISC: NSG (3) MONITOR SKIN TURGOR. DISC: NSG (4) ENCOURAGE ADEQUATE FLUID INTAKE DAILY. DISC: NSG D (5) OFFER FLUIDS OF CHOICE. DISC: ALL (6) INCREASE AMOUNT OF FLUID INTAKE TO 2500CC DAILY. DISC: NSG (7) CHECK MUCOUS MEMBRANE MOISTNESS Q SHIFT DISC: NSG (8) MONITOR VITAL SIGNS Q 4 HOURS AND PRN. DISC: NSG
(2) POTENTIAL FOR IMPAIRED SKIN INTEGRITY DUE TO DECREASED MOBILITY. ONSET TARGET RESOLVE 09/06/XX 12/05/XX / /	(1) FREE FROM RED OR OPEN AREAS. BEGIN TARGET RESOLVE 09/06/XX 12/05/XX / / (2) MAINTAIN SKIN INTEGRITY. BEGIN TARGET RESOLVE 09/06/XX 12/05/XX / /	(1) HAVE DIETICIAN CONSULT ABOUT DIET. DISC: D (2) INCREASE AMOUNT OF FLUID INTAKE DAILY. DISC: NSG (3) INCREASE MEAT/PROTEIN IN DIET. DISC: NSG D

PHYSICIAN / ALT. PHYSICIAN	PHONE NO.	ALLERGIES / NOTES				
SMART, NANCY D.O. KEELEY, SHAWN D.O.	(555) 888-1212					

RESIDENT	STATION / ROOM / BED	ADMISSION NUMBER / DATE	SEX	DATE OF BIRTH	CARE PLAN DATE	PAGE #
MARTIN, FRANK	WEST-322-B	23891 09/22/1995	M	08/04/1918	09/07/XX	1

Figure 2–3 Everyone caring for the resident follows the care plan. The plan is changed as often as necessary.

MARYSVILLE CARE CENTER	CARE PLAN	09/07/XX
		FORM # 280L

PROBLEM	SHORT TERM GOAL	APPROACH
(3) RES. INACTIVE, SITS IN CHAIR MOST OF DAY	(1) NO CONTRACTURES OR DEFORMITIES RELATED TO IMMOBILITY.	(1) AROM/PROM 5 REPS BID.
		(2) INCREASE FLUIDS.
ONSET TARGET RESOLVE	ONSET TARGET RESOLVE	(3) ENCOURAGE ACTIVITY. DISC: NSG
09/06/XX 12/05/XX / /	09/06/XX 12/05/XX / /	(4) KEEP BED LINEN OFF EXTREMITIES. DISC: NSG
		(5) KEEP EXTREMITIES IN PROPER ALIGNMENT & PROPERLY SUPPORTED. DISC: NSG
		(6) KEEP HEEL PROTECTORS ON AT ALL TIMES TO REDUCE PRESSURE. DISC: NSG
		(7) KEEP DRY AND CHANGE AFTER VOIDING. DISC: NSG
		(8) KEEP SKIN CLEAN, DRY AND FREE OF PRESSURE. DISC: NSG
		(9) TURN EVERY 2 HOURS AND PRN. MAINTAIN GOOD BODY ALIGNMENT WITH PILLOWS. DISC: NSG
		(10) MULTIVITAMINS WITH IRON AND VITAMIN C. DISC: NSG
		(11) SPENCO MATTRESS TO BED AND CHAIR. DISC: NSG

PHYSICIAN / ALT. PHYSICIAN	PHONE NO.	ALLERGIES / NOTES					
SMART, NANCY D.O. KEELEY, SHAWN D.O.	(555) 888-1212						

RESIDENT	STATION / ROOM / BED	ADMISSION NUMBER / DATE	SEX	DATE OF BIRTH	CARE PLAN DATE	PAGE #
MARTIN, FRANK	WEST-322-B	23891 09/22/1995	M	08/04/1918	09/07/XX	2

Figure 2–3, continued.

MARYSVILLE CARE CENTER	CARE PLAN	09/07/XX
		FORM # 280L

PROBLEM	SHORT TERM GOAL	APPROACH
(4) ALTERATION IN COGNITIVE SKILLS FOR DAILY DECISION MAKING:RES. RARELY OR NEVER MAKES DECISIONS	(1) RES. WILL MAKE ONE DECISION PER WEEK CONCERNING OWN CARE, INCREASED BY ONE WEEKLY UNTIL SEVERAL ARE BEING MADE DAILY	(1) CAPITALIZE ON RES'S STRENGTHS & MAXIMIZE INDEPENDENCE. DISC: NSG
ONSET 09/06/XX TARGET 12/05/XX RESOLVE / /	BEGIN 09/06/XX TARGET 12/05/XX RESOLVE / /	(2) WORK WITH RES. TO HELP RES. EXPRESS NEEDS. DISC: SS, ACT, NSG
		(3) ENCOURAGE RES. TO MAKE INCREASINGLY MORE & INDEPENDENT DECISIONS EACH DAY. DISC: NSG
		(4) ASK RES. OPINION IF POSSIBLE WHEN FACED WITH A CHOICE. DISC: NSG

PHYSICIAN / ALT. PHYSICIAN	PHONE NO.	ALLERGIES / NOTES					
SMART, NANCY D.O. KEELEY, SHAWN D.O.	(555) 888-1212						
RESIDENT	STATION / ROOM / BED	ADMISSION NUMBER / DATE		SEX	DATE OF BIRTH	CARE PLAN DATE	PAGE #
MARTIN, FRANK	WEST-322-B	23891	09/22/1995	M	08/04/1918	09/07/XX	3

Figure 2–3, continued.

MARYSVILLE CARE CENTER	CARE PLAN	09/07/XX
		FORM # 280L

PROBLEM	SHORT TERM GOAL	APPROACH

(5) INABILITY TO MAKE SELF UNDERSTOOD: RES. IS RARELY OR NEVER UNDERSTOOD
 	
ONSET   TARGET   RESOLVE
09/06/XX 12/05/XX / /
	(1) RES. WILL BE UNDERSTOOD BY OTHER RESIDENTS & STAFF BY INCREASED FREQUENCY AND MEANS OF COMMUNICATION
	
	BEGIN TARGET RESOLVE
	09/06/XX 12/05/XX / /
		(1) ALLOW TIME FOR RESPONSE.
		    DISC: NSG
		
		(2) ALLOW TIME; PRAISE ALL EFFORTS.
		    DISC: ALL
		
		(3) ALWAYS STAND IN FRONT OF RES. SO FACE AND MOUTH CAN BE WATCHED DURING VERBAL COMMUNICATION.
		    DISC: ALL
		
		(4) COMMUNICATION - WHEN YOU APPPROACH RES., IDENTIFY YOURSELF.
		    DISC: ALL

(6) ALTERATION IN BLADDER CONTINENCE: RES. EXPERIENCES MULTIPLE EPISODES OF BLADDER INCONTINENCE DAILY; RES. IS CONSIDERED INCONTINENT
 	
ONSET   TARGET   RESOLVE
09/06/XX 12/05/XX / /
	(1) WILL BE KEPT DRY.
	
	BEGIN TARGET RESOLVE
	09/06/XX 12/05/XX / /
		(1) ASSESS FOR BOWEL AND BLADDER TRAINING PROGRAM
		    DISC: NSG
		
		(2) CHECK FREQUENTLY FOR WETNESS; CHANGE CLOTHES & BED LINEN PRN.
		    DISC: NSG
		
		(3) DIAPER OR INCONTINENT PAD FOR PROTECTION, PRN.
		    DISC: NSG

		(4) STAFF TO ANTICIPATE AND MEET NEEDS PROMPTLY.
		    DISC: ALL
		
		(5) MONITOR FOR S/S BREAKDOWN DAILY AND REPORT.
		    DISC: NSG
		
		(6) PERICARE AFTER EACH INCONTINENT EPISODE.
		    DISC: N

PHYSICIAN / ALT. PHYSICIAN	PHONE NO.	ALLERGIES / NOTES				
SMART, NANCY D.O. KEELEY, SHAWN D.O.	(555) 888-1212					

RESIDENT	STATION / ROOM / BED	ADMISSION NUMBER / DATE	SEX	DATE OF BIRTH	CARE PLAN DATE	PAGE #
MARTIN, FRANK	WEST-322-B	23891 09/22/1995	M	08/04/1918	09/07/XX	4

Figure 2–3, continued.

MARYSVILLE CARE CENTER	CARE PLAN	09/07/XX
		FORM # 280L

PROBLEM	SHORT TERM GOAL	APPROACH
(7) MAINTENANCE OF NUTRITIONAL APPROACHES: RES. HAS MECHANICALLY ALTERED DIET.	(1) ABLE TO EAT A WELL-NOURISHED DIET. NO WEIGHT LOSS. NO EPISODES OF CHOKING.	(1) MONITOR FOOD INTAKE DISC: NSG.D
		(2) MONITOR MONTHLY WEIGHT. DISC: NSG
ONSET TARGET RESOLVE 09/06/XX 12/05/XX / /	BEGIN TARGET RESOLVE 09/06/XX 12/05/XX / /	(3) PROVIDE DIET AT CONSISTENCY RES. CAN TOLERATE. DISC: D
		(4) SUPERVISE CLOSELY AT ALL MEALS. DISC: NSG
(8) RES. AT RISK FOR DEHYDRATION DUE TO DIURETIC MEDICATION AND POOR ORAL INTAKE.	(1) WILL BE ADEQUATELY NOURISHED & HYDRATED.	(1) OFFER FLUIDS EACH TIME YOU ARE IN THE ROOM. DISC: NSG
ONSET TARGET RESOLVE 09/06/XX 12/05/XX / /	BEGIN TARGET RESOLVE 09/06/XX 12/05/XX / /	(2) MONITOR FOR S/S DEHYDRATION AND REPORT. DISC: NSG
		(3) INTAKE AND OUTPUT Q SHIFT AND EVALUATE. DISC: NSG
*** CURRENT MEDICATION ***		
*** WEIGHT HISTORY ***		
*** CURRENT DIAGNOSIS ***		

PHYSICIAN / ALT. PHYSICIAN	PHONE NO.	ALLERGIES / NOTES					
SMART, NANCY D.O. KEELEY, SHAWN D.O.	(555) 888-1212						
RESIDENT	STATION / ROOM / BED	ADMISSION NUMBER / DATE		SEX	DATE OF BIRTH	CARE PLAN DATE	PAGE #
MARTIN, FRANK	WEST-322-B	23891	09/22/1995	M	08/04/1918	09/07/XX	5

Figure 2–3, continued.

Although using the RAI is required, the government does not require specific care plan approaches. The approaches are developed by members of the interdisciplinary team. They are designed using all available resources to help the resident. You are an important team member. You may be invited to attend care conferences, or your supervisor will share information that you have provided.

Holistic Care

The care plan uses a holistic approach. **Holistic** means emphasizing the organic or functional relation between parts and the whole; in other words, looking at the entire person. **Holistic care** is designed to meet the resident's individual needs. This means that all factors affecting the resident's care are considered. The medical model focuses on physical factors only. The holistic approach causes us to consider mental, emotional, financial, spiritual, and other factors when planning resident care.

Using Triggers in Care Plan Development

The interdisciplinary team will determine if triggered conditions present a problem. If so, information about the condition is included in the care plan. The trigger may suggest that the resident will benefit from a restorative program. If so, team members further assess the resident and develop a program to meet his or her needs. The program may be used to assist the resident to learn new skills. It may also teach the resident skills that he or she has lost. Some programs maintain the resident at his or her present status and prevent declines. Some restorative programs are developed because of triggered conditions. Others are developed because staff identifies a need. The team feels that the program will benefit the resident.

Developing Realistic Goals

(SA) When developing the care plan, the team tries to develop realistic goals. A *realistic goal* is one that the resident will be able to meet. Goals must also be measurable. This means that you should be able to look at the goal and see if the resident is meeting it or making progress. (SA) Everyone working on the goal should be able to evaluate the resident's progress. Numbers are often used to make goals measurable. An example of a measurable goal is for the resident to walk 50 feet with the walker and a standby assistant. Team members can readily determine how many feet the resident walks. The best goals are functional or useful. Giving the resident a purpose to walk 50 feet is best. Walking to the dining room for meals or to the activity room for an activity is a purposeful goal. When developing goals, remember that the skill should be useful. For repetitive goals, have the resident do something like shine shoes or polish the

chrome on the wheelchair. Goals that make the resident feel useful, or through which he or she helps others, are good for developing satisfaction and self-esteem. Helping others is beneficial to most residents.

When a resident reaches a goal, the team uses it to build on the resident's success. Sometimes goals are very small. As the resident achieves a goal, another goal or step is added. This continues until the resident reaches his or her maximum potential. At this point, a maintenance program is developed. This helps the resident continue to function at the highest level possible.

As you can see, a great deal of time is spent on the RAI and care planning. The team lists approaches for all caregivers to follow. Using the approaches helps residents meet their goals. All staff caring for the resident must be familiar with, and use, the care plan. Using the plan ensures consistent care. The resident will benefit because all staff are working on the same problems using the same approaches.

Quarterly Care Plan Reviews

During the quarterly care plan reviews, the team evaluates the resident's progress. They decide if the resident has met or is making progress toward the goals. Each quarter, the team assesses goals the resident has met. As the resident meets small goals, new goals are added. Sometimes residents are not meeting the stated goals. In this case, team members attempt to find out why. They will modify the goal or the approaches so they are more realistic and achievable for the resident. Although the resident may be making progress, the care plan may be modified. This helps the resident slowly build on small successes, so that larger goals are gradually achieved.

Changes in Condition

(SA) The care plan is changed any time the resident's condition changes. It is not necessary to review the RAI for a minor change in condition.(SA) For example, a minor infection will not be permanent, so an RAI review is not done. The infection may change the resident's care, though, so the care plan is revised. Understanding this is important. If the resident meets the restorative care plan goals, inform your supervisor. He or she will change the goals and approaches or develop a maintenance program. Likewise, if a specific approach is not working, your supervisor will change the care plan.

Meeting Residents' Needs

You will help residents meet needs on many different levels. As the residents' conditions improve, they begin to meet more needs on their own. The ability to meet their own needs provides a sense of self-satisfaction and accomplishment. This keeps residents psychologically healthy. Residents who are physically dependent on others can still derive mental satisfaction from being in control of their care. Allow them to make decisions about their routines.

RISK FACTORS

You have learned that *risk factors* are conditions that may cause a resident's health to worsen. The RAI assists facility personnel to identify risk factors in advance so that a plan of care can be developed to prevent declines. For example, an incontinent, bedfast resident is at high risk of skin breakdown and other complications. The care plan will list actions to prevent skin breakdown. ⓢⒶ Preventive care and anticipating risk factors is an important part of the RAI and care planning process. This benefits both the resident and the facility. If the resident's medical record is involved in a lawsuit because of a decline, the preventive care plan proves that personnel anticipated the risk and took measures to prevent the decline.ⓢⒶ

Identifying New Risk Factors

Although the RAI identifies many risk factors, it does not identify all of them. If you believe a resident is at risk for an injury or decline, report this information to your supervisor. For example, Mrs. Long is sick and bedfast for 3 days. Before she became ill, you walked with her in the hallway daily. After her illness, you notice that her legs are stiff. Her balance is not as good. You will address these problems immediately in your daily care. Informing your supervisor is also important. The stiffness and difficulty balancing indicate that if Mrs. Long is not walked each day, she will decline rapidly. She may need range of motion or another program to prevent declines. Immobility, even for a few days, is a risk factor for this resident. As you can see from this example, risk factors are highly individualized.

When the interdisciplinary team reevaluates care plan goals, they look for other signs of decline. The team will plan ways to avoid them. Declines can occur rapidly. However, in the elderly, they can also occur slowly and may not be recognized. Knowing the residents you care for and communicating with other team members helps identify risk factors and prevents deterioration. Preventing declines is an important part of providing care in all health care settings.

KEY POINTS IN CHAPTER

Residents are assessed by a nurse immediately upon admission, and an interim plan of care is developed.

The RAI is an important document that must be completed accurately.

The RAI consists of the MDS 2.0, triggers, and RAPs.

The RAI must be completed within 14 days of admission. The interdisciplinary care plan must be completed within 7 days of completion of the RAI.

Triggers help identify real problems, potential problems, risk factors, and candidates for restorative programs.

All care begins with an assessment.

The nursing process is used by the interdisciplinary team to care for the residents.

The four steps of the nursing process are assessment, planning, implementation, and evaluation.

The resident must understand what is expected of him or her and what the expected outcome of a restorative procedure is.

Safety is a primary concern when providing restorative care.

Supporting resident rights during restorative care is very important.

The restorative assistant monitors the resident's response during and after restorative care.

Restorative programs are based on an assessment of the resident's needs. They begin with small goals. As each goal is met, another is added. Eventually the resident will be able to complete a larger skill.

CLINICAL APPLICATIONS

1. Mrs. Gonzalez was admitted to your facility 10 days ago. Your supervisor has developed an interim care plan. You are assigned to ambulate Mrs. Gonzalez 25 feet twice a day. You must check her blood pressure before and 10 minutes after ambulation. You have noticed that the resident becomes slightly short of breath when she ambulates. Her blood pressure usually rises during ambulation. It does not return to the original range for nearly an hour. Mrs. Gonzalez has a steady gait and can easily walk the 25-foot distance. She prefers to walk immediately before breakfast. She likes to take an afternoon nap. She wants to walk again immediately before your shift ends for the day. When Mrs. Gonzalez walks in the hallway, she prefers to wear her tennis shoes, with white socks. After her walk, she returns to her room and puts on nylon stockings and a pair of black pumps. What information is important to the care plan that you will share with your supervisor? Will the supervisor further assess this resident before the care plan conference?

2. Mrs. Garza is very modest. She tells you that she refuses personal care because she is embarrassed. What information will you report to your supervisor? How will the interdisciplinary team determine which restorative program to begin with?

3. Mr. Perry is a mentally confused resident with a diagnosis of congestive heart failure. You are assigned to do passive range-of-motion exercises twice a day. He always yells when you begin exercising him. You discover that he quiets down and cooperates if you ask him to sing a song with you. Because of the heart condition, Mr. Perry is on intake and output. His total oral intake averages about 700 cc a day on your shift. Mr. Perry had a stroke 20 years ago. He has no paralysis, but the left side of his face droops slightly when he tries to smile. Although he has full range of motion, his left side is weak. You observe that he cannot grasp a glass with his left hand without spilling. The right side of the bed is next to the wall. The overbed table, containing the water pitcher, is on the left side of the bed. Mr. Perry does not drink much water. What information about this resident is important to address at the care plan conference?

4. Mrs. Lund is weak and unsteady on her feet. She grabs objects and furniture as she walks in her room. Mrs. Lund's vision is poor. She does not recognize common items unless they are very close to her face. The resident's skin is very dry and she asks you to put lotion on her arms and legs each day. Mrs. Lund bruises and gets skin tears easily. She informs you she had a pressure ulcer when she was in the hospital for hip surgery. This information provides clues to four high-risk conditions for this resident. Identify them, and explain why including this new information on the care plan is important. Describe nursing measures you can take to prevent complications.

The Elderly in Long-Term Care

OBJECTIVES

After reading this chapter, you should be able to:

- *Spell and define key terms.*
- *Review the functions of each body system.*
- *List at least two aging changes that occur in each body system.*
- *List each level of Maslow's hierarchy and explain how the hierarchy relates to restorative programs.*

THE ELDERLY

At present, most residents in long-term care facilities are elderly. A basic understanding of the aging process, chronic disease, and the needs of the elderly are essential to your success.

AGING CHANGES

Aging begins at birth and continues throughout life. Aging changes affect the way residents react and adapt to their environment **(Figure 3–1).** Each body system has a specific function. You learned these functions in your nursing assistant program. These are summarized in **Table 3–1.** Every body system undergoes aging changes. People age at different rates. Some seem to age quickly. Others seem much younger than their chronological age. Heredity, lifestyle, disease, nutrition, and environment all affect the aging process. Aging changes to each body system are summarized in **Table 3–2.**

Effects of Aging Changes on Functional Status

Normal changes of aging affect body function. One weak system may affect the function of the entire body in various ways. For example, a resident with weakness of the legs may have trouble getting out of the chair to go to the bathroom. If the resident's knees are weak, he may not be able to walk to the bathroom. He may become incontinent. This causes odors, which affect self-esteem. The skin irritation may cause pressure ulcers. The weak knees have affected many systems. Assisting the resident to stand and walk to the bathroom solves the problem.

Healthy people do not realize that problems such as weakness in the knees may affect the control of

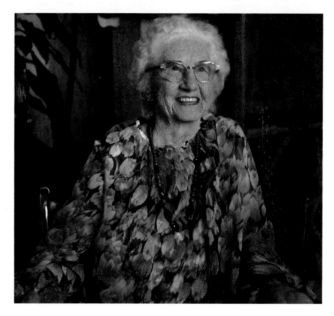

Figure 3–1 The way the elderly react to their environment is determined by their lifetime experiences.

urine. You must develop a sensitivity to things like this. Remember to look at each resident holistically. Realize that one problem can affect the whole person. Aging changes in vision and hearing may also cause the resident to lose contact with the environment and appear confused. The confusion disappears if hearing and vision are corrected. Changes in the environment or acute illnesses may cause:

- confusion
- changes in behavior
- feelings of loss of control
- stress
- sleep disturbances

Table 3–1 Function of Body Systems

System	Function
Circulatory	Carries oxygen and nutrients to the cells for nourishment, removes waste products
Respiratory	Takes in oxygen and eliminates carbon dioxide from the body
Integumentary	Covers and protects the body, regulates temperature, eliminates waste products, protects against infection, serves as a vehicle for sensory perception
Urinary	Maintains balance of liquid and electrolytes in the body, eliminates liquid waste products
Gastrointestinal	Transport and digests food, absorbs nutrients, eliminates waste products
Endocrine	Produces hormones that regulate many body functions
Reproductive	Reproduces, fulfills sexual needs
Nervous	Sends and receives messages between the brain and the body, controls all body functions and mental processes
Musculoskeletal	Provides support and protection for the body and internal organs, provides movement, provides shape

Table 3–2 Aging Changes

Body System	Aging Changes
Circulatory	■ Heart rate slows, causing a slower pulse and less efficient circulation. The resident has less energy and slower responses. He or she tires easily. ■ Blood vessels lose elasticity and develop calcium deposits, causing vessels to narrow. ■ Blood pressure increases because of changes to the blood vessel walls. ■ Heart rate takes longer to return to normal after exercise. ■ Veins enlarge, causing blood vessels close to the skin surface to become more prominent.
Respiratory	■ Lung capacity decreases as a result of muscular rigidity in the lungs. ■ The ability to cough effectively is reduced; this results in pooling of secretions and fluid in the lungs, increasing the risk of infection and choking. ■ Shortness of breath on exertion as a result of aging changes in lungs. ■ Gas exchange in the lungs is less effective, resulting in decreased oxygenation.
Integumentary	■ Skin thins and loses elasticity, wrinkles appear, skin becomes irritated and breaks, cuts, and tears easily. ■ Increased fragility of blood vessels that nourish the skin, causing bruising, senile purpura, and skin tears.

(continues)

Table 3–2 Aging Changes, *continued*

Body System	Aging Changes
Integumentary *continued*	■ Reduced blood flow in vessels that nourish the skin results in delayed healing. ■ Reduced secretion from oil glands that supply the skin causes dryness and itching. ■ Decreased perspiration, resulting in impaired ability to regulate temperature. ■ Subcutaneous fat diminishes, resulting in less protection and complaints of feeling cold. ■ Blood supply to the feet and legs is reduced, increasing risk of injury and ulcers, feeling of coldness. ■ Finger and toenail growth slows and nails become brittle. ■ Hair thins and turns gray.
Urinary	■ Bladder capacity decreases, increasing the frequency of urination. ■ Kidney function increases at rest, causing increased urination at night. ■ Weakening of bladder muscles, causing leaking of urine or inability to empty the bladder completely. ■ Enlargement of the prostate gland in the male, causing frequency of urination, dribbling, urinary obstruction, and urinary retention.
Digestive (Gastrointestinal)	■ Decreased saliva production in the mouth, causing difficulty with digestion of starches. ■ Taste buds on the tongue decrease, beginning with sweet and salt, changes in taste buds may result in appetite changes and increase in condiment use. ■ Gag reflex is less effective, increasing the risk of choking. ■ Movement of food into the stomach through the esophagus is slower. ■ Slower digestion of food in the stomach, so food remains there longer before moving to the small intestine. ■ Indigestion and slower absorption of fat as a result of decreased digestive enzymes. ■ Food movement through the large intestine is slower, resulting in constipation.
Endocrine	■ Delayed release of insulin, increasing blood sugar level; incidence of diabetes increases greatly with age. ■ Metabolism rate and body function slow, reducing the amount of calories needed for the body to function normally. This increases the risk of overweight and obesity.
Reproductive	Changes in the Male ■ Hormone production decreases, decreasing size of testes and lowering sperm count. ■ More time required for an erection. Changes in the Female ■ Fewer female hormones are produced. ■ Vagina becomes shorter and narrower. ■ Vaginal secretions decrease. ■ Breast tissue decreases and the muscles supporting the breasts weaken.
Nervous	■ Tasks involving speed, balance, coordination, and fine motor activities take longer because of slowed transmission of nerve impulses. ■ Balance and coordination problems as a result of deterioration in the nerve terminals that provide information to the brain about body movement and position.

(continues)

Table 3–2	Aging Changes, *continued*
Body System	**Aging Changes**
Nervous, *continued*	■ Visual changes result from decreased flexibility in the lens in the eye. ■ Dryness and itching of the eyes as a result of decreased secretion of fluids. ■ Difficulty hearing due to a decrease in the nerves and blood supply to the ears. ■ Risk of injury increases because of decreased ability to feel pressure and temperature changes. ■ Decreased blood flow to the brain, which may result in mental confusion and memory loss.
Musculoskeletal	■ Loss of elasticity of muscles and decrease in size of muscle mass result in reduced strength, endurance, muscle tone, and delayed reaction time. ■ Bones lose minerals, become brittle, and break more easily. ■ Spine becomes less stable and flexible, increasing the risk of injury. ■ Posture may become slumped over because of weakness in back muscles. ■ Degenerative changes in the joints cause limited movement, stiffness, and pain.

Restorative nursing involves understanding that these changes are beyond the residents' control. You will help them adapt to changes in their lifestyle. Residents become frustrated because they recognize these changes, but cannot stop them. Assisting residents to use their strengths will improve their self-esteem.

COMMON DISEASES AND CONDITIONS SEEN IN LONG-TERM CARE FACILITY RESIDENTS

The elderly often develop chronic diseases. A *chronic illness* or *disease* is one that lasts for a long time, often for life. The appearance of a chronic illness requires changes in lifestyle. The resident must make many mental adjustments. Some residents develop more than one chronic disease. This increases the residents' frustration and sense of loss. It may make self-care difficult or impossible. Many chronic illnesses cause pain and fatigue. Some limit mobility and activity. Some diseases interfere with sexual function. **Table 3–3** lists common diseases and conditions seen in long-term care facility residents.

BASIC HUMAN NEEDS

Helping residents meet their own needs is a very important responsibility. The resident's behavior may change if his or her needs are not met. When needs on a lower level are not met, you will notice physical problems. For example, a resident who is thin and weak needs food and fluids. These needs affect other body systems, causing the resident to be tired and have other functional problems. When needs on a higher level are not met, you may notice anger, withdrawal, or behavior problems **(Figure 3–2).** Likewise, this causes stress, which creates problems with other body systems. Your care and observations are important to the resident's success in meeting the care plan goals and overcoming or adjusting to the problems caused by aging and disease.

Understanding how one body system affects another and reviewing Maslow's hierarchy of needs

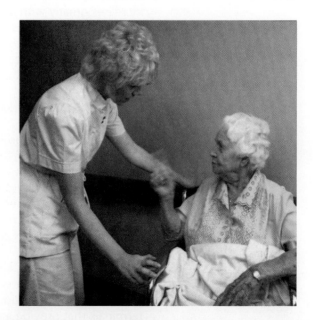

Figure 3–2 When residents' psychosocial needs are not met, they may lash out with anger.

Table 3–3 Common Conditions Seen in Long-Term Care Facility Residents

Disease or Condition	Description
Alzheimer's disease	A progressive disease resulting in deterioration of brain cells in which the resident gradually loses mental and physical ability. The disease is incurable and ends in death.
Amputation	Removal of an extremity. Amputation is usually performed because of trauma or gangrene.
Arteriosclerosis	A narrowing of the inside walls of the arteries, making them rigid and thick. The blood flow passing through the vessel walls is reduced, depriving the body of oxygen and other nutrients. Hypertension is common because the heart must work harder to force blood through the blocked vessels. Residents with this condition are at high risk of stroke and heart attack.
Arthritis	A painful inflammation of joints that results in limited movement and deformities.
Atherosclerosis	A buildup of plaque, calcium, and fat on the walls of the arteries, making them rigid and thick. The blood flow passing through the vessel walls is reduced, depriving the body of oxygen and other nutrients. Hypertension is common because the heart must work harder to force blood through the blocked vessels. Residents with this condition are at high risk of stroke and heart attack.
Cancer	A malignant tumor or new growth anywhere in the body. Cancer may spread slowly or rapidly.
Cerebrovascular accident (CVA)(stroke, brain attack)	An incident in the brain caused by a blood clot or bursting of a blood vessel, causing blood to spill into the brain cavity. Common effects of a stroke are paralysis on one side of the body, loss of bowel and bladder control, and speech impairment. The effects may be temporary or permanent.
Congestive heart failure	A condition in which the heart is unable to pump sufficient blood to meet the needs of the body. Characterized by hypertension and edema.
Diabetes mellitus	A disorder of the endocrine system in which the body cannot properly metabolize carbohydrates, proteins, and fat.
Emphysema	A disorder in which the alveoli of the lungs have stretched and lost their elasticity, causing them to be unable to contract to remove excess air. This condition causes a chronic shortness of breath and deprivation of oxygen needed for body functions.
Head injury	Caused by trauma; some head injuries are severe and cause permanent brain damage that results in loss of physical and/or mental function.
Hearing impairment	Difficulty hearing from a number of causes. May range from hard of hearing to complete deafness. Some residents may benefit from use of a hearing aid. Some types of deafness can be treated with a cochlear implant to restore hearing.

(continues)

Table 3–3 Common Conditions Seen in Long-Term Care Facility Residents, *continued*

Disease or Condition	Description
Heart attack (myocardial infarction)	A serious medical emergency in which the blood vessels that nourish the heart muscle are blocked or burst, disrupting the normal flow of blood through the heart.
Heart block	A condition that may require a pacemaker for treatment. Caused by a disruption in the conduction of impulses in the heart.
Hemiplegia	Paralysis on one side of the body; most common cause is CVA.
Hip fracture	A broken hip that is usually the result of a fall but can result from osteoporosis. The hip must be repaired surgically or by using traction to enable the resident to walk again.
Hip replacement	Removal of the entire hip joint and replacement with a synthetic joint. The resident usually requires skilled therapy and restorative nursing after surgery and will return to his or her former level of function after recovery.
Huntington's disease	A progressive, hereditary disease resulting in rapid, involuntary movements and progressive dementia.
Hypertension	High blood pressure. The resident may have no symptoms, or may develop dizziness, headaches, and fatigue. If undiagnosed for a long time, may cause permanent kidney damage.
Multiple sclerosis	A chronic, progressive disease marked by intermittent periods of remission. The resident has weakness, incoordination, speech, visual, and sensory disturbances.
Paraplegia	Paralysis below the waist. The condition is usually caused by trauma, but can be caused by tumors and other conditions.
Parkinson's disease	A neurological disorder that results in tremors, muscular rigidity, and shuffling gait.
Peripheral artery disease	A condition caused by atherosclerosis that results in insufficient blood flow to the legs. It may result in leg ulcers, gangrene, and amputation.
Peripheral vascular disease	A disorder that is frequently the result of varicose veins. Blood return from the legs is inadequate, frequently resulting in blood clots and leg ulcers.
Pneumonia and influenza	Serious infections of the lungs contracted by the droplet method of transmission.
Quadriplegia	Paralysis below the neck. The usual cause is trauma, but can result from tumors, infection, and other conditions.
Vision impairment	Difficulty seeing, caused by any of a number of causes. Sometimes vision can be improved with glasses or surgery. In some disorders vision cannot be restored.

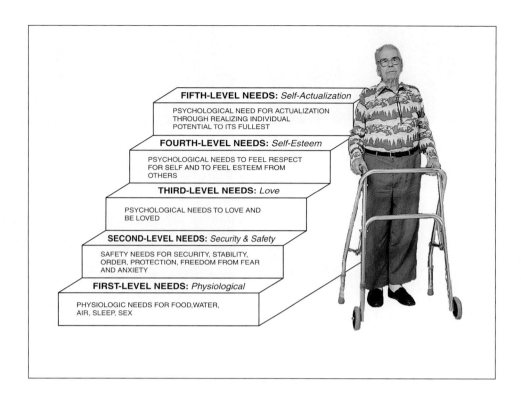

FIFTH-LEVEL NEEDS: *Self-Actualization*

PSYCHOLOGICAL NEED FOR ACTUALIZATION
THROUGH REALIZING INDIVIDUAL
POTENTIAL TO ITS FULLEST

FOURTH-LEVEL NEEDS: *Self-Esteem*

PSYCHOLOGICAL NEEDS TO FEEL RESPECT
FOR SELF AND TO FEEL ESTEEM FROM
OTHERS

THIRD-LEVEL NEEDS: *Love*

PSYCHOLOGICAL NEEDS TO LOVE AND
BE LOVED

SECOND-LEVEL NEEDS: *Security & Safety*

SAFETY NEEDS FOR SECURITY, STABILITY,
ORDER, PROTECTION, FREEDOM FROM FEAR
AND ANXIETY

FIRST-LEVEL NEEDS: *Physiological*

PHYSIOLOGIC NEEDS FOR FOOD, WATER,
AIR, SLEEP, SEX

Figure 3–3 Needs on the lower levels of Maslow's hierarchy must be met before higher-level needs become important.

will enable you to assist residents in meeting their needs. As the residents' conditions improve, they will begin meeting more needs on their own. Becoming independent provides a sense of satisfaction, accomplishment, and fulfillment. This helps meet psychological needs.

Maslow's Hierarchy of Needs

You learned about Maslow's hierarchy of needs in your nursing assistant program. To be a successful restorative nursing assistant, you must understand this theory. Maslow's theory is based on the belief that all human beings are good. Maslow says that self-actualization, or realizing one's full potential, is the goal of life. If something blocks the path to achieving self-actualization, the person becomes frustrated. Normal, healthy development enables people to realize their full potential. Behavior problems may result from frustration when the individual's needs are not met.

Maslow says that all human beings have the same basic needs. His theory is often described by using a pyramid or stairs **(Figure 3–3).** The figure reads from bottom to top. The needs at the bottom are the most urgent and essential to life. They are important for survival. As the physical needs are met, the higher-level psychological needs become important. Psychological needs must be met if a

person is to be emotionally healthy. Maslow writes that fulfilling the needs on the upper levels of the pyramid improves a person's quality of life.

Physiological Needs. Some residents may have diseases or conditions that make meeting lower-level needs difficult or impossible. Residents who are not receiving adequate oxygen and are struggling to breathe are using all of their energy to fulfill this one basic need **(Figure 3–4).** Until the breathing problem is resolved, other needs are not important.

Safety and Security Needs. When survival needs are met, safety and security become important. Residents must feel safe, secure, and protected from danger and hazards in the environment. They must also feel secure in family relationships. Financial security is important. If the illness strains family relationships or causes worry about paying medical bills, the resident's security needs are not met.

Love and Belonging Needs. The first two levels of Maslow's hierarchy involve physical needs. When these needs are satisfied, emotional needs become important. The most basic emotional need is to give and receive love. Strong family support will help meet this need. The way you interact with residents also affects this need. This is particularly true in the early stages of illness, when the resident

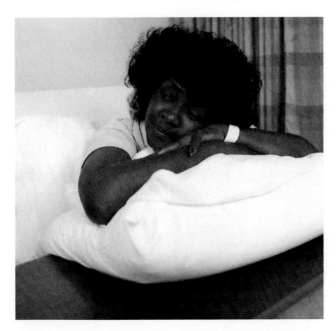

Figure 3–4 This resident is in the orthopneic position to enlarge her chest, making breathing easier.

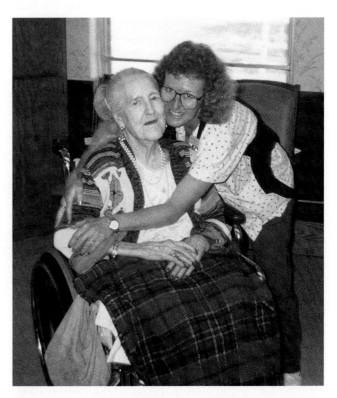

Figure 3–5 Giving a resident unconditional love shows that you accept and respect his or her identity as a person.

has not accepted his or her disability or disfigurement. Giving acceptance and support shows that you respect and accept the resident as a person. Your acceptance must be unconditional, regardless of disability, condition, appearance, or behavior **(Figure 3–5).**

Self-Esteem. **Self-esteem** refers to the mental image we have of ourselves. This is the image that we believe we project to others. Everyone has the need to feel important and worthwhile. Residents may feel they are not worthwhile because of their illnesses or disabilities. They often fear the outcome of the disease. They worry about how they will cope and how the condition will affect their lives and relationships. They are concerned about how they will appear to others. Many are fearful of dying and are afraid of the unknown. This threatens their self-image, causing a negative feeling.

Residents may not know or understand why they feel this way. For example, a resident who has had an amputation may believe that she is ugly and disfigured. She may be angry and complain about everything. Sometimes the resident criticizes you or other staff members. The resident is upset about the situation and is not mad at you. She is afraid of the outcome of her amputation, how she looks, and how she will cope. She reacts with anger because the amputation threatens her self-esteem.

Other residents may react in different ways. Allow residents to talk about what is bothering them. Avoid judging them for what they think, feel, and do. Show that you understand how they feel by showing concern. Many residents get pleasure from feeling as if they are needed. Activities in which residents provide a service or help others often improve their self-esteem.

Self-Actualization. **Self-actualization** means feeling a sense of accomplishment and success. You will help residents meet this need by recognizing improvements, even if they are small. Encouraging and assisting residents to return to self-care also helps meet this need. Sincerely compliment residents for their accomplishments. Self-actualization is promoted by helping the residents feel that they are overcoming a disease or disability.

DEVELOPMENTAL TASKS

All people have developmental tasks that must be completed throughout each stage of life. These are intellectual, social, and emotional skills that a person must accomplish at a certain age. The tasks are simple in childhood, but become more complex with age. Developmental tasks are listed in **Table 3–4.** Residents have developmental tasks that they must complete while living in the nursing facility. If they fail to complete these tasks, because of illness or facility admission, their emotional growth slows or stops. It remains at the level it was at before admission, until the resident completes the task.

Table 3–4 Developmental Tasks

Age	Stage of Development	Developmental Tasks
Birth to 1 year	Infant	Learns to trust self and others
Toddler	1–3 years	Learns to differentiate self from other people
Preschool	3–5 years	Develops initiative and is able to plan and initiate tasks
School age	6–11 years	Develops physical and mental ability, develops relationships with others
Adolescence	12–18 years	Develops a sense of identity and sexuality
Young adulthood	19–25 years	Establishes intimate relationships with a spouse or significant other
Middle adulthood	26–50 years	Self-realization in marriage and family; establishes a career
Late adulthood	51–65 years	Adjusts to the aging process, helps adult children
Old age	65+ years	Critically reviews the events and circumstances of life; develops feelings of fulfillment, acceptance, and self-worth

▬ RESIDENT COMFORT

Comfort is a state of well-being. The resident is not in pain or upset. He or she feels calm and relaxed. Many factors affect residents' comfort. Environmental factors include noise, odor, temperature, lighting, and ventilation.

Pain

Pain is a state of discomfort. It is unpleasant for the resident. Pain is a warning that something is wrong. Many factors affect residents' reactions to pain. The reactions may be different from one moment to the next. Four types of pain are listed in **Table 3–5.** Pain is common in the elderly. Research has shown that elderly residents in long-term care facilities are undermedicated for pain. Many will not ask for pain medication. They view discomfort as part of the aging process or chronic disease. Pain is a serious condition that affects the residents' well-being. Monitor the residents' body language for signs of pain. Ask residents if they are in pain.

Pain is a warning. It indicates a problem. Some elderly individuals do not feel pain. In some, the intensity of pain is less severe than it would be in a younger person. Some try to ignore the pain. This increases the risk of injury because the normal warning that pain provides goes unrecognized. Some residents may try to ignore or deny pain because they are afraid of what it means. Never ignore signs of pain in residents. Use nursing measures to make the resident comfortable. Always report pain to your supervisor.

Residents' Response to Pain.   Residents' responses to pain may be related to culture. People from some cultures are very emotional when they are in pain. Others are very stoic. Some think that showing pain is a sign of weakness. Some people believe that pain is a punishment from God.

Pain causes stress and anxiety. It interferes with comfort, rest, and sleep. Rest and sleep are necessary for the body to restore strength and energy and to repair itself. Inability to sleep may be caused by pain.

Table 3–5 Types of Pain

Type of Pain	Description
Acute pain	Occurs suddenly and without warning. Acute pain is usually the result of tissue damage, caused by conditions such as injury or surgery. Typically, acute pain decreases over time, as healing takes place.
Chronic pain	Chronic pain lasts longer than 6 months. It may be intermittent or constant. Chronic pain may be caused by multiple medical conditions.
Phantom pain	Phantom pain occurs as a result of an amputation. The resident has had a body part, such as a leg removed, but complains of pain in the toes. The pain is real, not imaginary.
Radiating pain	Radiating pain moves from the site of origin to other areas. For example, when a resident is having a heart attack, the pain may radiate from the chest to the jaw or arm.

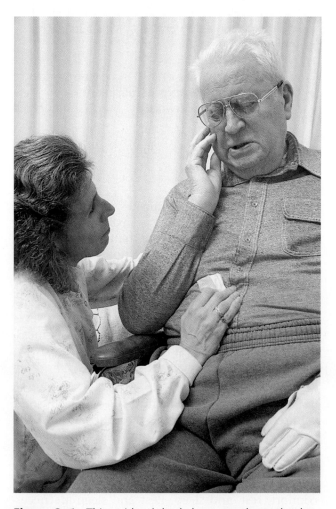

Figure 3–6 This resident's body language shows that he is in pain.

Signs and Symptoms of Pain. Pain always requires intervention. Be aware of signs and symptoms of pain in cognitively impaired residents. Facial expressions, moaning, refusing to move, limited movements, crying, yelling, or screaming may be clues that the resident is having pain **(Figure 3–6).** Report your observations to a nurse. Always report verbal complaints of pain to a nurse. Describe the pain in the resident's exact words. Additional information to report when a resident complains of pain includes:

- Pulse, respiration, and blood pressure
- Skin color
- Time of onset and duration of the pain
- Location of the pain and whether it radiates to another area
- Intensity and description of the pain, as described by the resident
- Any factors that improve the pain or cause it to worsen
- Other observations, such as facial expressions, movements, nausea, or vomiting

Restorative Comfort Measures. Basic nursing measures may make the resident more comfortable. Measures the restorative assistant can take to make the resident more comfortable include:

- Telling the resident what you are doing and how you will do it
- Assisting the resident to assume a comfortable position

PROCEDURE

1 RELAXATION ACTIVITIES

1. Perform your beginning procedure actions. These are explained in Chapter 5 and are listed on the inside front cover of this text.

2. Approach the resident in a calm, quiet manner. Provide emotional support.

3. Reduce noise and confusion in the environment. Provide low-level lighting unless the resident objects. These activities are most effective if done in a quiet, restful area.

4. Hold the resident's hand, use touch, or give a backrub.

5. Provide diversional activities or distraction, as directed. Examples of these techniques are humor, guided imagery, soft music, reading to the resident from a favorite book, or assisting the resident to focus his or her attention away from the source of pain or anxiety.

6. Assist the resident to sit or lie in a comfortable position, close eyes, and practice slow, deep breathing **(Figure 3–7)**.

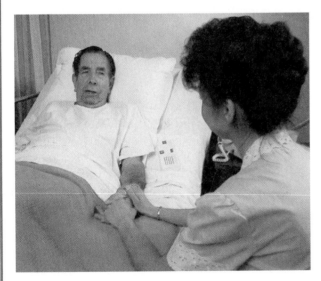

Figure 3–7 Assist the resident into a comfortable, relaxed position.

7. Remain with the resident, providing touch as appropriate. If the resident is combative or does not like to be touched, reassure him or her with eye contact, words, actions, and body language. Encourage the resident to verbalize concerns. Provide emotional support.

8. Assist the resident to meditate:
   a. Assist the resident to assume a comfortable position.
   b. Instruct the resident to close his or her eyes and relax the muscles. If the resident has difficulty relaxing, assist him or her to focus on and relax one area of the body at a time. Begin with the toes and move upward.
   c. Instruct the resident to select a one-syllable word, repeat it, and focus on it during exhalation.
   d. Continue this activity for the desired or designated length of time. After the activity, instruct the resident to remain quiet with eyes closed for a few minutes.
   e. Instruct the resident to repeat the procedure when needed.

9. Assist the resident with guided imagery:
   a. Assist the resident to assume a comfortable position.
   b. Instruct the resident to close his or her eyes and relax.
   c. Instruct the resident to think of a pleasant location or sensation. If a location is selected, the resident should imagine that he or she is there. Ask the resident to describe the location, then guide the images with a soft voice. Make suggestions about the sights, sounds, smells, and pleasant experiences. If the resident selects a sensation, guide the sensation in a soft voice. Describe sights, sounds, smells, taste, and feeling.
   d. Assist the resident to terminate the imagery after the specified time by suggesting that the resident take 10 deep breaths, then open the eyes.

(continues)

10. Assist the resident with relaxation therapy:
    a. Provide a quiet place and assist the resident to assume a comfortable position.
    b. Instruct the resident to close his or her eyes and relax the muscles.
    c. Speak in a low tone of voice.
    d. Use relaxation techniques specified in the care plan, such as deep breathing, abdominal breathing, or guided imagery.
    e. Use a relaxation tape with earphones, or verbally instruct the resident to relax all muscles, slowly and in sequence. Then, in sequence, contract and relax each muscle group. Begin at the toes and work upward to the feet, legs, abdomen, buttocks, fingers, hands, arms, shoulders, neck, and facial muscles. Remind the resident to breathe slowly and deeply throughout the activity.
    f. Avoid conversation. Assist the resident to focus on the technique to achieve a sense of relaxation.
    g. Terminate the activity at the designated time and allow the resident to rest.
11. Perform your procedure completion actions. These are explained in Chapter 5 and are listed on the inside front cover of this text.

- Avoiding sudden, jerking movements when moving or positioning the resident
- Using pillows to support the affected body part
- Maintaining a comfortable environmental temperature
- Giving a backrub
- Playing soft music to distract the resident
- Listening to the resident's concerns
- Providing emotional support
- Providing a quiet, dark environment

Your supervisor may direct you to apply warm or cold applications to make the resident more comfortable. These treatments are described in Chapter 6.

RELAXATION ACTIVITIES

You may assist residents with relaxation activities to relieve pain. The same techniques are used to relieve anxiety in residents who are not in pain. Relaxation activities include a combination of techniques. They reduce pain, anxiety, and fear, and promote a sense of well-being. Specific techniques are selected by the nurse or therapist. Relaxation activities are based on the resident's needs and a history of what has helped the resident in the past.

REST

Rest is a state of comfort, calmness, and relaxation. The resident's basic needs of hunger, thirst, elimination, and pain must be met before rest is possible. The resident may sit or lie down, or may do things that are pleasant and relaxing. The environment should be calm and quiet to promote rest. If basic care is tiring for the resident, allow him or her to rest before continuing. Some residents feel refreshed after 15 minutes of rest. Others need more time. Some residents must rest frequently throughout the day. Plan your schedule and activities to allow for rest periods. Providing a backrub or relaxation activities may assist the resident to rest. Follow the care plan and your supervisor's instructions.

SLEEP

Sleep is a basic need of all mammals. It allows the mind and body to rest. The body repairs itself during sleep. Adequate sleep is necessary for the body and mind to function properly. Sleep is a period of continuous or intermittent unconsciousness in which physical movements are decreased. Because movement and activity are minimized, the body's metabolic needs are reduced. The resident may need a blanket because he or she is not moving, and may become cold. Vital signs are lower during sleep. The need for sleep decreases as a person ages. Elderly residents require less sleep than young adults or middle-aged residents.

Many factors affect sleep. Obvious problems that interfere with sleep are:

- pain
- hunger
- thirst

- illness
- exercise
- noise
- temperature
- ventilation
- physical comfort
- medications
- caffeine intake
- anxiety

Sleep is important to prevent feelings of fatigue. Getting enough sleep and rest allows residents to function at the highest level possible. Moving through the stages of the sleep cycle is important. Residents who do not sleep well may become disoriented. This correctable condition is often mistaken for confusion! It is easily corrected by allowing them uninterrupted sleep. Use basic comfort measures, such as those used to relieve pain, to promote sleep. **Table 3–6** lists ways to promote comfort, rest, and sleep. Specific measures for the resident will be listed in the care plan.

Sleep has been studied extensively by researchers. Each person has a sleep-wake cycle. An internal biological clock tells the person when it is time to sleep and wake up. The sleep cycle is divided into two phases. **Rapid eye movement (REM) sleep** restores mental function. If you look closely, you will see the resident's eyes moving during this phase. Avoid awakening a resident in REM sleep, whenever possible. This is the part of the cycle in which dreams occur. **Nonrapid eye movement (NREM) sleep** has four phases, that progress from light to very deep. This part of the sleep cycle begins when the resident first falls asleep. In the first two phases, the resident is easy to arouse. As he or she progresses through each phase, arousal becomes more difficult as sleep becomes deeper. Within approximately 60 to 90 minutes, the resident passes through the stages into REM sleep.

Table 3–6   Measures to Promote Comfort, Rest, and Sleep

- Provide comfortable environmental temperature; give the resident a blanket if desired
- Eliminate unpleasant odors
- Assist the resident with toileting or incontinent care
- Eliminate noise
- Adjust the lighting to a comfortable level for the resident; darken the room as much as possible for sleep
- Eliminate pain, such as offering a backrub or repositioning the resident
- Keep bed linen clean and wrinkle-free
- Provide soft music to distract the resident
- Report pain to your supervisor or a licensed nurse
- If a resident is having pain, wait for at least 30 minutes after pain medication before performing procedures
- If a resident is anxious, listen to what he or she says; eliminate the cause of the anxiety if possible
- Avoid startling the resident
- Handle the resident gently during care
- Meet the resident's physical needs
- Assist the resident to put on comfortable clothing for rest and sleep
- Organize care to allow the resident uninterrupted sleep or rest
- Avoid physical activity or other activities that are upsetting to the resident before bedtime
- Assist the resident to perform personal bedtime rituals, if any
- Allow the resident to select his or her own bedtime
- Provide a warm bath or shower, if preferred
- Avoid serving beverages containing caffeine before bedtime
- Provide a bedtime snack, if desired
- Allow the resident to read, watch television, or listen to the radio, if desired
- Read to the resident from a favorite book
- Assist with relaxation exercises and activities, as ordered

KEY POINTS IN CHAPTER

- A basic understanding of the aging process and the needs of the elderly is essential to the success of the restorative nursing assistant.

- Aging changes affect the way residents react and adapt to their environment.

- One weak system affects the function of the entire body.

- Holistic care involves looking at the entire person and realizing that a condition that affects one part or system affects the whole person.

- Restorative nursing involves understanding that aging changes are beyond the residents' control and helping residents adapt as much as possible.

- Assisting residents to use their remaining strengths to meet their needs and maintain independence will improve self-esteem.

- Maslow's hierarchy of needs describes the basic needs of all human beings. According to Maslow, needs at the bottom of the pyramid are the most urgent and essential to life. As physical needs are met, the higher-level psychological needs become important.

- Psychological needs must be met for a person to be emotionally healthy.

- Developmental tasks are intellectual, social, and emotional skills that each person must accomplish at certain age levels throughout life.

- Elderly residents are at high risk of developing chronic diseases because of normal aging changes in the body.

- Chronic illness requires the resident to make mental adjustments and changes in lifestyle.

CLINICAL APPLICATIONS

1. Mrs. Bouzian takes pride in her appearance. She has a lovely wardrobe and takes a long time to apply makeup and style her hair each day. She was admitted to the hospital for a mastectomy because of a cancerous tumor in her breast. After several days in the hospital, she is readmitted to your facility. You are assigned to perform range-of-motion exercises on Mrs. Bouzian twice a day. You tell her you will assist her with her exercises after lunch. When you serve her lunch tray, she pushes it off the table and it flies across the room. She yells at you that she doesn't want her lunch. What do you think the problem is? How can you assist this resident? How will you know what type of exercises to do on the operative side of her body?

2. Mrs. Hayes must be spoon-fed. She is mentally confused and is supposed to wear glasses. However, she loses them frequently and cannot find them most days. One day Mrs. Hayes wears her glasses to the dining room. You observe another nursing assistant feeding her. Mrs. Hayes opens her mouth readily when she sees the spoon. You observe that she grabs the glass of milk and takes a drink without spilling. She also grabs a cookie and eats it. What do these observations tell you about Mrs. Hayes's need to be fed? What recommendations can you make? Should she be assessed for a restorative program?

3. Mrs. Shams is a resident who has chronic pain. She receives pain medication regularly, but often complains that her back and hips hurt. The resident tells you she is a "very nervous" person and that when she is anxious, her pain seems worse. When you have time, you give her a backrub. She thanks you sincerely each time and tells you how much it helps. What nursing comfort measures can you suggest to relieve Mrs. Shams's pain? Should she be evaluated for a restorative program?

Infection Control

After reading this chapter, you should be able to:

Spell and define key terms.

Describe the restorative assistant's responsibilities in preventing the spread of infection.

Describe and demonstrate standard precautions and transmission-based precautions.

List the three categories of transmission-based precautions and identify two diseases in each category.

List 10 times when the handwashing procedure should be performed.

Describe how and when to use personal protective equipment.

Demonstrate how to care for and clean equipment used in rehabilitation and restorative programs.

Demonstrate how to open a sterile package and apply sterile gloves.

OVERVIEW OF INFECTION CONTROL

You learned the principles of infection control in your nursing assistant class. They will not be repeated here. However, prevention of infection is an important responsibility. This is an area of ongoing research and study. Because of this, infection prevention practices change frequently. You may wish to review the chain of infection and medical asepsis in your nursing assistant text before beginning this unit. This chapter will provide you with an overview of the changes in practice that have occurred over the past few years. It also describes procedures specific to your responsibilities in keeping the equipment that you use free from pathogens.

Preventing the Spread of Infection

You will work with residents who have many diseases and conditions. The aging process weakens the immune system. Some residents have infections that may be spread to others. Others have diseases or conditions that increase the risk of infection. ⓢⒶ The most important way to prevent the spread of infection is by frequent, thorough handwashing.ⓢⒶ

Separation of Clean and Soiled Items and Equipment

ⓢⒶ To prevent infection, keep clean and soiled items separate.ⓢⒶ Clean items are either new, wrapped articles or reusable articles that have been cleaned by staff. Soiled items are things used by a resident or brought into a resident's room. They are considered soiled even if they were not used for resident care. They must be cleaned or disinfected when they are removed from the room. For example, linen is brought into a resident's room, but is not needed. It cannot be removed and used in the care of another resident. It must be washed before it is used.

STANDARD PRECAUTIONS

The Centers for Disease Control and Prevention (CDC) is a government agency that studies diseases and makes recommendations to prevent their spread. The CDC published guidelines for health care workers in the 1980s in response to the AIDS epidemic. These guidelines, called *universal precautions,* were designed to prevent the spread of bloodborne pathogens. A similar set of guidelines, called *body substance isolation,* was developed by a hospital. Both types of precautions were widely used by health care

General Guidelines for Preventing the Spread of Infection

- Wash your hands frequently.
- Use liquid soap for cleaning procedures and handwashing whenever possible. Avoid using antimicrobial soap unless the resident is in isolation or has an infection. Using this type of soap all the time increases the drug resistance of pathogens.
- Perform procedures in the way you were taught. Avoid taking shortcuts.

Food Handling

- Handle food properly. Cover food and beverages when you carry them in the hallway. Avoid returning used trays to the food cart until after all clean trays have been passed.
- Keep the food cart and clean linen cart separated from the soiled linen hamper and housekeeping cart by at least one room's width in the hallway.
- Remove the housekeeping cart and soiled linen hampers from the hallway when food trays are being served.
- Avoid storing lab specimens in the refrigerator with food or beverages. A separate, specially marked refrigerator or cooler is used for lab specimens.

Resident's Unit

- Bring only needed items and supplies into the resident's room.
- Keep residents' individual bars of soap separated. Store bar soap in a container that allows water to drain from the bottom of the bar. Follow your facility policy. Some facilities do not allow bar soap.
- Mark water pitchers, cups, and hygiene and grooming items with each resident's name.
- Keep clean and soiled items separate in the bedside stand and other storage areas.
- Wear gloves when necessary. Apply the principles of standard precautions in all resident care. Use standard precautions without regard for disease state or diagnosis.
- Avoid touching clean supplies, linen, equipment, or environmental surfaces with gloves that you have worn during resident contact.

- Dispose of used gloves according to facility policy. Generally they are not discarded in the open wastebasket in the resident's room. If you must throw soiled gloves or other contaminated items into the wastebasket, remove the bag. Tie it closed and take it with you when you leave. Replace it with a new bag after you have discarded the soiled items.

Environment

- Keep clean and soiled items separate in hallways, treatment rooms, work areas, and storage areas.
- Dispose of trash contaminated with blood or body fluids in covered containers. Containers will be marked with a biohazard emblem. Most facilities designate a special storage area for biohazardous waste.
- Cover bedpans, urinals, and other soiled items when carrying them.

Work Area

- Keep your work area neat, tidy, and sanitary.
- Handle clean and soiled items correctly. Carry these items away from your uniform.
- Handle and dispose of soiled material properly.
- Disinfect surfaces, such as mats and treatment tables, after each use.
- Clean equipment immediately after use. Follow your facility policies and manufacturers' directions for the chemicals you use. Affix a sticker to clean items showing the date of cleaning and your initials.
- Follow your assignment and department cleaning schedule for washing and disinfecting resident care items. Wash soiled items in the soiled utility room. The friction created by wiping is important to remove microbes. Supplies must be completely dry before they are stored. Permanent equipment may be packaged in paper, plastic, or mesh bags after cleaning. Affix a sticker with the date and your initials. Store clean supplies in a clean storage area.

Facility Pets

- Many facilities have pets. They should not enter areas where food is being prepared or served. If you feed or touch the pets, wash your hands.

workers. State survey agencies required long-term care facilities to use them in all resident care. In 1996, the CDC published a new set of infection control guidelines called **standard precautions (Figure 4–1).** ⓢⓐ Standard precautions are used in the care of all residents.ⓢⓐ The CDC developed standard precautions to replace universal precautions and body substance isolation. Standard precautions are now the standard of care for health care workers.

You may have learned universal precautions or body substance isolation in your nursing assistant class. Most facilities are no longer using these systems. They have been replaced with standard precautions. Standard precautions are easier to use. They provide a higher level of protection for both you and the residents. You are responsible for learning the principles of standard precautions. ⓢⓐ You must anticipate and select the correct type of personal protective equipment to use in resident care procedures.ⓢⓐ **Table 4–1** summarizes the CDC text for standard precautions.

Handwashing

Handwashing is still the most important method of preventing the spread of infection. It is also a very important part of standard precautions. Handwashing is done before all resident care and procedures. You must also wash your hands before applying and after removing gloves. Although gloves are worn, you can still pick up a microbe on your hands. This may happen because of microscopic defects in the gloves. You can accidentally contaminate your hands when you remove your gloves. Wash your hands immediately if you accidentally contact blood or any moist body fluid except sweat. Each resident care procedure begins and ends with handwashing.

ⓢⓐ Waterless hand cleaner may be used if you do not have access to a sink. Wash your hands with soap as soon as a source of running water is available. Before using a waterless agent, read the label on the bottle. To be effective, the solution must contain 60% to 70% ethanol or isopropyl alcohol. Isopropyl alcohol concentrations below 60% will not eliminate some pathogens.ⓢⓐ

▮▮▮ PERSONAL PROTECTIVE EQUIPMENT

ⓢⓐ Using personal protective equipment (PPE) **(Figure 4–2, p. 46)** is an important part of standard precautions. This involves wearing gloves for handling or touching blood, any moist body fluid (except sweat), secretions, excretions, mucous membranes, and nonintact skin.ⓢⓐ

Using Gloves

ⓢⓐ If your gloves become visibly soiled with infective material, remove them and wash your hands. Apply a clean pair of gloves before continuing. An important new practice in standard precautions

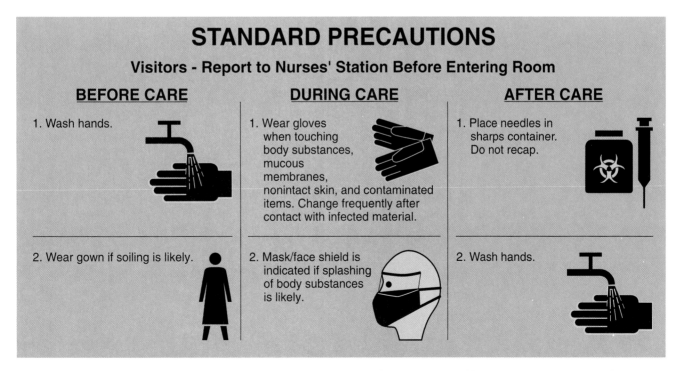

STANDARD PRECAUTIONS
Visitors - Report to Nurses' Station Before Entering Room

BEFORE CARE	DURING CARE	AFTER CARE
1. Wash hands.	1. Wear gloves when touching body substances, mucous membranes, nonintact skin, and contaminated items. Change frequently after contact with infected material.	1. Place needles in sharps container. Do not recap.
2. Wear gown if soiling is likely.	2. Mask/face shield is indicated if splashing of body substances is likely.	2. Wash hands.

Figure 4–1 Standard precautions were designed to replace universal precautions and body substance isolation. They are less confusing, and are used in the care of all residents. (Courtesy of Briggs Corporation, Des Moines, IA. (800) 247-2343)

Table 4–1   Summary of Standard Precautions

Summary of Standard Precautions

Handwashing is performed	Before and after resident contact.
	Before applying and after removing gloves.
	After contact with blood, body fluids (except sweat), secretions, excretions, mucous membranes, and nonintact skin, even if gloves were worn during the contact.
	After touching environmental surfaces, equipment, or other articles that may be contaminated with blood, body fluids, secretions, or excretions.
Soap for handwashing	A plain antimicrobial soap is used unless the resident is in transmission-based precautions (isolation).
	An antimicrobial soap or waterless antiseptic agent is used in transmission-based precautions or during outbreaks of infection.
Gloves	Provide a barrier against pathogens and prevent contamination of the hands when touching blood, body fluids (except sweat), secretions, excretions, mucous membranes, or nonintact skin.
	Reduce the possibility that pathogens on the hands of the health care worker can be transmitted to residents.
	Reduce the possibility that pathogens from another resident or piece of equipment will be transmitted via the hands of the health care worker to a resident.
	Are changed if they contact high concentrations of infective material.
	Are changed *immediately* before contact with mucous membranes or nonintact skin, if gloves are being worn during resident care.
	Wearing gloves does not replace the need for handwashing. Gloves can have defects that cannot be seen, but allow pathogens to enter. The hands can become accidentally contaminated when gloves are removed.
	Changing gloves and washing hands may be necessary several times during the course of caring for one resident, to prevent cross-contamination between body sites.
	Wearing gloves for all resident contact is not necessary or desirable if you understand and apply the principles of standard precautions.
Masks, respiratory protection, eye protection, and face shields	Worn during resident care and cleaning procedures that may generate splashes of blood, body fluids, secretions, or excretions.
	A surgical mask is usually used.
	Masks are worn for one use, then discarded.
	If a resident is in airborne precautions, a NIOSH-approved respirator filter is worn (HEPA respirator filter, N95, or PFR95).
	A surgical mask is worn when caring for residents in contact precautions.
	A face shield or protective eye goggles are never worn without a mask.

(continues)

Table 4–1   Summary of Standard Precautions, *continued*

Gowns and protective garments	Are worn to prevent contamination of the uniform and protect the skin from splashes of blood, body fluids, secretions, or excretions.
	May be cloth or paper, but must be resistant to liquids and prevent soaking of the clothing or skin.
	Protective leg covers, boots, shoe covers, and hats provide greater protection when large quantities of infective material are present or splashing of fluids is anticipated.
Sharps	Are not recapped, bent, broken, or cut.
	Are disposed of in a puncture-resistant container near the location of use.
	Broken glass is never picked up by hand. Use tongs, forceps, or another mechanical device and discard in a puncture-resistant container (OSHA).
Blood and body fluid spills	Are removed using an absorbent powder or disinfected according to facility policy using an approved disinfectant. Wear personal protective equipment appropriate to the procedure.
	Liquids contaminated with blood or body fluids can be discarded in a drain connected to a sanitary sewer.
Resuscitation	Resuscitation bags, face shields, mouthpieces, and other ventilation devices are used to minimize the risk of exposure to pathogens by mouth-to-mouth contact. The health care worker should be trained in the use of the device.
Equipment and other articles	Disposable equipment is discarded after use.
	Reusable equipment is disinfected after use.
	Equipment used for sterile procedures or to enter the body is washed and sterilized after use.
	Resident care equipment and supplies contaminated with blood or body fluids are single-bagged; double-bagging is unnecessary unless the outside of the bag becomes contaminated during the bagging process.
	Equipment is handled and transported in a manner that reduces the risk of transmission of pathogens and avoids environmental contamination.
Linen and laundry	No special handling is necessary. All soiled linen should be handled, transported, and laundered in a manner that avoids transfer of pathogens.
	Single-bagging is used unless the outside of the bag becomes torn or contaminated during the bagging process. Facilities that use water-soluble bags should double-bag with an outer plastic bag; contact with wet linen will cause the water-soluble bag to dissolve before it reaches the laundry.
Dishes, cups, glasses, and eating utensils	No special precautions are used. Proper technique in the dish room and the combination of hot water and detergent in the dishwasher destroys pathogens on these items.
Routine and terminal cleaning	All rooms are cleaned upon resident discharge using the same terminal cleaning procedures, unless the amount of infectious material or environmental contamination indicates that special cleaning is necessary. Adequate disinfection of bedside equipment, supplies, and environmental surfaces is critical. ⍾

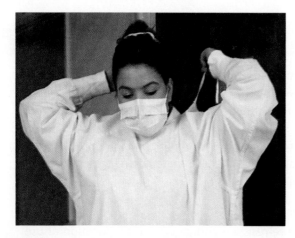

Figure 4–2 The restorative nursing assistant is responsible for selecting the correct personal protective equipment needed for the task.

 General Guidelines for Times to Wash Your Hands

At a minimum, handwashing should take 10 to 15 seconds. Take longer if your hands are soiled. Wash your hands:

▪ When coming on duty
▪ After picking up anything from the floor
▪ Before and after caring for each resident
▪ Before applying and after removing gloves
▪ Before handling a resident's food and drink
▪ After contact with anything considered soiled; or contaminated
▪ Before handling any supply considered clean
▪ Immediately before touching nonintact skin (skin that is broken, chapped, cut, or cracked); if you are already wearing gloves, change them
▪ Immediately before touching mucous membranes (tissues of the body that secrete mucus that open to the outside of the body); if you are already wearing gloves, change them
▪ After touching nonintact skin, mucous membranes, blood, or any moist body fluid, secretions, or excretions (human waste products eliminated from the body), even if gloves were worn during the contact
▪ Whenever your hands are visibly soiled
▪ After touching equipment or environmental surfaces that might be contaminated
▪ Any time your gloves become torn
▪ After personal use of the toilet or using a tissue to blow your nose
▪ After you cough or sneeze
▪ Before and after applying lip balm
▪ Before and after manipulating contact lenses
▪ Before and after eating, drinking, or smoking
▪ Before you go on break and at the end of your shift before you leave the facility ⓢ

involves removing your gloves, washing your hands, and reapplying clean gloves *immediately* before contact with mucous membranes and nonintact skin. This is done to avoid transferring a harmful microbe to a vulnerable area of the body. Mucous membranes and nonintact skin are areas that can readily acquire an infection. Mucous membranes are found in areas that open to the outside of the body. The eyes, nose, mouth, and genital area are lined with mucous membranes. When applying the principles of standard precautions, changing your gloves and washing your hands may be necessary several times during the care of one resident. Change gloves:

▪ Before each resident contact
▪ After each resident contact
▪ *Immediately before* touching mucous membranes
▪ *Immediately before* touching nonintact skin
▪ After you touch a resident's secretions or excretions, before moving to care for another part of the body
▪ After touching blood or body fluids, before moving to care for another part of the body
▪ After touching contaminated environmental surfaces or equipment
▪ Any time your gloves become visibly soiled
▪ If your gloves become torn

Wear gloves when touching dressings, tissues, infective items, and contaminated surfaces or equipment. Do not carry glove use to the extreme. Use gloves when necessary, but avoid wearing gloves for all resident contact. Using gloves at all times sends a negative message. It implies that the resident is untouchable. Touching is very important to all human beings. Use gloves only when contact with blood, moist body fluids, secretions, excretions, mucous membranes, or nonintact skin is likely. Wear gloves for resident contact if your hands are cut, cracked, or chapped. Be very careful not to contaminate clean equipment, supplies, or the environment with used gloves. If you must carry a soiled item, removing both gloves may not be possible. To avoid environmental contamination, remove one glove. Hold it in the other, gloved hand. Pick up the soiled item with the gloved hand. Use the ungloved hand to open doors, turn on faucets, and touch other environmental surfaces. If removing one glove is not possible, hold a clean paper towel or other clean item under your gloves. Use the paper towel to touch environmental surfaces. This is an important principle to remember. Health care workers unknowingly contaminate the environment with their gloves many times each day.

Gowns

(SA) Wear a gown if your clothing may contact blood or any of the body fluids listed. The gown may be cloth or paper, but it must be fluid-resistant. (SA) Many gowns are specially treated to keep fluid from soaking through. You may wear a gown when assisting with dressing changes and other procedures. Review the procedures for applying and removing the gown in your nursing assistant textbook.

Face Protection

(SA) Wear a face shield **(Figure 4–3A)** or goggles and a surgical mask **(Figure 4–3B)** during procedures in which body fluids or secretions may splash into your face. You can wear a mask without eye protection. However, you should never wear eye protection without a mask. A mask with an eye shield attached **(Figure 4–3C)** may be used. The facial barriers protect the mucous membranes in your eyes, nose, and mouth. Always try to anticipate what PPE you will need. Apply it before beginning a procedure. Check the equipment before using it. Replace items that are cut, torn, or cracked. They will not protect you. If you tear your gloves during a procedure, remove them as soon as possible. Wash your hands and put on a new pair of gloves before continuing. Your facility will have a policy for discarding, laundering, or decontaminating personal protective equipment after use. Replace what you have used so that it will be quickly available the next time it is needed.(SA)

Handling Needles and Sharps

Needle and sharp precautions are also part of standard precautions. You may handle these items when assisting with skilled procedures. (SA) Never replace the cap, bend, or cut a used needle. Leave the cap off. Handle needles, scalpel blades, razors, and other sharp objects with care. After using a sharp item, dispose of it in a puncture-resistant sharps container. Avoid overfilling the sharps container.(SA) Cap the container when it is three-quarters full. The cap is designed so it cannot be snapped back off after it is closed. The sealed container is stored until it is picked up with the biohazardous waste.

(SA) If you must clean up broken glass, always wear gloves. Avoid picking it up with your hands.

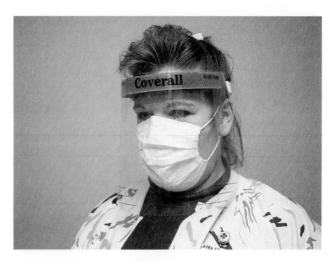

Figure 4–3A The face shield does not provide adequate protection against splashes, so a surgical mask is also worn.

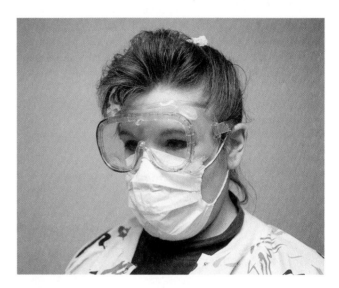

Figure 4–3B The goggles and face mask should fit tightly against the face.

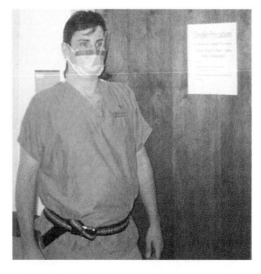

Figure 4–3C An alternate type of mask, to which eye protection is attached, is available in some facilities.

Use a broom and dustpan, forceps, or other mechanical method. Protect your hands from being cut. Discard the glass in a puncture-resistant container.

Cleaning Blood and Body Fluid Spills

Follow your facility policy for cleaning blood or body fluid spills. Many facilities use an absorbent powder **(Figure 4–4)** for cleaning body fluid spills. The powder turns the liquid into a solid, so that you can sweep it up. After sweeping the powder, wipe the floor with disinfectant. Some disinfectants must sit on the floor to kill pathogens. After the solution sits for the designated time, wipe it up. Follow manufacturers' directions. If your facility uses bleach as a disinfectant, mix it in a container using 1 part bleach to 100 parts of water. Previously, stronger bleach solutions were recommended. Research has shown that a concentration of 1:100 is all that is needed to eliminate bloodborne pathogens. Know and follow your facility policy. Label the container with the contents, the date it was mixed, and your initials. Bleach solution should be mixed at least every 24 hours.

Disposing of Biohazardous Waste

Items that have contacted blood or body fluids are biohazardous waste. Dispose of items contaminated with blood or body fluids according to your facility policy. Discard contaminated trash in containers marked with the biohazardous waste emblem. By law, this type of trash requires special handling in health care facilities. Store it in a designated holding area until it is removed from the facility. Having biohazardous waste removed is expensive. Avoid placing non-biohazardous materials into the container. For example, plastic outer wrappers, cardboard, plastic containers, and noncontaminated items are discarded in the regular trash.

Body fluids such as urine can safely be discarded in a drain connected to a sanitary sewer. Know and follow your facility policy.

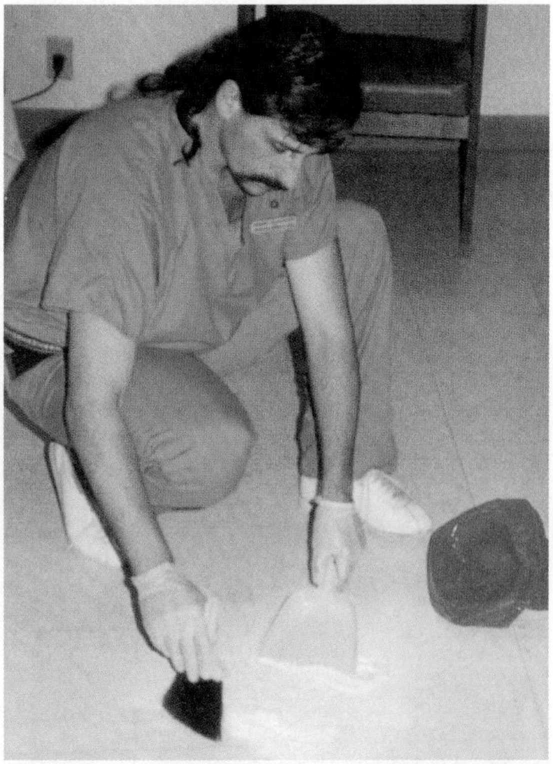

Figure 4–4 Special absorbent powder turns blood and body fluid spills into solid material that is easily cleaned. Wipe the floor with a facility-approved disinfectant after the powder is removed.

Cleaning Equipment

You may be responsible for cleaning equipment used in the therapy department. Wearing personal protective equipment when cleaning equipment is a good practice. Utility gloves may be better for cleaning than the exam gloves used for resident care. The chemicals used for cleaning enlarge the pores of disposable gloves. You will not see the defect, but the dilated pores allow microbes to pass through the gloves to your hands. Follow your facility policy for using gloves.

Latex Allergies

Hundreds of items used in health care are made of latex. Some health care workers and residents develop latex allergies because of repeated exposure to latex gloves and other latex supplies. Avoiding powdered gloves is an important way of reducing your exposure to latex. The powder in the gloves absorbs latex proteins. When the gloves are removed, the particles become airborne. Everyone in the room inhales them, increasing latex sensitivity. If you are allergic to latex, your employer must provide another type of glove. Glove liners and topical barriers may also be used. The liner or topical product forms a barrier. This prevents the latex from touching your skin. If you develop a latex allergy, avoid or cover other latex items so they do not contact your skin. Follow your physician's advice.

TRANSMISSION-BASED PRECAUTIONS

Isolation measures are used when a resident has a known or suspected pathogen. Using isolation prevents the spread of disease to others. The second tier of the 1996 CDC guidelines is called **transmission-based precautions.** These precautions were designed to replace the isolation categories used previously. The CDC recommends three types of transmission-based precautions. Standard precautions are used with transmission-based precautions.ⓈⒶ The type of precautions to be used is selected by the nurse manager and physician. The selection is based on the mode of transmission of the infection. Transmission-based precautions are used because normal cleanliness and standard precautions are not adequate to prevent the spread of infection with certain pathogens. A private room is used. This confines the pathogen to a single unit. In some situations, residents with the same pathogen will share a unit.

Airborne Precautions

Airborne precautions (Figure 4–5) are used for residents whose disease is spread by the airborne method of transmission (through the air). An example of a disease requiring airborne precautions is tuberculosis. The pathogen that causes this disease is very tiny and lightweight. It can be suspended on dust and moisture in the air. It travels for long distances throughout the facility in the ventilation system. ⓈⒶ Because of the mode of transmission, special precautions are taken to contain the microbe. A private room is essential. The room must have a special ventilation system that prevents the pathogen from escaping. In a normal facility room, the air is forced downward from the ventilation system. In an airborne precautions room, the ventilation is reversed and is drawn upward into the vents. This creates a **negative-pressure environment.** The ventilation is either specially filtered or exhausted directly to the outside of the building. This prevents the escape of pathogens. The room has 6 to 12 complete air changes per hour. The door to the room must be kept closed. The maintenance department checks the ventilation in the room daily to ensure it is working properly.ⓈⒶ

Respiratory Protection. ⓈⒶ Staff entering the airborne precautions room must wear a **NIOSH-approved respirator (Figure 4–6).** This type of mask is approved by the National Institute for Occupational Safety and Health (NIOSH).ⓈⒶ The masks have tiny pores that the pathogen cannot fit through. They are secured with two elastic straps on each side. The straps are positioned to hold the mask tightly to the face. The HEPA respirator filter, N95, and PFR95 respirator filter are examples of approved masks. To work in an airborne precautions room, staff must undergo mask fit testing. A medical examination is also required. No other personal protective equipment is necessary unless required to practice standard precautions.

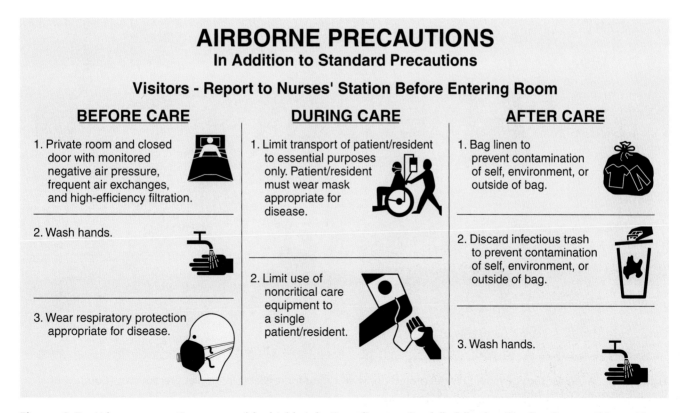

Figure 4–5 Airborne precautions are used for highly infectious diseases. Carefully following the directions on this card is very important. (Courtesy of Briggs Corporation, Des Moines, IA. (800) 247-2343)

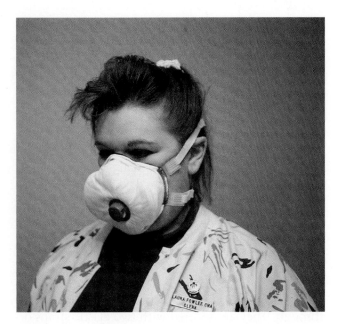

Figure 4–6 A NIOSH-approved respirator must be worn each time you enter an airborne precautions room. Before opening the door, check the respirator to make sure there are no air leaks.

Droplet Precautions

Droplet precautions (Figure 4–7) are used for infections that are spread in the air. An example of a disease for which droplet precautions are used is influenza. The pathogen is spread by the droplets in mucus from oral, nasal, and respiratory secretions. The droplets usually remain within 3 feet of the resident. The secretions containing the pathogen are too large and heavy to be carried in air currents. A private room is necessary, but special ventilation is not used. **SA** Surgical masks are worn when working within 3 feet of the resident.**SA** The pathogen is too large to fit between the pores of the surgical mask. The door to the room may remain open if the resident prefers. No other personal protective equipment is necessary unless it is needed to practice standard precautions.

Contact Precautions

Contact precautions (Figure 4–8) are used to contain pathogens that are spread by direct or indirect contact. The microbes are found in infections of the skin, wounds, mucous membranes, urine,

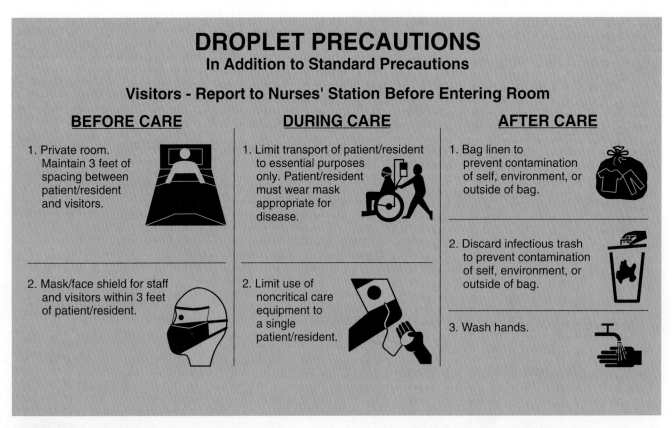

Figure 4–7 A regular surgical mask provides protection when caring for residents in droplet precautions. (Courtesy of Briggs Corporation, Des Moines, IA. (800) 247-2343)

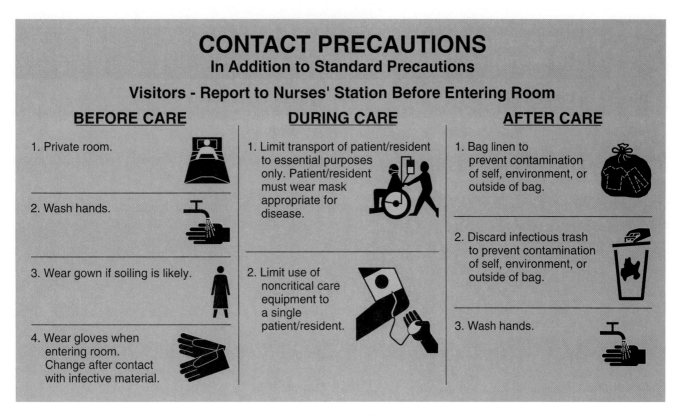

Figure 4–8 Contact precautions are used for residents with wound, skin, and urinary infections. (Courtesy of Briggs Corporation, Des Moines, IA. (800) 247-2343)

and stool. Standard precautions are used in addition to contact precautions. ⑤ Gloves are worn when you enter the room. No other personal protective equipment is necessary unless you will have direct contact with the resident, bed linen, or environmental surfaces. When contact is anticipated, wear a gown to cover your uniform. The principles of standard precautions are also used for residents in contact precautions.⑤ Use additional personal protective equipment if secretions may splash in the air. In this case, apply a face shield or goggles and a surgical mask. This will protect the mucous membranes in your eyes, nose, and mouth.

◼◼◼ SPECIAL CIRCUMSTANCES

Residents may have infections that are transmitted by more than one method. A resident may have an infection, such as a cold, that is spread by the droplet method. In addition, the resident may also have an infected pressure ulcer or urinary infection. Some diseases, such as chickenpox, are spread by more than one method. In this case, two types of isolation are used. Standard precautions are also

used. **Table 4–2** lists common diseases and the type of transmission-based precautions used for each.

Caring for Residents in Isolation

Most facilities post signs on the door to the room when a resident is in isolation. The sign lists personal protective equipment to wear and special precautions to take. ⑤ You must clearly understand the category of transmission-based precautions being used. Follow the precautions for that type of infection when entering the room.⑤ Check with your supervisor or the charge nurse if you have questions.

Transporting Residents in Airborne and Droplet Precautions

Occasionally, you must transport residents in respiratory isolation to other areas of the facility. ⑤ In this case, wear a mask when entering the room. Assist the resident to apply a surgical mask before leaving. Remove your mask and wash your hands when you leave the unit. The resident must wear the surgical mask when he or she is out of the room. Avoid removing the mask until the resident returns to his or her own room.⑤

Table 4–2   Diseases Requiring Standard and Transmission-Based Precautions

Disease or Condition	Type of Precautions
AIDS	Standard
Cellulitis with uncontrolled drainage	Contact
Chickenpox	Airborne and contact
Conjunctivitis, bacterial	Standard
Conjunctivitis, viral	Contact
Diarrhea	Standard
Drug-resistant skin infections	Contact
German measles	Droplet
Gonorrhea	Standard
Head or body lice (pediculosis)	Contact
Hepatitis A	Standard; use contact if diarrhea or incontinent resident
Hepatitis, other types	Standard
Herpes, oral or genital	Standard
Herpes zoster (varicella zoster) in immunocompromised resident or widely disseminated lesions	Airborne and contact
Herpes zoster (varicella zoster) in normal resident	Standard
HIV disease	Standard
Infected pressure sore with no drainage	Standard
Infected pressure sore with heavy drainage	Contact
Infectious diarrhea caused by a known pathogen	Contact
Influenza	Droplet
Measles	Airborne
Methicillin-resistant staphylococcus aureus (MRSA) in wounds and urine	Contact
MRSA in respiratory secretions	Droplet

(continues)

(SA) Table 4–2 Diseases Requiring Standard and Transmission-Based Precautions, *continued*

Disease or Condition	Type of Precautions
Mumps	Droplet
Scabies	Contact
Syphilis	Standard
Tuberculosis	Airborne (SA)

Transporting Residents in Contact Precautions to Other Areas of the Facility

Sometimes residents in isolation must go to the therapy department or another area for treatment. Usually, these residents need special treatment for infected wounds. The whirlpool is commonly used to **debride**, or clean, wounds covered with eschar **(Figure 4–9).** You may be responsible for giving a resident with an infection a whirlpool treatment. The best practice to follow is to treat the resident at the end of the day. You will need a great deal of time. In addition to bathing the resident, you must disinfect the therapy room and whirlpool. Doing the procedure at the end of the day prevents other residents from being exposed to the pathogen.

(SA) Before entering the contact precautions room, apply a gown and gloves. Assist the resident to dress, if necessary. Make sure that the infected area is covered with a dressing. The dressing should

be secure, with no leaks.(SA) If drainage is present, notify your supervisor before transporting the resident. Open a bath blanket and cover the wheelchair. After the resident is seated, wrap it around him or her **(Figure 4–10).** Before leaving the room, remove and discard your personal protective equipment. Wash your hands.

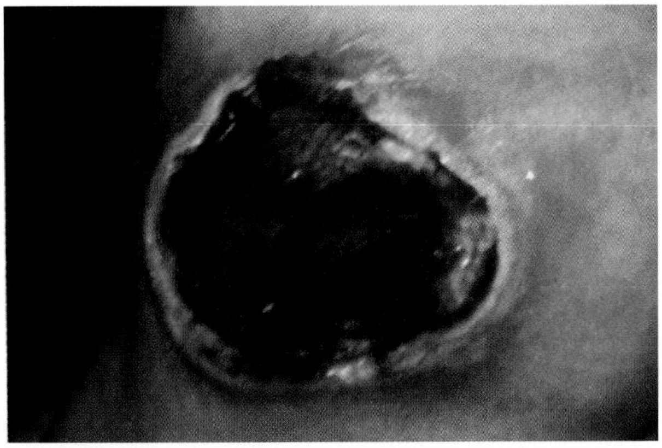

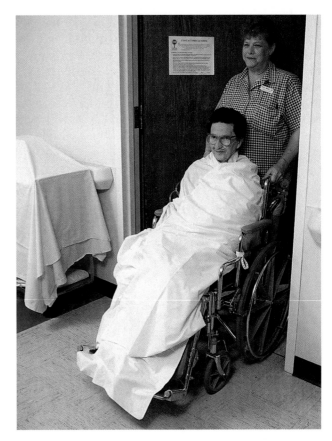

Figure 4–9 Eschar is thick, black, and leathery in appearance.

Figure 4–10 When transporting a resident in contact precautions, wrap her in a bath blanket before leaving the room.

Giving a Whirlpool Treatment to a Resident in Contact Precautions

The therapist or nurse will instruct you on specific solutions and techniques for the whirlpool treatment. Before beginning, clean the tub according to facility policy. Wash your hands, then apply a gown and gloves. The nurse or therapist removes the dressing. Give the whirlpool in the normal manner. The water should be 96°F. The treatment will last about 20 minutes. After the whirlpool, dry the resident. Apply gloves. Dry the wound with sterile gauze sponges. Remove the gloves. Assist the resident to put on a gown. Transfer him or her to a treatment table covered with a sheet. Cover the resident with a bath blanket.

Assisting with Mechanical Debridement

The therapist will perform **mechanical debridement.** This is done with sterile instruments. During the procedure, the therapist will remove nonviable, or dead, tissue. The treatment cleanses the inside of the wound and promotes healing. You will set up the tray **(Figure 4–11)** and assist with the procedure. If your gown or gloves contact drainage during the procedure, remove the personal protective equipment. Wash your hands, then reapply clean garments. You may be required to change your gown and apply sterile gloves before assisting with the debridement. You will be responsible for positioning the resident. If your hands are close to the treatment area, you will wear sterile gloves. After the treatment, the therapist or nurse will dress the wound with a sterile dressing. Assist the resident to dress and return him or her to the isolation unit. Ⓢ️ Before leaving the treatment area, remove and discard your personal protective equipment. Wash your hands. Reapply clean personal protective equipment before entering the unit. At a minimum, apply gloves. A gown is not necessary unless you will have direct contact with the resident or bed linen. Wear a gown if you will be transferring the resident. Remove and discard the protective attire. Wash your hands before leaving the room.Ⓢ️

Cleaning the Treatment or Therapy Room

After the treatment, you must clean the therapy room. This prevents the spread of the pathogen to others. Take this responsibility very seriously. Follow your supervisor's instructions carefully. The procedure for disinfecting the room depends upon your facility infection control policies. Ⓢ️ Wear personal protective equipment during this procedure. At a minimum, a gown and gloves are necessary. If you expect splashing, wear facial protection. Wipe down all areas that the resident contacted with disinfectant. Follow directions for the product you are using.Ⓢ️ The solution should sit for 5 to 10 minutes; then rinse and dry the area well.

Disinfecting the Whirlpool

Ⓢ️ The whirlpool tub is drained after each use and cleaned with disinfectant solution.Ⓢ️ Follow the manufacturer's directions for the type of tub and disinfectant you are using. Fill the tub with water and disinfectant. Turn on the whirlpool. Run the whirlpool action for 10 to 20 full minutes, or according to facility policy. Wipe areas that are not immersed in water with disinfectant solution. Let the full-strength solution sit on these areas while the whirlpool is running. Drain the tub while rinsing it well from top to bottom. Rinse the upper areas, working your way to the bottom of the tub. Rinse a second time from top to bottom. Dry the tub with a towel. As an extra safeguard, you may be assigned to disinfect the whirlpool a second time. You may be asked to disinfect it again the next morning before it is used.

Disposing of Trash

Ⓢ️ Discard the protective equipment, soiled dressings, and cleaning cloths in a sealed plastic bag. Dispose of them according to facility policy. Handle soiled linen as little as possible. Seal it in a plastic bag and transport to the laundry.Ⓢ️

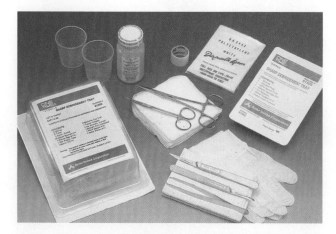

Figure 4–11 The sharp debridement tray is prepared using sterile technique. After use, discard the instruments in a sharps container. (Courtesy of Acme United Corporation, (800) 243-9852)

STERILE PROCEDURES

You may assist the restorative nurse or therapist with certain sterile procedures. You will wear sterile gloves if your hands are near the treatment area. You will set up trays and handle sterile supplies. Sterile technique is a pathogen-free technique. It is used for procedures within body cavities and during certain dressing changes. Sterile gloves are worn. Only sterile items contact the resident's body during the procedure. Most facilities purchase sterile supplies in disposable packages. Some facilities wash, wrap, and autoclave instruments and other sterile articles. A sterile package is double-wrapped in heavy cloth or paper fabric. Disposable packages are sealed in plastic. As long as the outer wrapper is intact, the items inside are considered sterile. Avoid using packages with a tear, crack, or opening in the outer wrapper. Items sterilized in an autoclave are sealed with special tape. The tape changes color **(Figure 4–12)** during the process. The tape color indicates that the contents of the package are sterile.

The nurse or therapist will advise you of your responsibilities for assisting with the procedure. You will set up the sterile instrument or supply tray and add items when necessary.

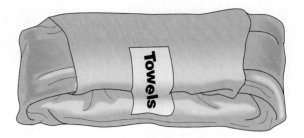
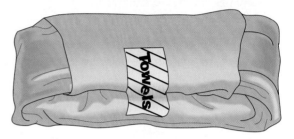

Figure 4–12 Autoclave tape is beige before processing. If the package has been processed correctly, black stripes appear on the tape.

(SA) General Guidelines for Assisting with Sterile Procedures

- If a sterile package is cracked, cut, or torn, it is contaminated and should not be used.
- Set up the sterile field or tray immediately before it is used; accidental contamination may occur if the tray is prepared before it is needed.
- Caution the resident and other staff to avoid touching the sterile field.
- Never turn your back on a sterile field.
- If you are interrupted or must leave the sterile supplies unattended, cover them with a sterile drape.
- The outside of a sterile wrapper is not sterile. You can touch it with your hands. Avoid touching the inside of the wrapper. Also, avoid touching items inside the package with your ungloved hands. Wear sterile gloves or use sterile forceps to touch the inside of the package.
- If you question the sterility of any item, consider it contaminated. Avoid using it.

- If a sterile item contacts an unsterile item, both articles are contaminated.
- If a sterile item or field becomes wet, it is contaminated.
- When placing instruments and supplies on a sterile field, place them in the center, as far from the edge as possible.
- Crossing over or touching a sterile field contaminates the entire field. If you must add an item to the sterile field, carefully drop it onto the field from the sterile package.
- Avoid passing contaminated dressings, instruments, or supplies over a sterile field.
- Avoid touching unsterile articles with sterile gloves. When wearing sterile gloves, keep your hands above your waist, away from your body. Anything below your waist is considered contaminated.
- Avoid coughing, sneezing, or talking directly over a sterile field. (SA)

PROCEDURE

2 OPENING A STERILE PACKAGE OR TRAY

1. Wash your hands.
2. Sanitize the tray or surface the package will be placed on. Thoroughly dry the surface.
3. Wash your hands.
4. Check the seal on the package to ensure that it is sterile.
5. Remove the tape or package seal.
6. Touch only the outside of the package.
7. Open the package away from your body.
8. Open the distal flap of the package by touching only the corner **(Figure 4–13A)**.

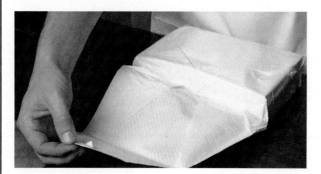

Figure 4–13A Opening a sterile tray. Carefully lift the top flap away from your body.

9. Open the right-hand flap by touching only the corner **(Figure 4–13B)**.

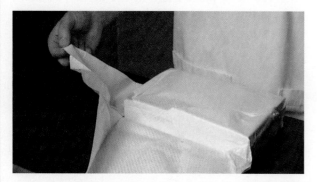

Figure 4–13B Grasping the edge, open the right side.

10. Open the left-hand flap by touching only the corner **(Figure 4–13C)**.

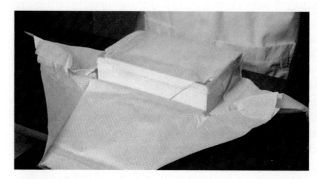

Figure 4–13C Open the left flap, taking care to avoid touching the inside of the package.

11. Open the proximal flap by touching only the corner, then lifting the flap up and pulling it toward you, allowing it to drop over the edge of the counter or table. Avoid touching the inside of the wrapper or the contents of the package **(Figure 4–13D)**.

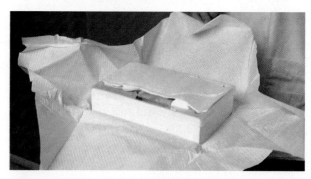

Figure 4–13D Cover your fingers with the edge of the flap, and open the side closest to you without contaminating the inside of the tray.

To add the item to the sterile field:

12. Open the sterile package using steps 4–11 above, or peel back the edges of the sterile package.
13. With your dominant hand, grasp the package from the bottom. With your free hand, pull the sides of the package away from the sterile field.
14. Drop the sterile item onto the sterile field. Avoid touching the sterile field with the package.
15. Discard the wrapper.

PROCEDURE

3 APPLYING STERILE GLOVES

1. Remove rings, watch, and jewelry that may puncture gloves. Pin jewelry to your uniform or place it in a safe area.

2. Wash your hands.

3. Check the glove package for sterility.

4. Open the outer package by peeling the upper edges back.

5. Remove the inner package containing the gloves. Place it on the inside of the outer package.

6. Open the inner package, handling it only by the corners on the outside **(Figure 4–14A).**

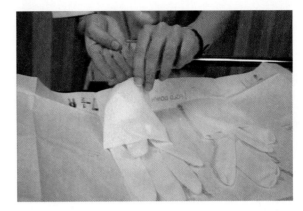

Figure 4–14B Lifting only the edges of the cuff, slide your hand into the glove.

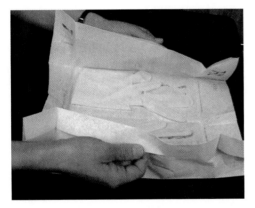

Figure 4–14A Opening a package of sterile gloves. Fold the edges of the package back without touching the inside of the wrapper or the gloves.

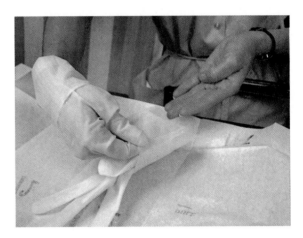

Figure 4–14C Place the fingers of your right hand under the cuff of the left glove.

7. Pick up the edge of the cuff of the right-hand glove using your left hand. Avoid touching the area below the cuff **(Figure 4–14B).**

8. Insert your right hand into the glove. Spread your fingers slightly. Insert them into the fingers of the glove. If the glove is not on correctly, do not attempt to straighten it at this time **(Figure 4–14C).**

9. Insert the gloved fingers of your right hand under the cuff of the left glove. Place your left hand into the glove. Avoid touching the gloved right hand with your skin.

10. Adjust the fingers of the gloves for comfort. Because both gloves are sterile, they may touch each other. Avoid touching the cuffs of the gloves.

(continues)

PROCEDURE **3** *continued*

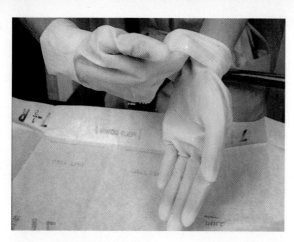

Figure 4–14D Adjust the cuffs for comfort without touching your wrists.

11. Insert your right hand under the cuff of the left glove. Push the cuff up over your wrist. Avoid touching your wrist or the outside of the cuff with your glove **(Figure 4–14D).**

12. Insert your left hand under the cuff of the right glove. Push the cuff up over your wrist. Avoid touching your wrist or the outside of the cuff with your glove.

13. You may now touch sterile items with your sterile gloves. Avoid touching unsterile items.

14. Hold your hands above your waist and away from your uniform.

After the sterile tray is set up, you will assist the resident with positioning. Provide emotional support during the procedure. At times you may be asked to assist the licensed health care worker. To do this, apply sterile gloves to avoid contaminating the sterile field.

◾ INFECTION CONTROL PRACTICES AND ROUTINE CLEANING PROCEDURES

You may assist with many procedures requiring the use of special equipment. Become familiar with and apply the principles of medical asepsis and standard precautions. You may also be responsible for cleaning and disinfecting the equipment after use. This is a very important responsibility. Take it seriously. Many residents participate in restorative programs. The potential to spread an infection throughout the facility is great.

Cleaning Procedures

Ⓢ Apply the principles of standard precautions during routine cleaning procedures. Follow the cleaning policies and procedures developed by your infection control committee. Your facility will provide special disinfectants to use for cleaning. These products are approved by the Environmental Protection Agency (EPA).Ⓢ They eliminate a wide range of microbes. Some are diluted. Some are used full strength. There is no one all-purpose disinfectant for health care facility use. Facilities will have several dif-

ferent products to be used for different purposes. Always follow the directions on the label. Wear utility gloves when using chemicals. Read the label before using the product to see if additional protective equipment is necessary. Make sure that all chemical residue is thoroughly rinsed from equipment. Allow items to dry completely before being stored.

Ⓢ Store chemicals in a locked cupboard away from food, beverages, and medications. Avoid skin contact with these products. If contact accidentally occurs, immediately wash the area well with soap and water. If mucous membrane contact occurs, flush the area well with cool, clear water. Check the Material Safety Data Sheet to see if additional action is necessary. Report the incident to your supervisor.Ⓢ

Routine Cleaning of Resident Supplies and Equipment

Procedures for using the equipment discussed in this chapter are described elsewhere in your book. Cleaning procedures are described here so you can find the information easily and use it as a reference. When cleaning supplies and equipment, avoid splashing as much as possible. After cleaning, wrap or package the item according to facility policy. Affix a sticker showing the date the item was cleaned and your initials.

Environmental Surfaces. Wipe the work surfaces in your department with a facility-approved disinfectant at least once a day. Usually, the housekeeping department will clean the area thoroughly. Disinfect the surface whenever you have reason to suspect contamination.

Refrigerators. Refrigerators are sometimes used to store supplies. (SA) Food and beverages are not stored in the same refrigerator as medications or treatment supplies. Food and beverages must be covered, labeled, and dated. A refrigerator thermometer must be in place at all times. The temperature must be 45°F or less, or according to the law in your state.(SA) The refrigerator must be defrosted periodically. Remove all food and beverages. Turn the refrigerator off until the ice melts. Wash the inside surfaces with an approved disinfectant. Remove all residue. Rinse the refrigerator well, and dry. Restock with food items.

Hydrocollator. The hydrocollator is a tank used to heat solution for hot packs. The packs are stored in the tank until use and returned after treatment. The procedure is described in Chapter 6.

The hydrocollator tank is emptied and disinfected every month. Unplug the tank and remove the packs. Carefully discard the hot liquid. Allow the tank to cool before touching the inside surface. When it is cool, scrub the inside with a facility-approved disinfectant. Rinse well to remove the chemicals. After cleaning, refill the unit with fresh distilled water.

Paraffin Treatments. Paraffin treatments are used for residents with arthritis of the hands. This treatment is described in Chapter 6. Monitor and record the temperature of the tank on a log daily. The temperature should be 110°F, or according to facility policy.

The paraffin tank is cleaned every 3 months, or according to facility policy. Unplug the tank. Carefully drain and discard the paraffin. After the tank cools, remove the residue by scrubbing with a brush. Wipe the tank with a facility-approved disinfectant. Rinse well. Dry with a clean towel. Refill the tank with a 5:1 solution. Use 5 pounds of clean paraffin to 1 pint of mineral oil, or follow the formula used by your facility. Most institutional tanks hold 15 pounds of paraffin and 3 pints of mineral oil.

Ultrasonic Treatments. **Ultrasonic treatments (Figure 4–15A)** are used to reduce inflammation. The treatment is never done on an area with a rash or broken skin. (SA) This procedure is performed only by a licensed person. You will assist with positioning, if necessary.(SA) You may also be responsible for cleaning the unit. A water-soluble lubricant is used on the skin during the treatment. Wipe the unit with a dry cloth to remove the lubricant. Next, wipe it with a disinfectant **(Figure 4–15B)**. Rinse the disinfectant off with a damp cloth. Dry with a clean towel. Avoid getting water inside the unit.

Walkers, Wheelchairs, and Canes. Your facility will have cleaning schedules for equipment used on the nursing units. Some equipment is stored in the

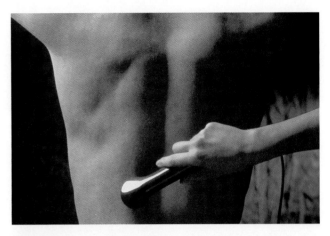

Figure 4–15A The licensed therapist performs the ultrasound treatment.

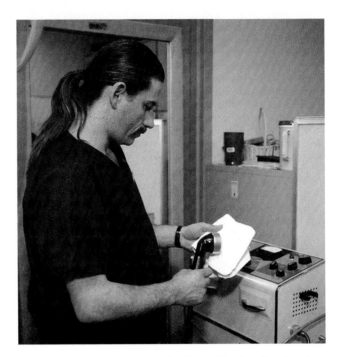

Figure 4–15B Follow your facility policy for cleaning the ultrasound unit after each treatment.

therapy department. The equipment is used intermittently, so separate cleaning schedules may apply. You may be responsible for keeping department utensils and equipment clean and sanitary. Walkers, wheelchairs, and canes are usually washed in the shower room, using liquid soap, water, and a soft scrub brush. Remove residue with a brush. Rinse, then wipe with a facility-approved disinfectant solution. Some disinfectants dry on the item and are not rinsed off. Follow the directions for the product you are using. After washing, dry the equipment and return it to the storage area.

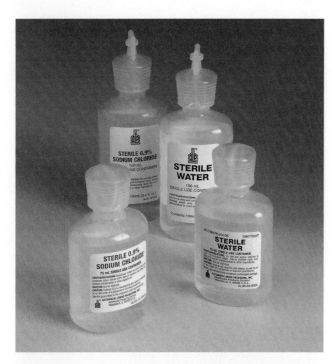

Figure 4–16 Single-use bottles of sterile water and normal saline are used to prevent contamination of larger bottles and avoid waste. (Courtesy of Briggs Corporation, Des Moines, IA. (800) 247-2343)

Basins, Bedpans, and Other Utensils Used in the Therapy Department. Utensils are scrubbed in the soiled utility room. Some facilities have special utensil washers and sanitizers. Never wash soiled utensils in the hand sink in the therapy department. Wash the articles with soap and water. Remove residue with a scrub brush. Rinse well. Soak the utensils in sanitizer solution for 10 minutes, or according to facility policy. Rinse and dry, or allow the disinfectant to air dry, following the directions for the product you are using. After utensils are thoroughly dry, bag them in clean paper bags. Ⓢ Affix a sticker with the date and your initials. Store them in a clean area.Ⓢ

Sterile Water and Normal Saline Solution. Many procedures involve the use of sterile water, distilled water, or normal saline. Most facilities use small containers of these solutions **(Figure 4–16).** These solutions do not contain preservatives, so microbes multiply rapidly in them. Ⓢ Date and time all liquid solutions when you open them.Ⓢ Write only on the label or a piece of tape. Some ink bleeds through plastic containers. The ink contaminates the contents. When opening the bottle, invert the cap so it is upright on the table. Water and normal saline are discarded within 24 hours of the time they are opened.

Oxygen Equipment

You may be responsible for cleaning and maintaining oxygen equipment. Take special care to prevent

pathogen growth. This equipment directly contacts mucous membranes. It has a high potential to spread serious infections. The type of equipment used and your state's requirements vary. Consequently, developing universal cleaning policies is impossible. Wear gloves when handling respiratory equipment that has touched mucous membranes. If you handle an oxygen cannula without gloves, avoid touching the nasal prongs.

Many facilities store equipment in plastic bags in cupboards after cleaning and disinfecting. Microbes grow best in a warm, moist, dark environment. The cupboard is warm and dark, providing an ideal medium for bacterial growth. Make sure that all equipment is dry before storage to prevent pathogens from growing. Many facilities use paper or mesh bags for storing respiratory equipment instead of plastic bags. The mesh bags are the same type you would use for washing delicate items such as lingerie. These bags keep dust off, but allow air to circulate, reducing moisture. Know and follow your facility policy for packaging these items after cleaning.

Oxygen Humidifiers. Use of oxygen humidifiers is a controversial subject. Cool mist humidifiers are rarely used in health care facilities, because of the high risk of pathogen growth in the container. The pathogens become airborne when the unit is turned on. Some facilities do not humidify oxygen. They prefer to administer it dry because of the high potential for infection when a humidifier is used, and the high cost of maintaining the equipment. Humidification of oxygen under 5 liters is not necessary. This is another reason that facilities do not routinely use humidifiers. Most provide humidification if the resident complains of irritation. If a humidifier is used, it must be regularly cleaned or replaced. The respiratory therapist and infection control committee will establish guidelines. Residents who use oxygen will need extra fluids because of the drying effect of the therapy.

Many facilities use disposable humidifiers **(Figure 4–17)** on oxygen tanks and concentrators. Ⓢ These are closed systems that are never opened or refilled. Check the water level daily. It must always be above the minimum fill line. Change the humidifier weekly, or according to manufacturers' directions and facility policy. To change the unit, remove the humidifier and discard it. Replace the humidifier with a new, sealed unit. Affix a sticker with the date and your initials.Ⓢ

Some facilities use refillable humidifiers. These are refilled with sterile distilled water. The sterile distilled water is dated when opened and discarded after 24 hours. Most facilities change the humidifier bottle every 24 hours because of the high risk for pathogen growth. The bottle is removed and

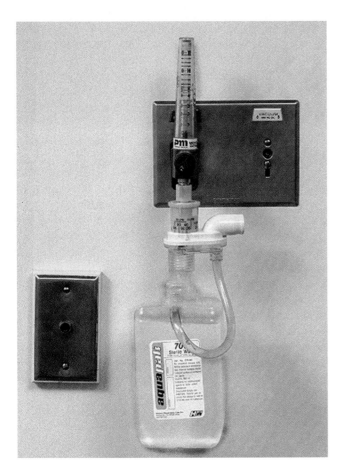

Figure 4–17 The disposable oxygen humidifier is changed weekly, or according to your facility policy.

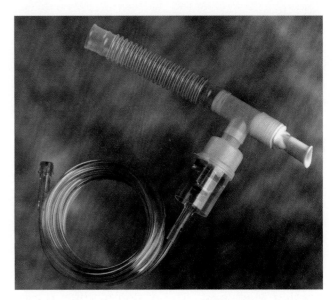

Figure 4–18 The nebulizer is used to administer inhalation medications. (Compliments of Hudson RCI, Temecula, CA, USA)

exchanged for a clean container. Empty the water in the humidifier into the sink. Pour a small amount of sterile water into the reservoir. Agitate gently to rinse all surfaces thoroughly. Discard the water. Fill a clean humidifier with sterile distilled water and replace the bottle on the tank or concentrator. Affix a sticker with the date, time, and your initials. Wash the soiled humidifier with soap and water. Disinfect it with a 2% alkaline gluteraldehyde solution or another facility-approved product. Some facilities sterilize humidifiers. After the unit is thoroughly dry, package it in a paper bag.

Oxygen Cannulas and Masks. Facility infection control policies vary for the frequency of oxygen equipment changes. Some facilities change masks and cannulas every 24 hours. Others change them in frequencies varying from 48 hours to 1 week. The infection control committee will develop policies. The cannula or mask is removed and replaced with a new, sealed item. Discard the used equipment according to facility policy. After replacing the equipment, affix a label to the tubing or other designated location. Write the date, time, and your initials on the label. Oxygen administration equipment must be covered when not in use. New,

unused equipment is covered with the original, sealed plastic bag. A cannula or mask that is used intermittently is covered with a mesh, paper, or plastic bag, according to facility policy.

Oxygen Tanks and Concentrators. ⑤ Dust should not accumulate on oxygen administration equipment.⑤ Wipe these items daily with a damp cloth, or other solution according to facility policy. Some facilities cover the oxygen tank and regulator with a pillowcase or plastic bag when not in use. This keeps them clean and free of dust. Remove the filter on the oxygen concentrator weekly. Wash it in soap and running water, or according to manufacturers' directions. Rinse well, squeeze dry, and replace the filter.

Medication Nebulizers. The respiratory therapist or nurse administers inhalation medications in a small hand-held unit called a **nebulizer (Figure 4–18).** The cup contains medication and sterile normal saline solution. Upon completion of therapy, empty the remaining liquid into the sink. Rinse the container well with sterile water. Tap water is not used because it increases the risk of Legionnaire's disease. Some facilities clean these units with 2% alkaline gluteraldehyde solution. Follow your facility policy. The cup is inverted onto a clean paper towel and allowed to dry. Some facilities use disposable units. After the cup is clean and dry, it is reconnected to the administration set. Wipe the mouthpiece with a damp paper towel or gauze sponge. Store the dry unit in a mesh, paper, or plastic bag, according to facility policy. Write the date, time, and your initials on the bag. Change the administration set every 24 hours, or according to facility policy.

Tubing. Many pieces of respiratory therapy equipment use large, corrugated tubing. You will not be responsible for manipulating this tubing when it is in use. You may be required to clean the used tubing. This tubing has a high potential to spread infection. The respiratory therapist will instruct you on your responsibilities. (SA) After cleaning the tubing, allow it to dry well before storage or reuse.(SA) This is difficult because the diameter of the tube is small and the corrugations retain moisture. Follow your facility policy for hanging the tubing to ensure that it is dry. Package it in a paper or mesh bag according to facility policy.

Suction Machines. The suction machine is used by the nurse or respiratory therapist to remove secretions from the resident's airway. (SA) Apply the principles of standard precautions when handling this equipment. The suction bottle is disinfected after each use. The tubing is disposable and is discarded and replaced.(SA) Avoid getting the pump wet. Check

with your supervisor if you believe the electrical pump needs cleaning. (SA) Suction machines at the resident's bedside are usually cleaned at the end of every shift. Like other respiratory equipment, it must be thoroughly dry before storage. Cover the suction machine with a pillowcase or plastic bag to keep it free of dust when not in use.(SA)

The suction catheter and tubing are disposable. Discard these items according to facility policy. Carefully empty the contents of the suction jar into the drain connected to the sanitary sewer. Avoid splashing. Fill the jar half full with water and disinfectant solution. Scrub the inside with a bottle brush. Rinse in clear water. Soak the suction jar, lid, and metal tubing in disinfectant solution for at least 1 hour, or according to facility policy. Remove the equipment and rinse well in clear water. Allow the equipment to dry thoroughly before reassembling the unit. Some facilities sterilize the bottle. Wipe the exterior of the unit with facility-approved disinfectant. Replace the plastic tubing with a new package of disposable tubing. Restock the drawer below the suction machine with gloves and other disposable supplies.

KEY POINTS IN CHAPTER

- *The restorative nursing assistant has an important responsibility in preventing the spread of infection.*

- *Handwashing is the most effective means of preventing the spread of infection.*

- *The Centers for Disease Control and Prevention introduced standard precautions in 1996; this system was designed to replace universal precautions and body substance isolation.*

- *Standard precautions are used in the care of all residents, without regard for disease or diagnosis.*

- *The restorative nursing assistant is responsible for selecting and using the correct personal protective equipment if contact with blood, body fluids, secretions, excretions, mucous membranes, or nonintact skin is likely.*

- *Transmission-based precautions are the second tier of the 1996 CDC recommendations; this system was designed to replace previously used isolation categories.*

- *Airborne precautions are used for diseases in which the causative agent is an airborne pathogen that is tiny and travels for long distances on dust, moisture, and in air currents; a NIOSH-approved respirator is worn.*

- *Droplet precautions are used for diseases in which the causative agent is spread on droplets that remain within 3 feet of the resident; a surgical mask is worn.*

- *Contact precautions are used for diseases in which the causative agent is spread by direct or indirect contact with blood, body fluids, secretions, excretions, mucous membranes, or nonintact skin; a gown and gloves are worn.*

- *Standard precautions are always used in addition to transmission-based precautions.*

(continues)

**KEY POINTS
IN CHAPTER
*continued***

A face shield or goggles and surgical mask are worn to protect the mucous membranes of the assistant's eyes, nose, and mouth if splashing or spraying of blood, body fluids, secretions, or excretions is likely.

The restorative nursing assistant must have a basic working knowledge of sterile technique.

The restorative nursing assistant is responsible for routine cleaning of restorative and rehabilitation equipment, to prevent the spread of infection.

CLINICAL APPLICATIONS

1. Mr. Torres has a skin condition called psoriasis. He has open, itchy areas on his forearms, scalp, and legs. Sometimes he scratches the lesions, causing them to bleed. You are assigned to work with this resident daily for the restorative dressing program. Is it necessary to apply personal protective equipment when assisting the resident to dress? If so, what equipment will you wear?

2. You have completed care for Mr. Torres. You are ready to assist Mrs. Hillman with passive range-of-motion exercises. You wash your hands when you leave Mr. Torres's room. Is it necessary to wash your hands again before assisting Mrs. Hillman with her exercises? Why or why not?

3. Mr. King is in droplet precautions. You must perform passive range-of-motion exercises on this resident. The resident has bowel and bladder control and does not have any open areas on his skin. What personal protective equipment will you wear? Explain your rationale.

4. Mrs. Day has a pressure sore infected with MRSA. You are assigned to give her a whirlpool bath daily. Following the whirlpool treatment, the therapist will debride the ulcer. Describe how you will prevent the spread of infection when transporting the resident to the tub room. What cleaning procedures will you perform after Mrs. Day has returned to her unit?

5. Miss Johnson is a mentally confused resident with a urinary tract infection. She is incontinent and resists personal hygiene care. She frequently removes her adult brief and throws it on the floor. Occasionally the resident smears feces on the bed, side rails, and wall. Miss Johnson is in contact precautions. She does not understand why she must stay in her room. How will you assist this resident?

6. The therapist has asked you to set up a sterile wound care tray in preparation for debriding Mr. Lincoln's pressure ulcer. You remove the last tray from the cupboard and set it up at the bedside next to the resident, who is confused and restless. He coughs and sneezes. You are not sure if he has contaminated the tray. What should you do?

Principles of Restorative Nursing and Rehabilitation

OBJECTIVES

After reading this chapter, you should be able to:

Spell and define key terms.

Describe how persons with disabilities are like you.

Demonstrate how to communicate with persons who are disabled.

Describe how the medical model of care is different from restorative care.

List the principles of rehabilitation and restoration, and explain how the care each service provides is similar.

Explain the purpose of teaching restorative care to the resident, family, and nursing staff.

Describe how to prepare the resident for restorative care.

Describe how to support resident rights during restorative procedures.

▉▉▉ THE PERSON WITH A DISABILITY

Disabilities can take many forms. Some, such as speech, hearing, or language problems, interfere with communication. Other problems, such as physical impairments, may make you uncomfortable. You may be unsure of what to say or do without offending the resident. Individuals who are newly disabled are more sensitive to their problems than persons who have lived with a disability for a long time.

Persons with disabilities are like you are. They have the same wants and needs. Their problems are no different from yours. However, having a disability makes living with these same problems much more difficult. It creates additional problems. Persons with disabilities can do many of the same things you can. However, they may need to adapt the environment to do them. **⑤** OBRA '87 encourages facilities to adapt the environment to promote independence. Changing things to meet a resident's needs is called providing **reasonable accommodation (Figure 5–1).** Changes can be simple, like adding a raised toilet seat to a low toilet. A **restorative environment** encourages and enables residents to be independent **(Figure 5–2).⑤** Persons with disabilities may perform a task differently than you do. However, the outcome of a task is the same. Their bodies just work differently!

As a rule, persons with disabilities do not want to be treated differently from anyone else. Many are self-sufficient and lead productive lives. Individuals with disabilities are valuable and equal members of society. They may be physically or mentally challenged, but most have other talents and abilities. Disabled residents may enter the facility for rehabil-

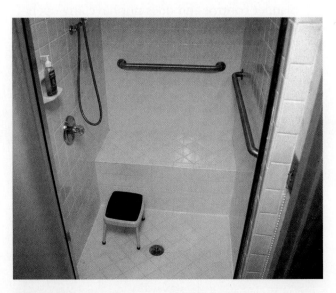

Figure 5–1 The shower in a resident's room has a built-in bench and a foot stool, enabling the resident to bathe independently.

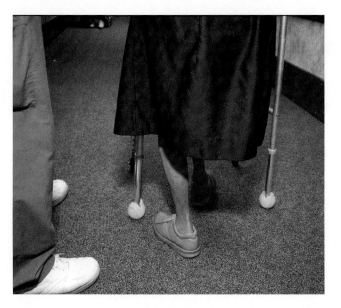

Figure 5–2   This resident had difficulty moving her walker on the carpeted floor of the facility. Staff cut tennis balls and slipped them over the rubber tips, enabling her to be independent using her walker instead of a wheelchair.

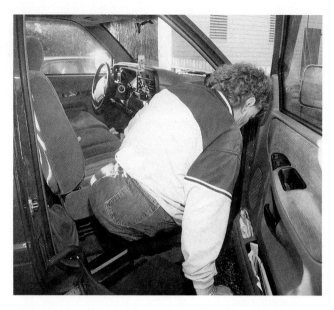

Figure 5–3   This gentleman is a below-the-waist amputee who lives independently in the community. He propels the wheelchair to his truck, then transfers, pulling the chair in behind him. (Courtesy of Skip Baker Photography)

itation and restorative care, then return home. Many live independently **(Figure 5–3).** They will not be institutionalized for life because of their disability.

Nursing Assistant Responsibilities

Emphasize the uniqueness, value, and worth of all persons. Avoid comparing the differences between people. Your efforts on behalf of the disabled will help eliminate the "them-versus-us" attitude that prevents acceptance of persons with disabilities. Treat those with disabilities the way you like to be treated.

Communicating with Residents with Disabilities

Sensitive communication is important. You will use the same principles of communication you learned in your nursing assistant class. However, some additional guidelines are necessary:

- Always be polite and use good manners.
- Avoid referring to the resident as a condition, such as "the multiple sclerosis resident in 221." Say instead, "Mrs. Smith in 221." Always emphasize the person over the condition.
- Use common sense. Talk to the resident the same way you would anyone else. Avoid treating the resident differently.
- Some medical conditions are severely disabling, but the person may appear healthy. Avoid assuming that someone is *not disabled* because the disability is not visible. Never assume that a

person with a nonvisible disability is pretending. Heart disease and other conditions can cause severe problems, but are not visible.
- Shaking hands is appropriate with residents who have upper extremity disabilities, limited movement, or a prosthesis. Shake hands gently with a person who has arthritis.
- Avoid assuming that a person with a disability needs help, unless he or she is struggling. Always ask before assisting. Asking is not offensive.
- When caring for a resident with a disability, ask before providing care. Never assume that the resident can or cannot do something.
- It is all right to ask residents about their disabilities. Many are comfortable and will talk about them. Some look at this as an opportunity to teach others about their condition. Many know a great deal about their own health. However, it is all right if they do not want to talk about it. People who are newly disabled may not have reached a point of acceptance yet. They may be uncomfortable speaking about their problem. Accepting and learning to live with a disability takes time.
- Always stress the resident's ability and not the disability.
- Avoid making assumptions about residents who use wheelchairs, canes, walkers, and crutches. These individuals have a visible disability, but most are not sick.

Table 5–1 Terms to Use in Conversation

Offensive and Unacceptable— Do Not Use in Conversation	Acceptable Use This Instead
Disabled person	A person with a disability
Blind person	A person who is vision-impaired
Deaf person	A person who is hearing-impaired
A hunchback	A person who has curvature of the spine
The disabled	People who are disabled; the disabled community
He is a cripple (or gimp)	He has a disability
Dumb (or deaf and dumb)	A person who has a speech or hearing impairment
She is nuts, crazy	She has an emotional disability or mental illness
Retard	A person who is mentally retarded
Birth defect	A person who is disabled from birth
Fit	Seizure
Normal person instead of a disabled person.	A person who is not disabled as compared with a person who is
Confined to a wheelchair	A person who uses a wheelchair

Remember: Always emphasize the person over the disability or condition.

- Avoid treating individuals in wheelchairs as if they are mentally impaired. Talk to the person in the wheelchair, not a companion. When speaking, position yourself at the other person's eye level whenever possible.
- Excuse yourself if you walk in front of a resident in a wheelchair.
- Avoid standing in front of a person in a wheelchair; it blocks the view.
- Avoid leaning or hanging on the wheelchair. The chair is an extension of the resident's body. Hanging on it is an invasion of the resident's personal space.
- Words such as "see," "hear," "run," and "walk" can be used when speaking with persons with disabilities.
- Choose words that are positive and nonjudgmental. Avoid using demeaning, negative words like "cripple," "gimp," "spastic,"

"retard." **Table 5–1** gives examples of unacceptable terms. Remember, always emphasize the person first; emphasizing the disease is demeaning. **Table 5–2** lists phrases to use when speaking to others about persons with disabilities.

- Service animals, such as seeing-eye dogs, hearing-ear dogs, and others are on duty. Do not feed them or pet them without the owner's permission. This distracts the animals and prevents them from doing their job.
- Do not park in spaces reserved for persons who are disabled. They need them more than you do. Avoid parking in a space reserved for persons with disabilities while a companion runs into a store. A person with a disability driving in right behind you will have nowhere to park. This happens more often than you may think.

Table 5–2 Words to Avoid When Speaking with or about Persons with a Disability

Abnormal	Imbecile
Afflicted	Maimed
Burden	Moron
Cerebral palsied	Normal
Confined to a wheelchair	Palsied
Cripple	Poor
Crippled	Retard
Deaf and dumb	Retarded
Deaf mute	Spastic
Defect	Stricken with
Defective	Sufferer
Deformity	Suffers with
Diseased	Suffering
Epileptic	Unfortunate
Gimp	Victim
Invalid	

HISTORY OF RESTORATIVE CARE

The OBRA legislation of 1987 had a sweeping impact on the entire health care industry. The law was written specifically for long-term care. However, it has had a domino effect on care in many other settings. An example is restraint reduction. OBRA requires long-term care facilities to reduce restraint use. Shortly after this became law in long-term care, the organization that accredits hospitals also began requiring restraint reduction.

OBRA '87 focuses on eliminating the **medical model** of care in which the focus is on the illness or condition. Instead, OBRA '87 emphasizes rehabilitation, restoration, and holistic care. If one body sys-

tem becomes weak, initially the other systems will compensate for it. However, one weak system will, over time, cause declines in all other body systems. The physical condition also affects many areas of the resident's life. Remember this when delivering restorative care. When we look at the whole person, we see a complex being with many strengths and needs, both physical and mental. Each resident is an individual, a member of a family and a community. They all were children once. They have a past. They have people who love them. No two persons are exactly alike. Everyone has strengths and weaknesses.

Declines

An important part of OBRA '87 addresses declines in condition. Before OBRA, health care workers accepted declines as a normal part of the aging process and the effects of chronic illness. Some declines are obvious immediately. However, many are subtle. They are not readily apparent because they occur gradually, over a long period of time. Think of how residents were several years ago. Are they the same today? Better? Worse?

(SA) Remember that OBRA requires us to use all of our resources to assist residents to attain and maintain the highest level of function possible in their situation. Resources can be both within and outside of the facility. As you can see, what OBRA requires is *almost identical* to the definition of rehabilitation and restoration. In long-term care, we comply with this section of OBRA '87 by providing restorative care and preventing declines. Because each person is different, the highest level of function is highly personalized. Remember that mental, social, financial, family, and spiritual needs must also be considered. In doing this, we are treating the whole person and delivering holistic, restorative care.(SA)

PRINCIPLES OF REHABILITATION AND RESTORATION

The principles of rehabilitation and restoration are the same, and apply to all residents. They are:

- *Begin treatment early.* Starting restorative care early in the course of the disease or admission will improve the outcome.
- *Activity strengthens and inactivity weakens.* Keep the resident as active as possible, considering his or her medical condition. Encourage residents to be as independent as possible. For example, giving passive range-of-motion exercises prevents deformities and complications. However, active range-of-motion exercises done by the resident will prevent deformities *and* strengthen muscles **(Figure 5–4)**.
- *Prevent further disability.* Follow the care plan to prevent injury and deformity. Practice safety.

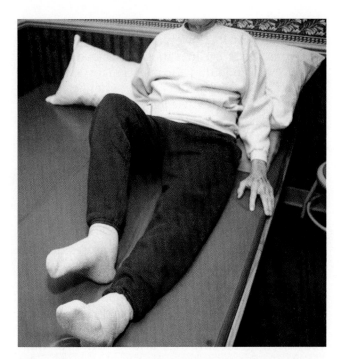

Figure 5–4 Active exercises strengthen the resident's legs.

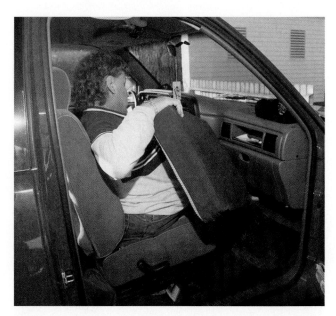

Figure 5–5 After transferring to the truck seat, this man lifts the wheelchair cushion into the truck. He uses this to sit on, enabling him to see over the steering wheel. He uses his arms and upper body strength to overcome the loss of his lower body. (Courtesy of Skip Baker Photography)

▓ *Stress the resident's ability and not the disability.* Emphasizing what the resident can do gives the resident confidence and provides hope. Instead of saying, "You can't use your right arm," say, "You can use your left arm."

▓ *Treat the whole person.* You have learned that you cannot isolate the medical problem from the rest of the person. Consider all of the resident's strengths and needs. Use and build on the strengths to overcome the needs **(Figure 5–5).** Communicate strengths so that others can use them to help the resident as well.

The care plan will guide you in the approaches to use. If you discover something that works for the resident, share this information with your supervisor. He or she will add it to the care plan. Good communication is also an important part of restorative care.

▓ REHABILITATION AND RESTORATIVE CARE

Many individuals assist residents to attain and maintain their maximum potential. The therapy departments provide skilled physical care.

Licensed therapists design **rehabilitation programs.** These programs help residents regain lost skills or teach new skills. The therapist provides skilled therapy for a certain period of time. Therapists teach others techniques for reinforcing and maintaining what the resident has learned. The

therapist or restorative nurse designs a restorative nursing program to complement the therapy program. Combining rehabilitation and restoration helps the resident master new skills more quickly. Using both programs provides more opportunities for practice and repetition.

Skilled therapy is treatment by a licensed therapist **(Figure 5–6).** It is usually designed to restore recently lost function. Sometimes, though, function cannot be restored. In these cases, the therapist designs programs that teach the resident to perform ADLs safely. The resident may need to learn a new way of completing certain tasks. His or her body may work differently as a result of some medical conditions. Safety is a major factor.

Skilled programs are not designed to restore function that was lost many years previously. For example, if a resident has used a wheelchair for 15 years, a therapist will not design a program to teach the resident to walk again. He or she may teach the resident another way of moving about. In some cases, the therapist will not provide skilled therapy. He or she will make recommendations for a nursing program to keep the resident at his or her present level of function.

Maintenance Programs

To participate in a skilled therapy program, the resident must qualify for Medicare Part A coverage. To do this, the resident must make fairly rapid, measurable progress. In some situations, the resident has potential for more improvement, but, progress is

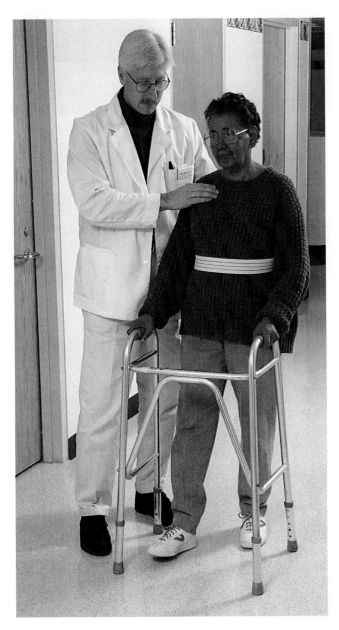

Figure 5–6 The licensed therapist works with the resident to restore function lost as a result of a recent illness. When the resident reaches her maximum potential, she will begin a restorative nursing program to maintain her ability.

very slow. Such a resident will not qualify for further Medicare Part A services. In this instance, the therapist will develop a restorative program. He or she will teach nursing personnel activities to use to help the resident. In this way, the resident continues to work toward the goal. Care is turned over to nursing and therapy is discontinued. The therapist acts as a consultant and answers questions as needed.

Therapists develop functional maintenance programs when a resident reaches his or her highest potential in therapy. The resident is then discharged from therapy to restorative nursing. The functional maintenance program provides repetition. This helps the resident maintain what he or she has learned. The objectives of functional maintenance programs are to:

- Maximize the resident's current level of function
- Maintain the resident at this level, preventing declines
- Keep the resident as safe as possible

ESTABLISHING THE RESTORATIVE NURSING PROGRAM

Restorative nursing care involves using basic nursing measures. The residents' success should not be limited by a health care worker's preconceived ideas. For example, do not feel that because the resident has a serious medical condition, he or she will never improve. Give the resident an opportunity to try. He or she may surprise you! Encourage the resident to keep trying every day.

The restorative nursing program begins with an assessment by the restorative nurse. The nurse will determine the resident's ability to perform each step of a procedure. For example, there are at least 25 separate and distinct steps involved in brushing one's teeth. If the resident cannot complete one step, he or she will be unable to complete the task. The restorative nurse will determine which steps the resident can do. You will begin the program with the first step the resident cannot complete. As you can see, each restorative program is highly individualized because of the type of assessment used. The **task analysis** in **Table 5–3** will give you an idea of the assessment. As the resident completes each step, the care plan is revised. You will work on each consecutive step until the resident masters the procedure.

Other Restorative Programs

Other qualified health care professionals may design restorative programs. The dietitian may design special nutrition or hydration programs. Nursing implements the program for residents who are underweight or at high risk of dehydration. Regardless of who develops the program, you play a critical role in its success. Everyone involved with the program must believe that the resident has the ability to succeed. The residents must believe that they can become more independent. Maintaining motivation is important. Daily routine, structure, and consistency are key to a successful program.

Teaching Residents, Family Members, and Staff

The licensed professional who develops the restorative program teaches residents and staff how to

Table 5–3   Toothbrushing Task Analysis

Key: **+ = Resident can complete task**
              0 = Resident cannot complete task
          N/A = Not applicable

Date	Key	Initial	Step
			1. Identifies equipment for toothbrushing.
			2. Gathers equipment.
			3. Removes cap from toothpaste.
			4. Turns on cold water.
			5. Wets toothbrush.
			6. Squeezes tube slowly and applies toothpaste to toothbrush.
			7. Places cap on toothpaste.
			8. Fills a cup with water for rinsing mouth.
			9. Turns off water.
			10. Grasps toothbrush handle.
			11. Turns bristles upward and brushes chewing surfaces of upper teeth.
			12. Brushes upper teeth beginning at one side, moving across front teeth, and ending on opposite side.
			13. Turns toothbrush and brushes inside of upper teeth.
			14. Brushes lower teeth beginning at one side, moving across front teeth, and ending on opposite side.
			15. Turns toothbrush and brushes inside of lower teeth.
			16. Brushes tongue.
			17. Turns bristles upward and gently brushes roof of mouth.
			18. Takes sip of water from cup.
			19. Rinses mouth.
			20. Spits water from mouth.
			21. Turns on cold water.
			22. Rinses toothbrush.
			23. Turns water off.
			24. Dries face with towel.
			25. Returns toothbrushing supplies to storage area.

implement the program. Family and staff are taught how to reinforce and support the resident. The resident benefits because everyone uses the same techniques and provides support. For example, the restorative nurse teaches a resident to pick up the washcloth, wet it, squeeze the water out, and use it to wash one cheek. The staff washes the remainder of her face. All staff use the same approaches when working with the resident. This repetition is important. When the resident washes one cheek independently, the goal will advance to washing both cheeks. You will build on this ability until she can wash her entire face. Beginning with small goals helps the resident learn each part of the skill. The larger goal builds on the smaller goals. All ADLs begin with small tasks. Like building blocks, each new step is built on mastery of the previous step. The resident's confidence improves with each step as positive reinforcement is provided. Providing restorative care may take longer initially. However, it takes less time as residents assume more responsibility for their own care. The investment is worthwhile for staff and residents!

▌▌▌ PREPARATION FOR RESIDENT CARE

Before beginning restorative procedures, a certain amount of preparation is necessary. You must prepare both the physical environment and the resident. Preparation for the next treatment starts as soon as you finish the current treatment. **SA** Clean equipment and dispose of soiled linen and trash **(Figure 5–7)**. Return reusable supplies to their proper location. If you are using a treatment room, disinfect the treatment table or mat. **SA** Remember the principles of good organization. Gather your equipment and supplies before beginning the procedure. By doing this, you will not have to leave the resident alone to obtain forgotten items. Good organization is safer for the resident and saves time for you.

If you will be using equipment, supplies, or adaptive devices, always explain the purpose to the resident. Demonstrate how to use the item. Do not expect the resident to remember the first time. The explanation familiarizes the resident with the item and describes safety precautions. He or she may need the directions repeated several times before understanding and remembering them.

You will care for residents in many areas of the facility. Some care is given in residents' rooms. Sometimes the therapy room, dining room, hallway, or other location is used. **SA** Check the area for safety. **SA** If you are working in a community treatment area, prepare the room first. Make sure that you have adequate linen, supplies, and other

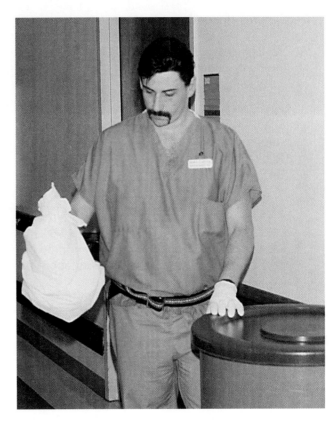

Figure 5–7 Clean the treatment area, and begin to prepare for the next treatment as soon as you have finished.

necessary items. Make sure that the path is clear and unobstructed before transporting the resident to the area. Supplies and equipment in your path make navigating a wheelchair difficult. These items also interfere with safe transfers and ambulation. Pay particular attention to furnishings and other items on wheels, such as overbed tables. If they will not be used, remove them. They present a safety hazard if residents try to hold them during transfers and ambulation. In some programs, you will not be attending the resident for the entire treatment. For example, residents may exercise independently using pulleys or a pedaler **(Figure 5–8, p. 74)**. If you will be leaving the area, make sure that the call signal is within reach and is in working order.

Beginning and Ending Procedure Actions

Review the beginning procedure actions and procedure completion actions from your nursing assistant class. Beginning actions are listed in **Table 5–4**. Ending actions are listed in **Table 5–5**. These are also listed in the inside covers of this text for your convenience. These steps are important and are appropriate for all of the procedures in this text.

Table 5–4 Beginning Procedure Actions

Beginning Procedure Actions	Rationale
1. Assemble equipment and take to resident's room.	Improves efficiency of the procedure. Ensures that you do not have to leave the room.
2. Knock on the resident's door and identify yourself by name and title.	Respects the resident's right to privacy. Notifies the resident who is giving care.
3. Identify the resident by checking the identification bracelet.	Ensures that you are caring for the correct resident.
4. Ask visitors to leave the room and advise them where they may wait.	Respects the resident's right to privacy. Advising visitors where to wait demonstrates hospitality.
5. Explain what you are going to do and how the resident can assist. Answer questions about the procedure.	Informs the resident of what is going to be done and what to expect. Gives the resident an opportunity to get information about the procedure and the extent of resident participation.
6. Provide privacy by closing the door, privacy curtain, and window curtain.	Respects the resident's right to privacy. All three should be closed even if the resident is alone in the room.
7. Position the resident for the procedure. Ask an assistant to help, if necessary, or support the resident with pillows and props. Make sure the resident is comfortable and can maintain the position throughout the procedure. Drape the resident for modesty.	Ensures that the resident is in the correct position for the procedure. Ensures that the resident is supported and can maintain the position without discomfort. Respects the resident's modesty and dignity.
8. Wash your hands.	Applies the principles of standard precautions. Prevents the spread of microorganisms.
9. Set up the necessary equipment at the bedside. Open trays and packages. Position items within easy reach. Avoid positioning a container for soiled items in a manner that requires crossing over clean items to access it.	Prepares for the procedure. Ensures that the equipment and supplies are conveniently positioned and readily available. Reduces the risk of cross-contamination.
10. Apply gloves if contact with blood, moist body fluids (except sweat), mucous membranes, secretions, excretions, or nonintact skin is likely.	Applies the principles of standard precautions. Protects the nursing assistant and the resident from transmission of pathogens.
11. Apply a gown if your uniform will have substantial contact with linen or other articles contaminated with blood, moist body fluids (except sweat), secretions, or excretions.	Applies the principles of standard precautions. Protects your uniform from contamination with bloodborne pathogens.
12. Apply a gown, mask, and eye protection if splashing of blood or moist body fluids is likely.	Applies the principles of standard precautions. Protects the nursing assistant's mucous membranes, uniform, and skin from accidental splashing of bloodborne pathogens.
13. Raise the bed to a comfortable working height.	Prevents back strain and injury caused by bending at the waist.
14. Lower the side rail on the side where you are working.	Provides an obstacle-free area in which to work.

Table 5–5   Procedure Completion Actions

Procedure Completion Actions	Rationale
1. Check to make sure the resident is comfortable and in good alignment.	All body systems function better when the body is correctly aligned. The resident is more comfortable when the body is in good alignment.
2. Remove gloves.	Prevents contamination of environmental surfaces from the gloves.
3. Replace the bed covers, then remove any drapes used.	Provides warmth and security.
4. Elevate the side rails, if used, before leaving the bedside.	Prevents contamination of the side rails from gloves. Promotes resident's right to a safe environment. Prevents accidents and injuries.
5. Remove other personal protective equipment, if worn, and discard according to facility policy.	Prevent unnecessary environmental contamination from used gloves and protective equipment.
6. Wash your hands.	Applies the principles of standard precautions. Prevents the spread of microorganisms.
7. Return the bed to the lowest horizontal position.	Promotes resident's right to a safe environment. Prevents accidents and injuries.
8. Open the privacy and window curtains.	Privacy is no longer necessary unless preferred by the resident.
9. Leave the resident in a safe and comfortable position, with the call signal and needed personal items within reach.	Prevents accidents and injuries. Ensures that help is available. Eliminates the need to call or stretch for needed personal items.
10. Wash your hands.	Although the hands were washed previously, they have contacted the resident and other items in the room. Wash them again before leaving to prevent potential transfer of microorganisms to areas outside the resident's unit.
11. Inform visitors that they may return to the room.	Demonstrates courtesy to visitors and resident.
12. Report completion of the procedure and any abnormalities or other observations.	Informs the supervisor that your assigned task has been completed so further care can be planned and you can be reassigned to other duties. Notifies the licensed nurse of abnormalities and changes in the resident's condition that require further assessment.
13. Document the procedure and your observations.	Ongoing progress and care given is documented. Provides a legal record. Informs other members of the interdisciplinary team of the care given.

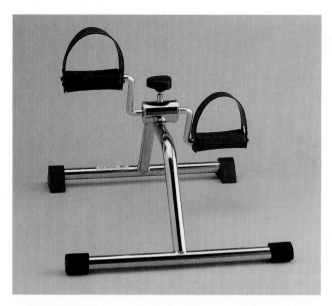

Figure 5–8   The resident can sit in a wheelchair and use the pedaler independently to exercise the legs. (Courtesy of Briggs Corporation, Des Moines, IA. (800) 247-2343)

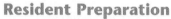

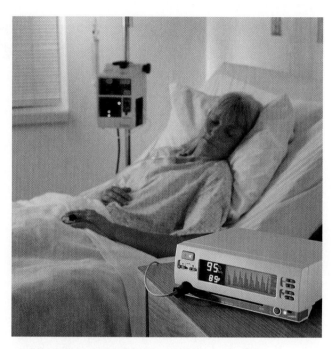

Figure 5–9   Avoid pulling, obstructing, or disconnecting electronic care and monitoring devices. (Courtesy of Ohmeda, Louisville, CO)

Resident Preparation

Prepare the resident for the procedure. Offer to take him or her to the bathroom before beginning. Whenever possible, dress the resident in slacks or shorts. Make sure that the pants are not too long. This is a safety hazard during transfers and ambulation. Socks are worn for comfort, personal hygiene, and to prevent injury to the feet. The resident should wear nonslip footwear for transfers and ambulation.

Timing.   Many residents have limited energy and strength. Timing the procedure is critical to success. Plan your care so the resident is well rested and comfortable. Before beginning, make sure that physical needs are met. If the resident is in pain, notify the nurse. Wait at least 30 minutes after the resident receives pain medication before beginning. ⓈⒶ The resident should not be hungry, thirsty, tired, in pain, or in need of toileting when you begin restorative care.ⓈⒶ These things distract the resident and affect his or her ability to learn.

Transfers.   Transfers move the center of gravity away from the base of support. Always use a transfer belt and good body mechanics. This ensures safety for you and the resident. Teach the resident what is expected and how he or she can assist. Before beginning, get feedback to determine the resident's understanding. Lock the brakes to the wheelchair. Move the leg rests of the wheelchair during transfers. Position the small front wheels to face forward. The largest part of the wheels should be in front. The position of the small wheels keeps the chair stable and prevents tipping.

Tubes and Equipment.   Residents may be using a variety of tubes. These are often connected to treatment or monitoring equipment **(Figure 5–9)**. Use caution when transferring or treating the resident. You must avoid dislodging tubes or disrupting a treatment. Find out in advance how to move the resident and how much movement is permitted. ⓈⒶ You will not be permitted to disconnect the tubing or turn equipment off.ⓈⒶ Repositioning tubes, containers, or other equipment may require the help of another assistant. Plan for and schedule this assistance in advance. Tubing and lines limit the resident's movement. Avoid allowing the tubes to become obstructed, kinked, tangled, stretched, or removed. In most cases, tubing should be secured to the resident's body with tape or a Velcro(®) strap before the procedure **(Figure 5–10)**. Position the resident so that he or she is not lying on the tubing.

ⓈⒶ Intravenous containers must remain above the resident's body. Catheter drainage bags must remain below the level of the bladder.ⓈⒶ If the resident is using a ventilator, or has chest tubes inserted, obtain specific directions from your supervisor before beginning. Disrupting either of these can create a life-threatening crisis. It is best to have an assistant when caring for residents with this equipment. ⓈⒶ If a tube accidentally becomes dislodged or an equipment alarm sounds, notify your supervisor or a nurse immediately.ⓈⒶ

ⓈⒶ **Draping the Resident.**   Drape the resident during transport and treatment to prevent exposure. Although no one else is present in the treat-

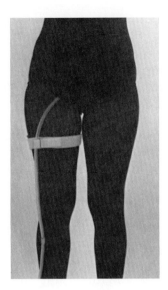

Figure 5–10 The catheter should be secured to the leg at all times. (Courtesy of Skil-Care Corporation (800) 431-2972)

ment area, this is a dignity and modesty issue. Close the door, window, and privacy curtains. Expose only the part of the body you will be working on. The purpose of draping a resident is to:

- Provide comfort and warmth
- Protect modesty
- Prevent scars, wounds, stumps, and undergarments from showing
- Expose a specific area of the body for treatment

If the resident is not dressed, drape him or her during transportation and transfers. Hospital gowns do not provide effective covering. If the resident is wearing a gown, consider putting a second gown on backward. This covers the resident in front and back. Assist the resident to put on underwear before the treatment. Cover the resident with a bath blanket during transport. Keep the resident draped as much as possible during care. Maintaining dignity and modesty are an important part of restorative care.

Maintaining a Restorative Attitude. Your attitude affects the resident. It also has a major effect on the care you provide. You must believe that restorative care works and that it is good for the resident. Do not judge the value of restorative care by the results you see today. It may take a long time to see results. However, when you see results, you will be just as excited as the resident! View restorative care as a positive process that is best for the resident. Understanding this will help you avoid discouragement. Be patient, sincere, tactful, sensitive, and empathetic. Explain the importance of the program to the resident. Provide encouragement and support. Learning new skills is not easy. Show the resident that you are pleased with his or her success.

THE RESTORATIVE NURSING ASSISTANT'S RESPONSIBILITIES

You will perform certain activities with the residents. Learn the cause of the resident's **self-care deficit** before beginning. This will help you to understand the problem you are working on. A self-care deficit is a state in which a resident cannot perform or complete an activity. You will receive verbal directions and follow the care plan. Check the care plan frequently. As the resident progresses, his or her goals and approaches will change. Likewise, if progress is stalled, the nurse may change the goals and approaches to meet the resident's needs. When developing a restorative program, the nurse tries to write goals that are as realistic as possible for the resident. The goals are designed because the nurse believes, based on the assessment, that the resident is physically and mentally able to achieve them.

Each program is designed to meet the resident's needs, so the approaches are personalized. Develop a sensitivity to the resident's abilities. Provide what the resident needs, but avoid doing more than necessary. Be available to assist, but do not help until you are certain the resident cannot accomplish the task. It may be difficult to watch, but the only way the resident will learn the skill is by doing it. The task may be simple for you, but it is a great deal of work for the resident.

Approaches Used in Providing Restorative Care

Consistent care is very important to the success of restorative programs. The care plan will list certain common approaches to use. These approaches are used both individually and in combination. Approaches you may see in the care plan are:

- **Set up** means preparing equipment and supplies for the activity.
- **Verbal cues** are hints that prompt the resident to do something. A cue is a brief, clear, and concise direction. You may need to repeat each cue several times.
- **Demonstration** is showing the resident what you want him or her to do. Show the resident how to do the skill. Simultaneously, give simple verbal directions. You will find methods of demonstration that work best for each resident. Some residents will require a demonstration of each individual step of the procedure. Others will be able to remember and follow more complete directions.
- **Hand-over-hand technique** means placing your hand over the resident's hand and guiding him or her to perform the desired action **(Figure 5–11).**

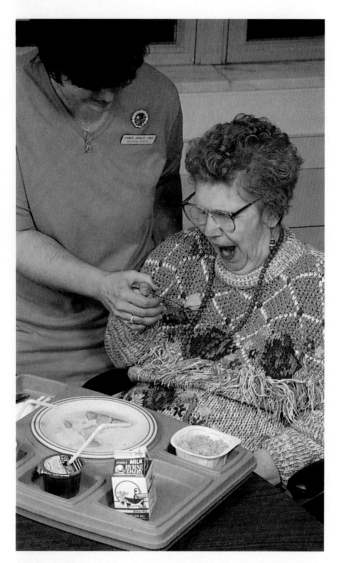

Figure 5–11 If the resident does not respond to verbal cues, use hand-over-hand technique.

Instructions, Verbal Cues, and Commands

To participate effectively, the resident must know what to do and what is expected. Residents must understand the *need to learn* the procedure. They must also be willing to invest the time and energy needed to learn. Give simple directions that the resident understands. Avoid using medical terms. Before beginning a procedure, describe the general sequence of events. Describe the expected response. After explaining the procedure, allow the resident to ask questions. Ask the resident if he or she understands. Asking the resident to repeat the steps of the task reinforces learning. It also provides an opportunity for you to evaluate the resident's understanding. Demonstrate the procedure several times, if necessary. People remember more of what they see than of what they hear. Stress that you will help and provide support.

Make sure the resident can hear your directions. Speak clearly and distinctly. Vary your tone of voice when appropriate. A sharp, quick command will cause the resident to react quickly. For example, if you say, "Watch out!" the resident will react quickly. He or she will react more slowly to a soft, slow command.

Verbal cues are short, simple, specific commands. They are things that the resident must act upon during the procedure. To be effective, cues must be properly timed. Avoid giving a long series of instructions at one time. Cues must specify the action required. For example, if the resident must move to the left, count to three and say, "Move left," or "Move to the left." Using this type of command enables the resident to respond without translating the word "three" into the action. Time each cue to occur in the proper sequence at the proper time. Cues are important to assist residents to complete the procedure safely and efficiently. Repeat them as often as necessary to prompt the resident to do the task. If the resident does not respond to cues, use hand-over-hand technique to help the resident begin the task. Remove your hand and allow the resident to complete the step, if possible. If he or she does not respond, put your hand back on the resident's hand and guide him or her through the task.

Monitoring the Resident's Response to Care

You must observe how the restorative program affects the resident. This is particularly true in the early stages of an illness. The resident may become easily frustrated. Allow him or her to struggle a little, but intervene before the resident reaches the point of frustration. Remind him or her that learning takes time. Practice empathy. Tell the resident you understand how frustrated he or she feels. Be aware of the resident's fears. A fear of falling or spilling may prevent the resident from participating.

Early in the restorative program, the resident may have a physical response. You have learned that bed rest, even for a short time, has a negative effect on the body. Any physical activity may cause a change in physical condition. Monitor for signs of fatigue. Be alert for changes and report them to your supervisor. A good practice is to take the resident's pulse before beginning. Then perform the activity. Monitor the pulse every 5 minutes during the activity. Normally, the pulse increases slightly with activity. Assuming the pulse is under 100 during the activity, continue. If the rate is more than 100, or if the resident develops other problems, such as pain, shortness of breath, nausea, or perspiration, stop the activity. If the resident is standing, assist him or her to sit down. Notify your supervisor or a nurse immediately. Pull the call signal or

- Become familiar with the resident's condition.
- Provide restorative care at the usual time of day for the activity.
- Make sure that the treatment area is ready, equipment is gathered, and the resident's physical needs are met before beginning.
- Follow the instructions on the care plan. Check frequently for changes.
- Provide privacy. The resident will make mistakes and become frustrated. Avoid embarrassing the resident in front of others.
- Eliminate as many distractions as possible.
- Apply **orthotic** and **prosthetic devices** as ordered. These will be listed on the care plan. Orthotic devices improve function and prevent deformities **(Figure 5–12).** Prosthetic devices are replacements for body parts, such as the eye, breast, hand, leg, or foot.
- Modify the environment to promote independence, if necessary.
- Practice good body mechanics for yourself and the resident.
- Practice safety and teach the resident safety measures.
- Remember that all ADLs have many steps. If the resident cannot complete one step, he or she will not be able to complete the activity.
- Treat the resident with dignity.
- Be positive and encouraging. Stress what the resident can do.
- Give the resident as much control as possible by allowing him or her to make choices and decisions.
- Allow enough time for the activity. Be patient and avoid rushing the resident.
- Work on one step at a time. When the resident masters one step, move to the next.
- Remember that the resident's progress may be inconsistent from one day to the next.
- Provide frequent, positive feedback during the procedure.
- Be patient.
- Provide adequate directions. Keep directions as clear and simple as possible. If the resident does not understand, demonstrate.
- Give verbal cues, whenever necessary, to describe what you want the resident to do.
- If the resident does not respond to verbal cues, use hand-over-hand technique. Place your hand on top of the resident's hand and guide him or her to begin the activity. If he or she does not respond, replace your hand and guide the resident through the activity.

- Allow the resident to do as much self-care as possible. Show the resident that you are confident of his or her ability.
- Use adaptive devices, if necessary **(Figure 5–13).**
- If the resident cannot complete an ADL, praise his or her accomplishment. Complete the task without comment or complaint.
- Report your observations to your supervisor. Notify the proper person if you think the resident's condition requires evaluation.
- Document care immediately after providing it. Avoid documenting in advance.🅢🅐

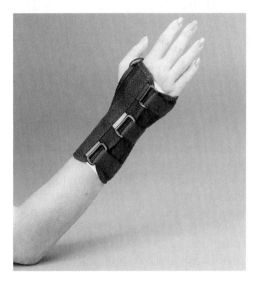

Figure 5–12 Splints are orthotic devices that improve function and prevent deformities. (Cock-up wrist splint is provided by Dammons Preston, Inc., A Bissell® HealthCare Company. Reprinted with permission.)

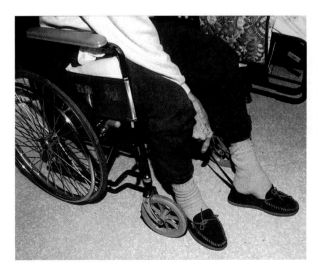

Figure 5–13 This resident uses adaptive devices to put on his shoes and socks independently.

send someone else to get help. Do not leave the resident alone. After you complete the activity, check the pulse again. It should return to within 10 beats of the resting pulse rate within 5 minutes.

Precautions and Special Situations

Residents with certain conditions require special care and handling. Avoid exercising extremities with fractures or dislocations. The bones of residents with osteoporosis or bone cancer break easily. **Osteoporosis** is a condition in which bone mass decreases, leading to fractures with little or no trauma. Check with your supervisor and the care plan before continuing. Notify a nurse if the resident has a wound, red, or open area on the joint you are exercising. Inquire if exercise will be harmful before continuing. If a resident is combative or resists care, explain why it is important. Try to coax him or her into participating. Try singing an old-time song with the resident for distraction. Avoid forcing him or her. Notify your supervisor if the resident continues to refuse.

Resident Rights

When transporting residents and performing treatments, remember the residents' rights. Unless you are working with a group of residents in an exercise or feeding activity, perform procedures in a private area. Other residents and unnecessary staff should not be present. Relearning old skills and learning new skills may be a very difficult, frustrating process for the resident. Allowing others to see him or her make mistakes, spill liquids or foods, become angry, or cry is demeaning. You are responsible for meeting the resident's need for privacy and emotional support.

During a treatment, allow the resident personal choices and control. Being unable to control movement and other bodily functions is very upsetting. Allowing residents to make decisions and control other aspects of their lives promotes dignity and self-esteem.

Remember that rehabilitation and restoration may take a long time. The treatment may take longer for an elderly person to complete than it would a younger person. Likewise, learning new skills or relearning previously used skills will take longer. Remind yourself and the resident of this. Providing restorative care takes a great deal of patience. We did not learn to care for ourselves overnight. Think about how long it takes a small child to learn to take a bath and get dressed. When adults lose the ability for self-care, it takes time to restore. The process can be frustrating for both you and the resident. Being patient, positive, and supportive is the best approach. Avoid becoming frustrated and impatient with the resident. If frustration or impatience are a problem for you, consult the RN, your supervisor, clergy, or another person qualified to give advice. Request assistance in dealing with your feelings. Remember that the resident is probably twice as frustrated as you are. Always treat residents with empathy, kindness, respect, and compassion.

KEY POINTS IN CHAPTER

Persons with disabilities are like you are. Residents with disabilities can do many of the same things you do. They may need to adapt the environment or their lifestyle in order to do the activity.

Use common sense when interacting with residents who have disabilities. Treat them the way you like to be treated.

The medical model of care treats a specific health condition. Holistic care is designed to treat the whole person.

A strength or weakness in one area can affect the resident's entire state of well-being.

Rehabilitation programs are designed and implemented by licensed therapists. These programs help residents regain lost skills or teach residents new skills.

Some restorative programs are designed to complement programs that therapists are working on. These programs reinforce learning and enable residents to progress more rapidly.

Restorative nursing involves using basic nursing measures to assist the resident to attain and maintain the highest degree of independence and self-care possible.

Most restorative programs are designed to assist the resident to become independent with activities of daily living.

(continues)

KEY POINTS IN CHAPTER *continued*

— *Maintenance programs help the resident remain at the present level of function.*

— *Declines in condition must be prevented whenever possible.*

— *The resident is the most important member of the interdisciplinary team.*

— *Restorative programs are designed with a specific functional purpose in mind. They are not designed to create more work for staff.*

CLINICAL APPLICATIONS

1. The licensed therapist feels that Mrs. Nguyen has reached her maximum potential. He discharges the resident from therapy services. The resident is in denial about her condition and overestimates her ability. Mrs. Nguyen had a CVA and has left hemiparesis. She wears a left hand splint and left leg brace when she is up. The licensed therapist recommends a range-of-motion program. She also teaches staff to apply the splint and brace. Safety is an important part of this program. What type of safety problems could this resident have?

2. Mrs. Long is a 72-year-old resident with chronic obstructive pulmonary disease (COPD). She ambulates to the activities room (150 feet) twice a day with minimal assistance of one staff member and a rolling walker. Mrs. Long must rest for 1 to 3 minutes after every 50 feet due to shortness of breath. The physical therapist informs the restorative nursing assistant that Mrs. Long's standing balance is good. However, her endurance, transfers, and turns are unsafe. Because of the resident's weakness and unsteady gait, you must use a gait belt for ambulation. What safety precautions will you take? Do you think that you can ambulate this resident without help? Why or why not? What will you do to prepare before caring for Mrs. Long?

3. Mr. Hall has a poor attention span and forgets to eat. He can pick up his utensils and feed himself. The occupational therapist instructs you to set up his tray. You are instructed to provide verbal cues for each bite of food. Mr. Hall stands up frequently during each meal. If no one intervenes, he will leave the room. How can you assist this resident?

4. The speech therapist is working with Mrs. Tsai to tuck her chin under to swallow. Mrs. Tsai uses a thickener for liquids. The restorative nurse instructs you to thicken all of this resident's beverages. How will you know the correct consistency for mixing the thickener? In addition to the supervisor's verbal directions, where would you expect to find written directions?

5. Mr. Stanislawski is a bedfast resident who had a CVA with left hemiparesis. He has a Foley catheter connected to a closed drainage bag. The resident is fed by gastrostomy tube, which is connected to a pump. He uses oxygen at 2 liters per minute through a nasal cannula. The resident appears to be mentally alert, but cannot speak. You are assigned to provide passive range-of-motion exercises to his affected side. He requires active assisted range-of-motion exercises to his unaffected side. Describe how you would prepare Mr. Stanislawski for the procedure. Describe how to ensure that the resident's rights are not violated. How will you manage the various tubes and pieces of equipment?

Caring for Residents with Musculoskeletal, Neurological, and Integumentary Conditions

Restorative Care of Residents with Musculoskeletal System Conditions

OBJECTIVES

After reading this chapter, you should be able to:

Spell and define key terms.

List three types of arthritis and describe how they are similar.

Describe osteoporosis and explain why this condition increases the risk of fractures.

Define fracture. List the types and patterns of fractures.

Describe the care of residents with casts and traction.

Describe the care of residents with hip fractures and hip replacement surgery.

Describe the care of residents with amputations.

State the purpose and benefits of heat and cold treatments.

ARTHRITIS

Arthritis is a common condition in long-term care facility residents. There are many different types of arthritis. The most common are osteoarthritis, rheumatoid arthritis, and gout, or gouty arthritis. Arthritis can cause mild discomfort to severe deformities and disability **(Figure 6–1).** Residents with arthritis are at high risk of contractures. If permitted by your facility, place residents with this condition in the prone position periodically. This reduces the risk of contractures of the hips and knees. Avoid placing pillows under the knees or elevating the knee area of the bed. Using a small, flat pillow under the head and neck is best. A large pillow pushes the neck into a position of flexion. Be very gentle when you perform range of motion on residents with arthritis. Avoid moving joints past the point of resistance.

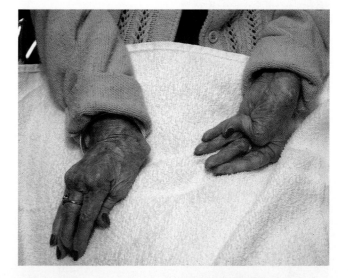

Figure 6–1 These deformities, caused by rheumatoid arthritis, make movement of the hand difficult.

Osteoarthritis

The most common type of arthritis is **osteoarthritis** (OA). This is a chronic condition that causes deterioration of the joints. Many factors cause OA, including chemicals, genetic factors, and metabolic and mechanical factors. Secondary osteoarthritis is common after trauma or a major injury to the body.

Signs and Symptoms. The most common symptom of osteoarthritis is pain. This is usually described as a deep, aching pain that occurs after exercise, weight bearing, or exertion. It is often relieved by rest. Changes in the weather may also cause pain. Other symptoms include limited ability to move and stiffness, particularly upon arising in the morning. This also may occur after strenuous exercise or physical overactivity. In some individuals, an audible grating sound can be heard in the joints during movement. Osteoarthritis may cause redness and swelling in the joints. Conditions such as obesity and stress aggravate the symptoms.

Treatment. The goals of treatment are to relieve pain, limit disability, and maintain or improve joint mobility. A combination of methods is used to treat arthritis. Drugs are available to decrease pain and joint inflammation. Splints, braces, and other adaptive devices may be used to relieve stress on the joints. Other measures include massage, heat applications, whirlpool, paraffin therapy, and range of motion exercises. You may assist residents with arthritis with **fine motor exercises.** These are done to develop skill using small muscles. Threading a needle and buttoning buttons are fine motor skills.

Rheumatoid Arthritis

Rheumatoid arthritis (RA) is a systemic, inflammatory condition that attacks muscles, tendons, ligaments, and blood vessels in the joints. The exact cause is not known. It causes severe deformities. This disorder requires lifelong treatment. It usually follows an intermittent course. RA has **exacerbations,** or times in which the condition seems to worsen; and **remissions,** or times in which the disease appears stable. It is more common in women than in men.

Signs and Symptoms. The onset of RA is usually gradual. Occasionally it occurs in childhood. Initially, RA produces symptoms such as fatigue, loss of appetite, low-grade fever, weight loss, and vague aches and pains in the joints. Later, more localized pain in the joints develops. The condition commonly begins in the fingers, but spreads to the wrists, elbows, hips, knees, and ankles. The joints become stiff when the resident is at rest. Edema, pain, and tenderness initially occur upon movement. As the disease progresses, these conditions are also present while the resident is at rest. The involved joints may feel hot to the touch. The condition causes reduced joint function and deformities. These can be severe and disabling.

Treatment. Treatment for RA ranges from drug therapy to surgery. Some residents benefit from wearing copper bracelets and jewelry. Range of motion and other individualized exercise programs are normally part of the plan of care. Therapy with heat and cold is used depending on symptoms. The goal of therapy is to maintain as much joint function as possible, prevent deformity, and relieve pain.

Gout (Gouty Arthritis)

Gout is a metabolic disease that can be severely disabling. It is caused by increased uric acid, which deposits in the joints and causes pain. It can occur in any joint, but is most common in the feet and legs. Gout also follows a course of remission and exacerbation. It can lead to complete disability, hypertension, and chronic renal disease. The cause is unknown, but it is thought to be caused by a genetic defect in the ability to metabolize uric acid.

Signs and Symptoms. Gout occurs in four stages. There are no symptoms in the first stage, but the uric acid level in the blood rises. The onset of gout is usually signaled by sudden, severe pain in one or more joints. The affected joints are hot and painful to touch. They may be red or cyanotic in appearance. The resident may have a low-grade fever during this time. The great toe is often the first joint affected.

After the initial, painful period, symptoms subside. The resident may be pain-free for a period of time, commonly 6 months to 2 years. The next attack is usually more painful and severe than the first. Eventually, chronic disease sets in. It is marked by constant pain, tenderness, and swelling in the joints. Other body systems may be affected in this stage.

Treatment. Treatment involves medication, resting the inflamed joint, and local heat and cold applications. Dietary restrictions are used to reduce the uric acid level in the blood. The dietitian will plan a diet that restricts the amount of red meat and foods rich in purines. Alcoholic beverages should be avoided.

▄▄ OSTEOPOROSIS

Osteoporosis is a metabolic disorder of the bones. It is most common in elderly females. Bone mass is lost, causing the bones to become porous and spongy. Bones affected are at very high risk for fracture. Fractures can occur spontaneously, such as when the resident is walking. They can also occur by turning the resident in bed or during transfers.

The cause of osteoporosis is unknown. It is thought to result from years of inadequate calcium intake. Other potential causes are declining adrenal function, faulty protein metabolism, estrogen deficiency, and lack of exercise or activity.

Signs and Symptoms. The first sign of osteoporosis is usually a fracture. Commonly, the resident moves or lifts something. He or she hears a "pop" or snapping sound in a bone. This frequently occurs in the lower back or hip. Sometimes the resident is walking and falls. This fall is the result of the fracture. In most falls, the opposite is true. After the initial incident, the area is very painful, particularly upon movement. Sometimes the onset of osteoporosis begins with a curvature of the spine and loss of height. The back progressively weakens, straining the neck, hips, and low back. Spontaneous fractures may occur on movement or as a result of a minor injury.

Treatment. The goals of treatment are to prevent further fractures and control pain. Gentle range of motion and other exercises may be used. Splints, braces, and other devices may be ordered to support weakened bones. Residents are given estrogen replacement and other drugs to replace calcium and bone mass.

▨ FRACTURES

Many residents are admitted to the long-term care facility to recover from the effects of fractures. Fractures are a condition in which treatment is usually successful. The resident is usually able to return home following intensive rehabilitation and restorative programs. A **fracture** is a break in the continuity of a bone. It occurs as a result of fall, trauma, or any condition in which more stress is placed on the bone than it can absorb. Other structures, such as muscles, tendons, ligaments, nerves, and blood vessels, may also be injured in the area of the fracture.

Types of Fractures

Fractures are classified by the type of break in the bone and whether the skin is broken.

▨ A **complete fracture** involves a break across the entire cross-section of the bone. It is often **displaced,** or improperly aligned, and must be reduced and straightened.

▨ An **incomplete fracture** involves only part of the cross-section of the bone.

▨ A **closed or simple fracture (Figure 6–2A)** occurs when the skin is intact and not broken.

▨ An **open** or **compound fracture (Figure 6–2B)** occurs when the skin over the fracture is broken. The bone may or may not protrude.

▨ A **pathologic fracture** is a fracture in a diseased bone. It occurs as a result of osteoporosis, a tumor, or cancer.

Patterns of Fractures

The pattern of a fracture describes the manner in which the bone is broken.

▨ A **greenstick fracture (Figure 6–2C)** occurs when only one side of the bone is broken and the other side is bent.

▨ A **transverse fracture (Figure 6–2D)** breaks completely across the bone.

▨ An **oblique fracture (Figure 6–2E),** is a fracture that runs at an angle across the bone.

▨ A **spiral fracture (Figure 6–2F)** twists around the bone.

▨ A **comminuted fracture (Figure 6–2G)** involves shattering and splintering of the bone into more than three fragments.

▨ A **depressed fracture (Figure 6–2H)** is seen only in fractures of the skull and face. This type of fracture depresses the bone and drives fragments inward.

▨ A **compression fracture (Figure 6–2I)** is seen only in the vertebrae of the spine. This type of fracture collapses the bone inward.

▨ An **avulsion fracture (Figure 6–2J)** occurs when a bone fragment is pulled off at the point of ligament or tendon attachment.

▨ An **impacted fracture (Figure 6–2K)** occurs when the fragment from one bone is wedged into another bone.

Signs and Symptoms. Signs and symptoms of fractures will vary with the location. Fractures are painful. Either movement is limited or the resident will be unable to move the injured area at all. The skin surrounding the fracture may appear deformed. Edema is common. **Ecchymosis,** or bruising, may occur. Some parts of the body, such as the area over the femur, are very **vascular.** They bleed readily under the skin. An area that is vascular contains many blood vessels. An ecchymosis the size of an adult's fist over the femur indicates loss of approximately one pint of blood.

Treatment. A new fracture is usually treated in the hospital emergency department. Admission for surgical correction of the fracture may be necessary. The resident is admitted or readmitted to the long-term care facility after hospital treatment. The immediate goals of care are to:

▨ Control pain

▨ Prevent complications of immobility

▨ Prevent or reduce edema

▨ Keep the fracture in good alignment

▨ Keep the fractured extremity immobile

You will assist residents who have fractures with range of motion exercises several times each day. Check with your supervisor for specific instructions. In most cases, you will not exercise the fractured extremity. You may be assigned to exercise the resident's joints above and below the cast to keep them mobile. For fractured arms and legs, you may be permitted to exercise fingers and toes. Exercising the rest of the resident's body is important. The exercise prevents complications related to immobility and inactivity.

You may also assist the resident with coughing and deep breathing exercises to prevent pneumonia. These are described in Chapter 16. When working with residents with fractures, encourage ade-

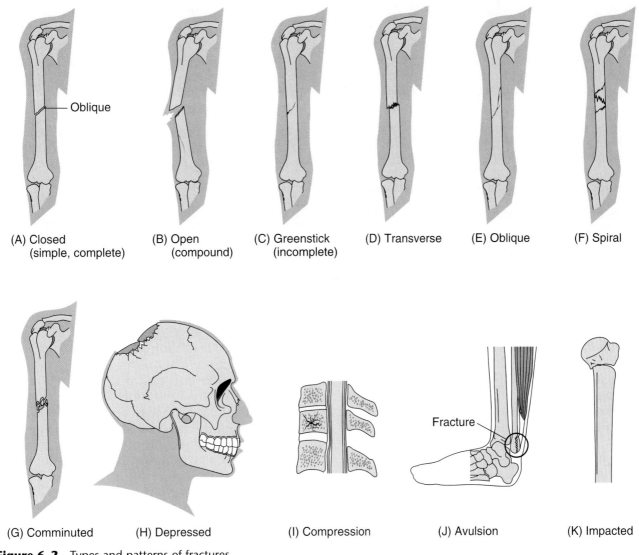

(A) Closed
(simple, complete)

(B) Open
(compound)

(C) Greenstick
(incomplete)

(D) Transverse

(E) Oblique

(F) Spiral

—Oblique

(G) Comminuted

(H) Depressed

(I) Compression

(J) Avulsion

(K) Impacted

Fracture

Figure 6–2 Types and patterns of fractures.

quate fluid intake. The increased fluid liquefies secretions that accumulate in the lungs. Coughing and deep breathing exercises are the same as those used in postoperative care. A **trapeze (Figure 6–3)** will be applied to the bed to assist the resident with movement.

Treatment for residents with fractures begins soon after admission. The type of treatment is determined by the location and type of fracture and the method of fracture reduction. For example, some fractures are treated with traction. The method of treatment for residents with this type of fracture will be significantly different from the treatment used for a resident whose fracture is treated with a cast. Your supervisor will teach you how to move and reposition the resident without interfering with the traction. The casted extremity is elevated on pillows if traction is not used.

Residents with fractures will be evaluated by the physical and occupational therapists. Therapists

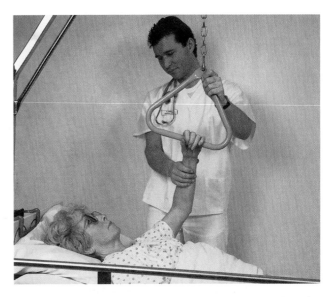

Figure 6–3 The trapeze is fastened to the bed so that the resident can move independently.

will design rehabilitation programs to meet their needs. These begin with bed mobility, or teaching the resident to move independently in bed. The resident is taught to turn by pulling on a trapeze or the side rails. The program may progress immediately to transfer training and ambulation. This is determined by the type of fracture and the physician's activity order. The restorative nurse or therapist will design a complementary restorative program. Residents with upper extremity fractures may also participate in ADL retraining programs, if their dominant hand and arm are affected by the fracture.

Care of a Resident with a Cast

Some fractures are immobilized with a cast **(Figure 6–4).** Monitor the skin around the edges of the cast for redness, irritation, or breakdown. Casts are made of fiberglass or plaster. They are applied wet and require a period of time to dry. Handle a new cast carefully to avoid pressure that will cause dents or deformities. Indentations cause pressure on the skin inside the cast. Skin breakdown under a cast causes severe problems. The lesions may not be detected for a long time because of the cast. To avoid pressure, handle the cast gently with the palms of your hands. Avoid positioning the cast against the footboard or side rail. Leaving the cast open to air until it dries is best. If the resident is cold, cover the cast loosely with a sheet. Avoid tucking the sheet under the mattress. A bed cradle may be used, if necessary. The greatest area of heat loss is the head. Covering the upper body and back and top of the head with a blanket may help keep the resident warm.

Elevate the casted extremity on a pillow. When positioning a resident with a leg cast, elevate the foot higher than the hip. An arm cast may be elevated in a sling **(Figure 6–5).** The fingers should be higher than the elbow. Avoid placing the cast on a flat surface. Avoid placing anything plastic under a wet cast. Check the skin distal to the cast frequently. Notify a nurse immediately if any of the following are noted:

- Pallor, gray, or cyanotic color in fingers or toes, which is an indication of decreased circulation
- Temperature changes; skin feels cool or cold distal to the cast
- Edema
- Complaints of excessive pain or tingling

Changes may occur after the cast dries that indicate infection or ulceration under the cast:

- Odor from the cast
- Drainage through the cast

After the cast dries, the resident may complain that the edges are irritating the skin. The upper and lower edges of the cast can be taped or padded to prevent irritation.

The casted extremity should remain elevated to prevent edema. A sling may be used to elevate an arm cast when the resident is out of bed. A wheelchair with an elevated leg rest is used for residents with leg casts. Cover the cast with plastic during bathing. Keep small objects from getting inside the cast. The resident may complain of an itching sensation under the cast. Discourage him or her from pushing objects down the cast to scratch. This could cause a skin injury and infection. Report complaints of itching to your supervisor.

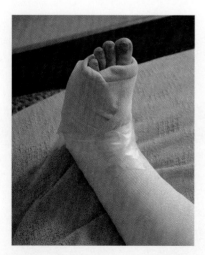

Figure 6–4 Avoid handling the plaster cast with your fingers until it is completely dry. Monitor the toes for color, temperature, movement, pressure, and sensation.

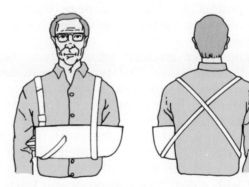

Figure 6–5 The arm sling may be used to elevate the cast, or for residents with injuries who must keep their fingers elevated.

PROCEDURE

4 APPLYING AN ARM SLING

1. Perform your beginning procedure actions.
2. Gather equipment:
   arm sling or triangular bandage
   padding for neck, if needed
3. Position the affected arm at a 90° angle.
4. Apply the sling:
   - If a triangular bandage is used, place one end of the triangle over the unaffected shoulder. Position the point of the triangle under the affected elbow. Bring the other end of the triangle over the shoulder on the affected side, covering the arm. Adjust the bandage so the fingers are elevated, and tie the ends of the bandage in back. Pad the skin under the knot to prevent pressure and irritation. Fold the extra fabric over at the elbow. Secure it on the inside with pins or tape.
   - If a commercial sling is used, support the affected arm. Guide the sling up over the hand until the elbow is covered and the fingers are exposed. Wrap the strap around the resident's neck, then fasten it to the buckle on the sling. Adjust the strap so the fingers are elevated. Pad the strap under the neck to prevent pressure and irritation.
5. Perform your procedure completion actions.

Caring for Residents in Traction

Some fractures are treated with **traction.** The bone ends are pulled into place with ropes and weights. The resident's body weight stabilizes the upper part of the bone. A bag of water or metal disks are attached to pull on the opposite end of the fracture. This stabilizes the lower part of the bone, bringing it into good alignment. **Skin traction (Figure 6–6)** involves applying a halter or belt of foam rubber, a boot, or other device to the injured extremity. The belt is attached to ropes and weights. **Skeletal traction (Figure 6–7)** involves surgically placing a wire, pin, or tongs into or through the fractured bone. The pin protrudes through the skin, where ropes and weights are attached.

Traction may be used as a temporary measure until the fracture is surgically repaired. It may be used until the fracture completely heals in residents who are not good candidates for surgery. Placement of the straps and the amount of weight used for

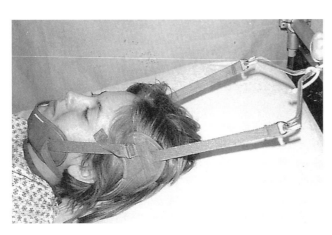

Figure 6–6   This cervical traction is an example of skin traction.

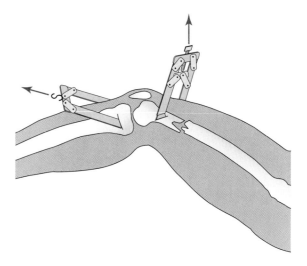

Figure 6–7   Skeletal traction is attached to surgically inserted pins. Monitor the insertion site for redness, drainage, or other signs of infection.

traction are prescribed by the physician. When caring for residents in traction, you should:

- Review the correct placement of straps and weights with the therapist or nurse.

- Avoid moving, dropping, or releasing the weights. They should not touch the bed, swing freely, or rest upon any object or surface. The weights hang still at the end of the bed.

- Position the resident in the center of the bed in good body alignment. The feet should not rest against the end of the bed.

- Keep the traction straps smooth and free from wrinkles. Monitor the position of the straps each time you are in the room.

- Monitor the skin under the straps for signs of irritation or breakdown.

Disc problems in the back and some other conditions may be treated with traction **(Figure 6–8).** This is an older form of treatment. In recent years the use of the traction for disc problems has decreased. In these conditions, the traction may be used intermittently. You will manage the traction in the same manner as if the resident had a fracture. Your supervisor will provide specific directions.

External Fixation Devices

External fixation devices (Figure 6–9) are metal appliances. They are sometimes used to treat fractures and other orthopedic conditions. The adjustable nuts on the appliance are moved periodically by the physician or licensed personnel to accomplish the desired result. You will not be responsible for caring for the metal appliance or adjusting the nuts. However, you may be responsible

for cleansing the skin at the insertion point daily with an antiseptic agent. Notify your supervisor immediately if redness, drainage, or other signs of infection are present.

Other Devices Used in the Treatment of Fractures

In addition to casts and traction, fractures are sometimes treated with splints. Splints keep the fracture

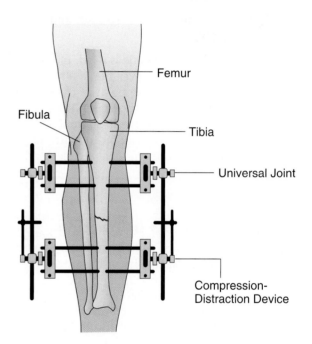

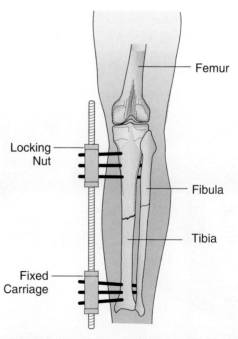

Figure 6–9 The external fixation device is adjusted by the licensed health care professional. Monitor the insertion site for redness, drainage, or other signs of infection.

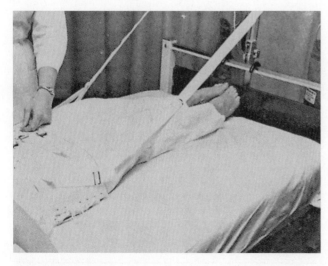

Figure 6–8 Pelvic traction is used occasionally to treat disc problems.

PROCEDURE

5 | APPLYING A CLAVICLE STRAP

1. Perform your beginning procedure actions.
2. Gather equipment:
   clavicle strap
   talcum powder
3. Assist the resident to sit (or stand) with the back straight.
4. Remove the resident's shirt.
5. Apply a light layer of talcum powder to the shoulders, back, and axillae to prevent skin irritation. Avoid using talcum powder near residents with respiratory disorders.

6. Place the strap on the resident, with the apex in the center of the back, between the shoulder blades.
7. Place the straps over the shoulders, with one strap under each arm. Place the end through the loop, adjusting the strap for comfort and support.
8. Secure the Velcro® on the straps to hold them in position.
9. Assist the resident to dress.
10. Perform your procedure completion actions.

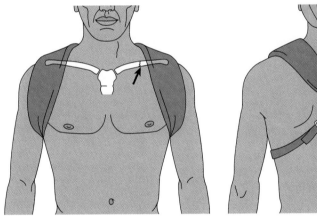
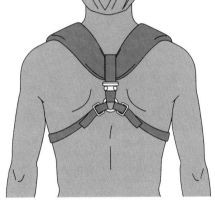

Figure 6–10 The clavicle strap immobilizes the shoulder and arm to promote healing.

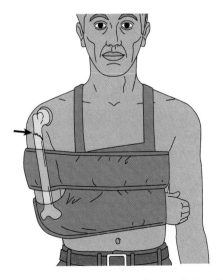

Figure 6–11 Because a cast cannot be applied to the upper humerus, the sling and swathe is used to immobilize it.

immobilized. You care for the resident with a splint in the same manner as you would one with a cast.

A **clavicle strap (Figure 6–10)** may be used if the resident has a clavicle fracture. A **sling and swathe (Figure 6–11)** is used to treat fractures of the humerus, in the upper arm. The nurse or therapist will instruct you regarding your responsibilities with these devices. Always make sure the straps are smooth and not binding or pinching. Check the skin around the straps daily for signs of irritation or skin breakdown.

▬ HIP FRACTURES

Hip fractures are the most common type of fracture in the elderly. The most common cause of hip fractures is falls, but they may also occur because of osteoporosis. In that condition, the resident may hear a popping sound in the bone, then fall. An x-ray will reveal a fracture. The term "hip fracture" really is not accurate. This term refers to a fracture anywhere in the upper third or head of the femur.

Signs and Symptoms of Hip Fracture

A resident with a fractured hip is usually found on the floor. He or she will be unable to get up or move the injured leg. The leg on the affected side may be shortened and in a position of **external rotation.** In this position, the toes point outward. The shortening and rotation occur because the strong muscles in the upper leg contract. This causes the bone ends to override each other. The resident will complain of severe pain in the hip. The pain of a hip fracture is usually localized in the hip. However, some residents complain of pain in the knee. This may be confusing or misleading. Edema and ecchymosis may be present in the hip, thigh, groin, or lower pelvic area.

SA Treatment. Avoid moving the resident until you are instructed to do so by a nurse. You will use a sheet, backboard, or other device to move the resident. Avoid excessive movement, which can worsen the injury. Moving a resident with a hip fracture requires four or five individuals. The resident is logrolled onto the lifting device. The device is then lifted to the bed or stretcher.SA Some facilities leave the resident on the floor and wait for an ambulance. Leaving residents on the floor prevents pain and further injury during a transfer. Cover the resident with a sheet or blanket. Place a pillow under the head for comfort. You may be assigned to monitor the resident's vital signs and check for signs of shock. The resident will be transported to the hospital for treatment, which usually involves surgical repair. Some residents are returned to the facility and treated with Buck's traction **(Figure 6–12).**

Open Reduction Internal Fixation

The most common treatment for a fractured hip is a surgical procedure called **open reduction internal fixation (ORIF).** This procedure is performed in the hospital under anesthesia. The resident is admitted or readmitted to the long-term care facility several days to several weeks after the procedure. The ORIF procedure involves reducing the fracture through a surgical incision. The fracture is stabilized with a metal plate, screws, nails, or pins.

Hip Replacement

A hip replacement **(Figure 6–13)** is sometimes performed after a fracture. The procedure is done for residents with severe arthritic deterioration of the hip. Hip replacement is the most common surgical procedure in the elderly. Selection of hip replacement as treatment for a fracture depends on the location of the fracture and the condition of the bone. Hip replacement prostheses are metal and plastic, and are fixed to the bone with a special cement.

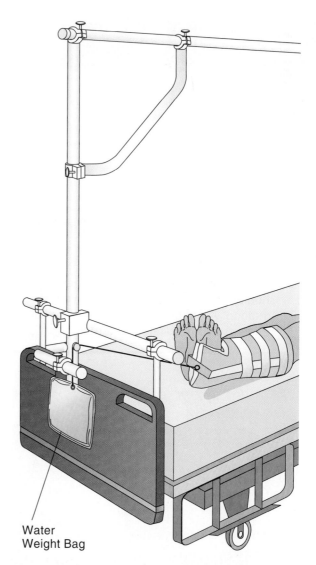

Water
Weight Bag

Figure 6–12 Buck's traction is used to stabilize a fractured femur before surgery. It is used until the fracture is healed in residents who are poor surgical risks.

Caring for the Resident with Hip Surgery

When the resident is admitted or readmitted to the long-term care facility following hip surgery, the following general procedures will be ordered:

▪ A trapeze is attached to the bed to assist with movement. The resident is instructed not to press down on the foot of the affected leg when using the trapeze.

▪ Anti-embolism stockings are applied

▪ A fracture bedpan is initially used for elimination. When the resident is able to use the toilet, an elevated toilet seat is used.

▪ The head of the bed is not elevated more than 45 degrees.

▪ Avoid acute flexion of the hip and legs. The therapist will give directions for positioning and the degree of flexion permitted.

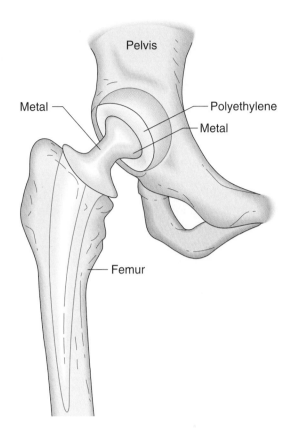

Figure 6–13 The hip prosthesis is used to replace the joint if it is worn and painful. It is sometimes used as treatment for a fractured femur.

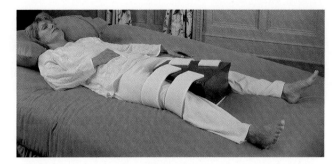

Figure 6–14 Residents often use the abduction pillow upon their return to the facility following hip surgery. The pillow prevents the resident from crossing the ankles, and holds the hip in proper alignment, preventing contractures. (Courtesy of Sammons Preston)

■ Residents who have had hip replacement surgery will use a special pillow, called an **abduction pillow**, to keep the legs apart **(Figure 6–14).** This is particularly important when the resident is turned on the side. The resident will be instructed to avoid crossing the legs, which can cause a dislocation.

Rehabilitation and Restoration Following Hip Surgery

The physician will specify how long the resident must avoid weight bearing after surgery. Some residents are able to ambulate shortly after admission. Some physicians do not permit ambulation for as long as 4 to 6 weeks. Initially, you will assist with procedures to prevent the complications of immobility. These include range of motion exercises, turning and repositioning, and coughing and deep breathing exercises. An incentive spirometer may also be used. The respiratory procedures are described in Chapter 16.

The resident will receive skilled physical therapy upon return to the facility. A progressive mobilization program will be initiated even if the resident is not allowed to ambulate. The physical therapist will begin with simple skills to increase the resident's independence. As the resident masters these skills, he or she will build upon them to become progressively more independent. An example of a progressive mobilization program is shown in **Table 6–1.**

■ AMPUTATION

Amputation of an extremity involves special resident care. Amputation is commonly done to treat trauma or gangrene **(Figure 6–15A** and **6–15B).** Residents with diabetes have a very high incidence of amputation. This is why you learned the importance of diabetic foot care in your nursing assistant class. Residents may complain of **phantom pain** after surgery. This is pain that seems to be present in the extremity that has been removed. The pain is real, not psychological, and is related to the nerves severed by the surgery. Many residents are fitted with a prosthesis following surgery.

Care of the Resident with an Amputation

A trapeze will be attached to the bed. Special positioning techniques will be used. Residents with amputations of the lower extremities are at high risk of developing flexion contractures of the hips and knee. To prevent flexion contractures:

■ Avoid placing pillows under the amputated extremity. Position the leg flat on the bed.

■ Avoid elevating the head of the bed for prolonged periods of time.

■ Keep the legs in a position of adduction. A trochanter roll is helpful. Avoid positioning the resident with pillows between the legs.

■ Assist the resident to lie in the prone position twice a day, if permitted.

■ Encourage and assist the resident to move in bed frequently.

You may be assigned to wrap the resident's stump with an elastic bandage. Wrapping reduces edema and shapes the limb for a prosthesis. The technique for wrapping the stump is shown in **Figure 6–16 (p. 93).**

Table 6–1   Example Progressive Mobility Program

Program Task	Purpose and Implementation of Task
Bed mobility	■ Increases ability to move independently in bed ■ Prevents skin breakdown, pneumonia, and other complications related to lack of movement ■ Teaches resident how to move and turn using side rails and overbed trapeze ■ Teaches resident principles of positioning and body alignment to prevent complications, deformity, and injury, as well as promote comfort
Transfer training	■ Teaches resident to transfer from bed to chair and back ■ Teaches resident how to transfer without weight bearing on affected leg ■ Teaches staff members how to assist resident using transfer belt and no weight bearing on affected leg
Strengthening	■ Increases arm strength in preparation for learning to walk with a walker ■ Increases strength in unaffected leg ■ Involves a series of exercises at the parallel bars and no weight bearing on affected leg; gait belt may be used to support resident during exercise
Ambulation with walker and no weight bearing	■ This step is not always used, but some programs teach the resident how to ambulate with a walker and no weight bearing on the affected leg to improve independence and ambulate short distances
Ambulation with walker and weight bearing	■ Weight bearing on affected leg begins at parallel bars ■ Resident initially begins to stand and balance at parallel bars ■ When resident can safely stand and balance, he or she is taught to walk holding parallel bars ■ Resident progresses to using walker, gait belt, and one assistant to walk short distances; distance is gradually increased
Progressive independence	■ If the resident is able, he or she will be taught to use a cane or to walk without assistive devices

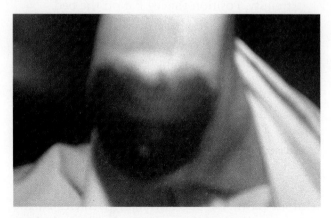

Figure 6–15A   This Caucasian resident has severe gangrene, which was treated by amputating the leg below the knee.

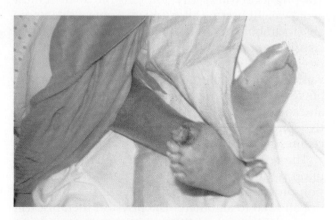

Figure 6–15B   This African American resident has gangrene of her great toe. The toe was amputated and the foot was saved.

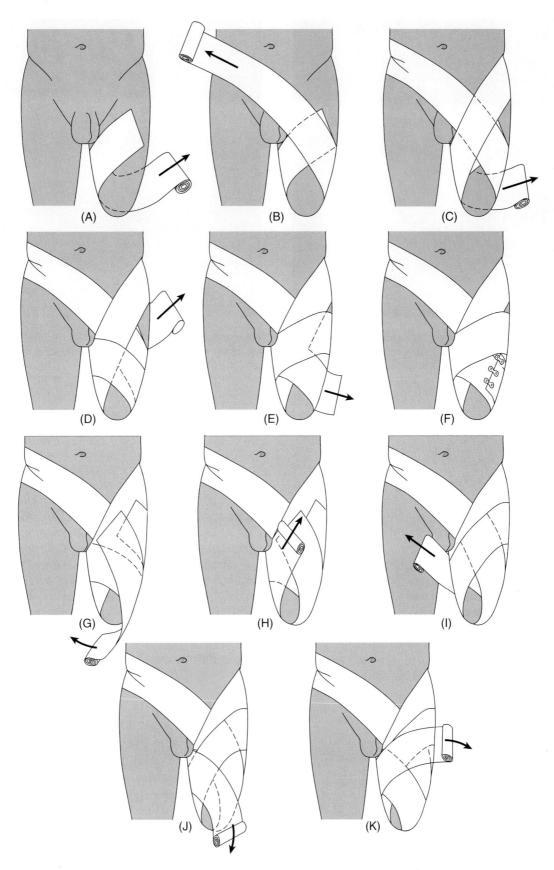

Figure 6–16 Wrapping the stump prevents edema and shapes the extremity for a prosthesis.

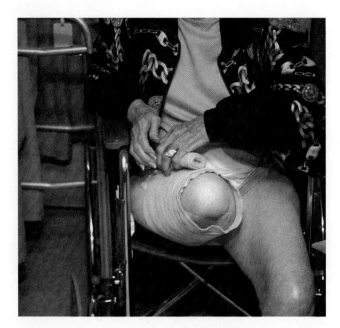

Figure 6–17A Whenever possible, residents are taught to wrap their stumps independently. This resident is wrapping her stump before applying the prosthesis.

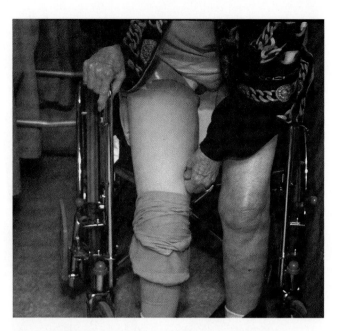

Figure 6–17B The resident applies the prosthesis and removes the bandage after the prosthesis is secured to her leg.

When caring for the resident with an amputation, check the stump daily for signs of redness, bleeding, irritation, or infection. Wash the area with a mild soap and pat it dry. Dry the stump well before wrapping it or applying a stump sock. Avoid applying lotion to the stump. Lotion softens the skin, making safe prosthesis use difficult. After the wound has healed completely, the resident will wear the prosthesis most of the time. Apply the prosthesis immediately upon rising to prevent edema. Whenever possible, residents are taught to wrap their own stumps **(Figure 6–17A)** and apply the prosthesis **(Figure 6–17B)**.

Wipe the inside of the prosthesis daily with a damp, soapy cloth to remove sweat and body oils. Rinse with a second damp cloth. Dry the inside of the socket well. Avoid placing a damp prosthesis on a resident. Never attempt to adjust the prosthesis. Consult your supervisor if you believe an adjustment is necessary.

The resident who has had a lower extremity amputation will participate in a progressive mobility program. This program is similar to the ones used for fractures and hip surgery. You will assist the resident to learn these new skills to restore independence and dignity.

▬ HEAT AND COLD TREATMENTS

Heat treatments (**thermotherapy** or **diathermy**) and cold treatments (**cryotherapy**) are commonly used to treat musculoskeletal conditions. Cold is applied after an injury. This may be changed to heat later. Many types of applications are used. Moist applications can be hot or cold. Water touches the skin during a moist application. Dry applications are those in which no water touches the skin. Some dry applications such as a hot water bottle, have water inside, but the outside of the application stays dry. Moist applications conduct heat or cold better than dry applications. Dry applications may be used to maintain the temperature of moist applications.

A **localized application** delivers heat or cold to a specific area. An ice bag to a sprained ankle is an example of this type of application. A **generalized application** delivers heat or cold to the entire body. A cooling bath or hypothermia blanket to reduce a fever is a generalized application. Heat **dilates** or enlarges blood vessels, bringing oxygen and nutrients to the area. This action relieves pain and speeds healing. Local cold applications relieve pain and prevent or relieve edema. Cold applications are also used to control bleeding. Cooling reduces the blood flow to the area and **constricts** blood vessels, making them smaller.

Principles of Using Heat and Cold Applications

㊐Follow your facility policies for using heat and cold. Some facilities do not allow unlicensed staff to perform these procedures.㊐ Localized heat and cold applications that contact the skin must be covered. This protects the skin from frostbite and burns. Covers are usually made of flannel. Pillowcases, towels, or a thin layer of foam are also used. If the device has a metal cap, face it away from the resident. The metal conducts heat or cold, which can injure the resident. When performing heat and cold treatments, assist the resident into a comfortable position. He or she must be able to maintain the position for the duration of the treatment. Expose only the part of the body that you will be treating.

Follow all safety rules to prevent spills and falls. If the resident has a dressing covering the area to be treated, consult your supervisor for directions. Apply the principles of standard precautions if your hands will contact blood, moist body fluids (except sweat), secretions, excretions, nonintact skin, or mucous membranes. Check the temperature of the solution with a thermometer. You may need to add more liquid during the treatment to maintain the temperature. Avoid pouring hot or cold liquid directly over the resident. For example, if you are performing a foot soak, remove the foot before heating the solution.

The elderly are very sensitive to heat and cold. Many residents have impaired sensation and fragile skin because of aging and disease. The skin in the elderly begins to burn at 115°F, on average, but in some residents this figure could be a little more or less. Check the skin under the application every 10 minutes, or according to facility policy. If the skin under a heat application appears red, or a dark area appears, stop the treatment. Notify your supervisor immediately. Stop a cold application and notify your supervisor if the resident's skin appears cyanotic, pale, white, or bright red, or if the resident is shivering. Cover the resident with a blanket.

Heat and cold applications are not left in place longer than 20 minutes, according to the purpose and type of treatment. When you are done, pat the skin dry. Make the resident comfortable. Clean and store used equipment. Remove gloves, if worn, and dispose of them according to facility policy. Wash your hands. Report to your supervisor that the procedure was completed and the resident's reaction.

Heat Treatments

Heat is used to relieve muscle spasms, pain, and inflammation. It may be ordered to increase drainage from an infected wound. Heat increases circulation and speeds healing. Heat can cause serious complications. It should not be used if bleeding or edema are present.

Hot Soaks. Administering hot soaks involves immersing part of the resident's body in water. The treatment should last no more than 20 minutes. The water temperature should not exceed 110° F.

Hot Compresses. Hot compresses are soaks used for treating small areas. Gauze sponges or washcloths are warmed in hot water and squeezed out. Fold the cloth and place it over the affected area. The com-

press cools quickly, so you must change it frequently. A hot water bottle or an aquathermia pad may be used to cover the application to keep it warm.

Heating Pads. The **aquathermia pad (Figure 6–18)** may also be called by the brand name K-Pad®, or Aquamatic K-Pad®. The plastic pad has coils on the inside. Distilled water circulates through the coils. The circulating water maintains a constant temperature. The pad is attached to a pump at the bedside. The temperature of the unit is preset between 95°F and 100°F. If you are responsible for setting the unit, you will adjust the temperature with a key. Remove the key before leaving so that the temperature cannot be changed. Like other heat applications, the plastic aquathermia pad should not contact the skin directly. Cover it with a pillowcase or flannel cover. Some facilities use two pillowcases to cover the pad. This provides extra protection against injury.

Hot Packs. Hot water bottles and chemical hot packs **(Figure 6–19)** are commonly used heat treatments in the long-term care facility. The temperature of the water inside the bottle should not exceed 110°F. The chemical hot pack is activated by squeezing or striking it. Always strike it away from your face, as leakage of chemicals can occur. The chemical hot pack feels very warm when you first activate it. Use caution when applying it to

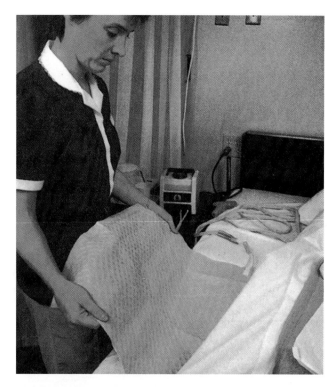

Figure 6–18 The aquathermia pad is a safe, effective heat treatment. Always cover the pad before using it. Make sure the key has been removed from the control box before leaving the room.

General Guidelines for Using Heat and Cold Applications

Before using a heat or cold application, you should know the:

- Type of application
- Area of the resident's body to be treated
- Length of time the application is to remain in place
- Proper temperature of the application
- Safety precautions to use
- Side effects to watch for

Other precautions:

- Remove all metal jewelry, buttons, or zippers that could conduct heat or cold, injuring the skin.
- Check residents frequently during the treatment.
- Always cover applications before using them.
- Avoid using heat treatments with temperatures over 110° F. Temperatures greater than this can cause burns in the elderly.
- Avoid using heat to treat the abdomen if appendicitis is suspected.
- Avoid using heat in the first 48 hours after an injury.

residents who have circulatory or neurological problems. Cover both the water bottle and chemical pack with fabric. The aquathermia pad is a safer, easier treatment that can be used in place of hot packs.

Moist Hot Packs. The **hydrocollator** is a rectangular tank containing very hot water. Hot packs are placed between dividers in the tank. You may be responsible for applying the hot packs to residents' skin. They are commonly used on the back and neck. Some facilities do not permit the restorative assistant to perform this procedure. Know and follow your facility policy.

The hot packs **(Figure 6–20)** are very hot to touch. Use tongs to remove them from the tank. Cover the pack with special, thick, terrycloth covers. The thick cover maintains a barrier between the pack and the resident's skin. The packs are applied

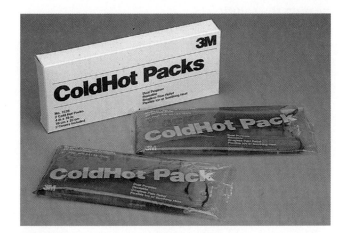

Figure 6–19 This gel pack can be used for heat or cold applications. It is disinfected and reused for the same resident. (Courtesy of Briggs Corporation, Des Moines, IA. (800) 247-2343)

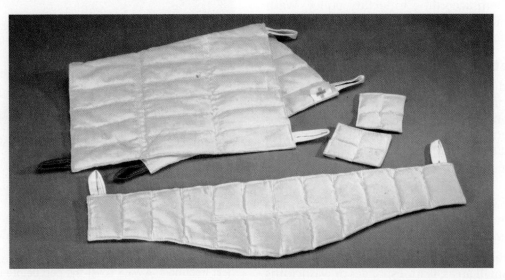

Figure 6–20 Select the hot pack that best conforms to the part of the body that you are treating. (Courtesy of Briggs Corporation, Des Moines, IA. (800) 247-2343)

for 20 minutes, or as ordered. Avoid placing the hot pack under the body, as it can cause serious burns.

After the treatment, remove the terrycloth cover. Place it in the soiled linen hamper so it can be washed before it is used again. The hot pack is returned to the hydroculator to reheat.

Paraffin Wax Bath. The paraffin wax bath **(Figure 6–21A)** is used for treating the hands. This is a common, comforting treatment for residents with arthritis and other joint diseases. Paraffin solution is mixed by adding 1 pint of mineral oil to 5 pounds of paraffin, or according to facility policy. The paraffin is heated to between 110°F and 120°F. (Temperatures may be as high as 130°F. However, most facilities use 110°F to prevent burns. Follow your facility policy.) Remove all rings and metal jewelry, to prevent conduction burns. Wash and dry the resident's hands before immersing them in the tank. Dip the hand in the wax, then remove it. The wax begins to harden immediately when removed from the tank. Dip the hand into the wax again, adding another layer. Repeat the procedure as directed, or until a thick coat of wax builds up **(Figure 6–21B)**. Remove the hand and wrap it in plastic wrap or towels to maintain warmth. The wax is left on for 30 minutes, or the designated length of time, then removed. Peel it off and discard it **(Figure 6–21C)**. The skin will feel soft, and the resident will have less pain. He or she will have more mobility in the joint for several hours. Paraffin may be used before exercising a resident. You may not be permitted to perform this procedure in some facilities. Know and follow your facility policy.

Ultrasound. **Ultrasound** uses high-frequency sound waves to treat pain and injuries **(Figure 6–22)**. This procedure reduces muscle spasms and speeds healing. You will not be permitted to perform this procedure. A licensed therapist will perform the procedure, but you may be asked to assist with positioning the resident. A conductive gel is applied to the skin before the treatment, which will last from 5 to 15 minutes. Following the treatment, remove the gel. Assist the resident to dress, if necessary. Follow your facility policy for cleansing the ultrasound unit.

Cold Applications

Cold treatments are used to relieve pain and edema and to reduce inflammation. Cold is also used to reduce bleeding and drainage. It is a common treatment in the first 48 hours after a musculoskeletal injury.

Ice Packs and Chemical Cold Packs. Ice and chemical cold packs **(Figure 6–23)** are the two most common types of cold treatments. An ice pack is made by filling a hot water bottle or ice collar one-half to three-quarters full with crushed ice.

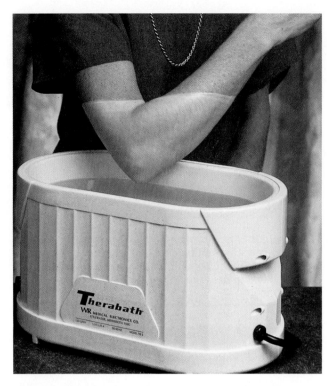

Figure 6–21A The paraffin bath is used for arthritic treatments of the hands. (Courtesy of Briggs Corporation, Des Moines, IA. (800) 247-2343)

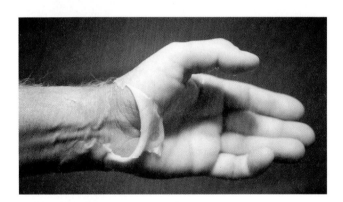

Figure 6–21B Dip the hand into the wax until a thick layer forms. Wrap it with plastic wrap and towels to maintain heat.

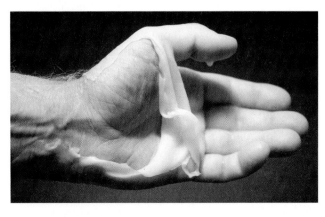

Figure 6–21C Peel the wax off the hand and discard it.

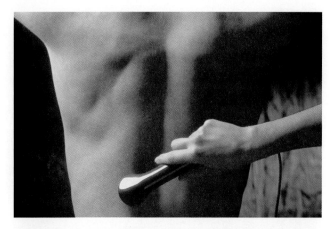

Figure 6–22 The ultrasound is applied only by a licensed therapist. The skin must be clear, with no rashes or open areas present. The restorative nursing assistant will assist with positioning the resident and cleaning the unit after the treatment.

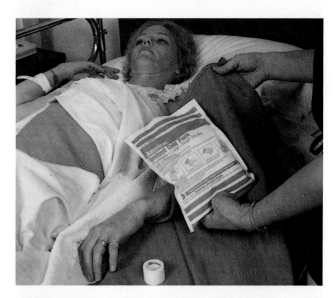

Figure 6–23 Cover the chemical cold pack before applying it to the resident's skin.

Avoid sharp edges. After filling the container, lay it flat on the counter. Press to remove the excess air. Activate the chemical pack by squeezing or striking it away from your face. Chemical packs are available in different sizes. The small packs do not stay cold for long, and may have to be replaced during the treatment. The larger packs stay cold for 20 to 30 minutes. Cover both types with fabric.

Cold Compresses and Soaks. Like heat, cold compresses are soaks used for treating small areas. Gauze sponges or washcloths are placed in a basin of ice and water, then squeezed out. Fold the cloth and place it over the affected area **(Figure 6–24).** The compress warms quickly, so you must change it frequently. An ice bag or chemical cold pack may be used to cover the application to keep it cool. Compresses are not used for more than 20 minutes.

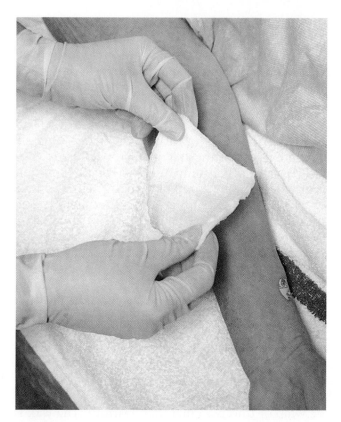

Figure 6–24 Wet the compress, wring out the excess water, and apply it to the area to be treated. Apply the principles of standard precautions if you are treating an open area.

 General Guidelines for Monitoring Hydrotherapy Equipment

- The temperature gauge should be within 2 degrees of the thermometer reading. Hot water in the tank should never exceed 105°F. Most tanks are set at 95°F to 97°F.
- The hydraulic lift is secured to the floor. Check the floor for hydraulic fluid or oil leaks.
- The bolts holding the seat to the lift should not be corroded.
- The seat belt should lock securely. Belts must be working and in good repair. Always lock the belt before lifting the resident to the tank.
- Check the sides of fiberglass tanks for cracks.
- Spray hoses must be crack-free. Hot water leaks can cause burns.
- The operating instructions should posted by the unit. SA

Hydrotherapy

Hydrotherapy is water therapy. You may be asked to perform range of motion exercises on some residents in the whirlpool. The warm, circulating water relieves pain and muscle spasms, making movement easier. This type of water therapy is called **hydromassage,** because of the massaging effect of the agitating water. Basins and small whirlpools may be used to perform hydrotherapy and hydromassage on extremities. Portable whirlpool units may be placed in the bathtub. Follow all safety precautions you learned in your nursing assistant class for bathing residents and using the whirlpool.

Hydrotherapy equipment has the potential to seriously injure residents if it malfunctions. Occasionally, the internal thermometer fails. The water comes out very hot. Always check the temperature with a thermometer. Test the water before moving the resident to the tank. The equipment should be checked weekly. Report problems to your maintenance department or appropriate person in your facility.

KEY POINTS IN CHAPTER

- *Arthritis is a chronic condition. It causes problems ranging from mild discomfort to severe disability. The most common forms are osteoarthritis, rheumatoid arthritis, and gouty arthritis.*

- *Osteoporosis is a metabolic disorder of the bones in which bone mass is lost. The condition causes the resident to be at very high risk for fracture.*

- *A fracture is a break in the continuity of a bone. It results from any condition in which more stress is placed on the bone than it can absorb. Muscles, tendons, ligaments, nerves, and blood vessels may also be injured in the area of the fracture.*

- *Fractures are classified by the type of break in the bone and whether the skin is broken.*

- *The pattern of a fracture describes the manner in which the bone is broken.*

- *Fractures are treated with casts, surgery, splints, clavicle straps, sling and swathe, and traction.*

- *Skin traction involves applying a halter or belt of foam rubber, a boot, or other device to the injured extremity and attaching a belt, ropes, and weights.*

- *Skeletal traction involves surgically placing a wire, pin, or tongs into or through the fractured bone, then attaching the metal to ropes and weights on the outside of the body.*

- *Hip fractures are the most common type of fractures in the elderly.*

- *The term hip fracture refers to a fracture anywhere in the upper third or head of the femur.*

- *Hip replacement surgery is done for residents with severe arthritic deterioration of the hip. It is sometimes performed after hip fracture. The hip replacement prosthesis is metal and plastic. It is fixed to the bone with special cement.*

- *Residents who have had hip fractures, hip replacement surgery, or amputations require special positioning to prevent deformity.*

- *One of the primary goals of restorative nursing care for residents with injuries of the musculoskeletal system is to prevent complications from immobility.*

- *Thermotherapy is treating an area with heat.*

- *Cryotherapy is treating an area with cold.*

- *Hydrotherapy is treating an area with water.*

- *Hydromassage is hydrotherapy performed in the whirlpool. The circulating water has a massaging action.*

- *The restorative assistant must take safety precautions when applying heat and cold applications.*

CLINICAL APPLICATIONS

1. You are assigned to apply hot packs to Mrs. Diaz's coccyx for low back pain. When you undress the resident, you notice a stage II pressure ulcer over the coccyx. What will you do?

2. Mr. Isaac was recently admitted to your long-term care facility. He has rheumatoid arthritis and his joints are deformed. The restorative nurse tells you that she will be evaluating this resident and writing a program to help maintain his independence. You notice that if the supplies, grooming articles, clothing, and other items Mr. Isaac needs are set up, he is able to perform self-care with bathing and dressing. Mr. Isaac is not able to put on his shoes without assistance. You notice that he is tired and must rest after performing his early morning ADLs. What information will you give the restorative nurse to help with her assessment? What suggestions do you have?

3. Mrs. Lyons has a long leg cast on her left leg. You notice an odor from the cast. The resident complains of a new pain in her ankle. Her toes appear edematous. What do you think is causing the problem? What action should you take?

4. Mr. Brown has difficulty walking and maintaining his balance. He is not able to stand for long periods of time. You notice that his oral hygiene is poor. The resident confides in you that he has difficulty standing at the sink to brush his teeth, so he has not brushed them lately. When he does stand at the sink, his legs are shaky and he bumps his teeth with the toothbrush. How is the problem with Mr. Brown's legs affecting his ADLs? Do you think that the problem affects other areas of his life? How can you assist this resident?

5. Mrs. Marshall had hip replacement surgery. You are assigned to assist her with learning independent bed mobility. When you enter her room, you notice that she has her legs slightly crossed at the ankles. You know that crossing the legs is contraindicated with hip replacement surgery. What will you teach Mrs. Marshall? Why?

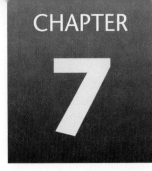

CHAPTER 7

Restorative Care of Residents with Common Neurological Conditions

COMMON NEUROLOGICAL PROBLEMS

Many residents in long-term care facilities are affected by neurological conditions. These conditions are severely disabling. They may affect both mental and physical function. The results are often not reversible. Neurological problems can affect the resident's ability to see, hear, touch, taste, and smell. Many neurological conditions affect movement and bowel and bladder control. Residents with neurological conditions need many restorative services.

CEREBROVASCULAR ACCIDENT

Cerebrovascular accident (CVA) is a common condition in the long-term care facility. A CVA may also be called a *stroke*. A newer term is *brain attack*. A CVA is caused by a sudden interruption of blood to the brain. This can be caused by a blood clot that blocks a small vessel. Sometimes a vessel bursts, causing blood to spill out into the brain cavity. Both conditions decrease blood supply and may cause permanent damage. CVA is the third leading cause of death in the United States. It strikes about 500,000 people annually. About half of these die. About half of those who survive develop a permanent disability. This group usually experiences a recurrence some time later in life. This could be days or weeks later; it could also be many years after the initial CVA. Risk factors for CVA are:

- hypertension
- diabetes
- high cholesterol and triglycerides
- lack of exercise
- cigarette smoking
- use of oral contraceptives
- family history of CVA

Signs and Symptoms

Signs and symptoms of a CVA vary. They depend on the area of the brain affected and the severity of damage **(Figure 7–1).** A CVA on the left side of the brain causes symptoms on the right side of the body. A CVA on the right side of the brain causes symptoms on the left side of the body. **Table 7–1** lists signs and symptoms of right- and left-sided CVA. Early signs and symptoms include drowsiness, dizziness, headache, and mental confusion. These may progress to seizures, vomiting, disorientation, mental impairment, and coma. One side of the body becomes weak or paralyzed. Paralysis on one side of the body is called **hemiplegia.** The paralysis may be temporary or permanent. The ability to speak or understand the spoken word may be affected, depending on the location of the attack in the brain. The resident may develop **hemianopsia,** or loss of half of a visual field **(Figure 7–2).** Other similar visual losses may also occur. Recognizing the effects of a CVA on vision is important.

Some residents lose the ability to differentiate right from left or up from down. This is called a **spatial-perceptual deficit.** Some residents show signs of **unilateral neglect.** In this condition, the resident ignores the affected side of the body. Stroke may also cause **emotional lability.** Residents

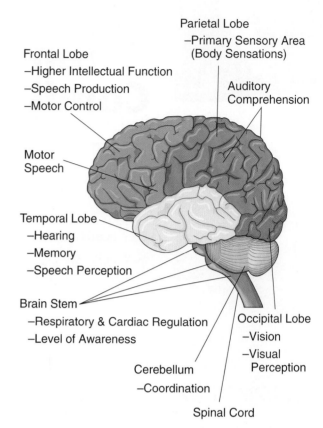

Figure 7–1 A brain attack or head injury in the areas of the brain shown will result in loss of ability.

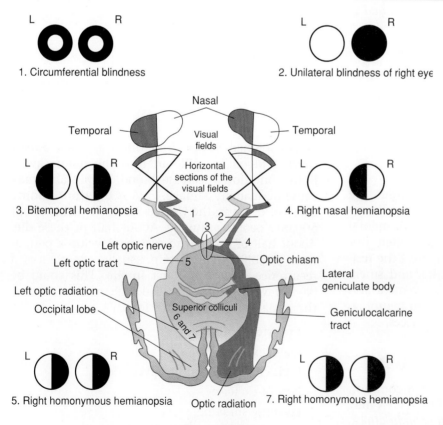

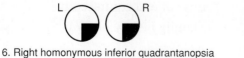

Figure 7–2 Remembering the names of the visual disturbances is not important, but understanding the effect they have on the eyes is.

Table 7–1 Comparison of CVA

Right Hemiplegia	Left Hemiplegia
Aphasia; impaired ability to understand directions	Little or no difficulty speaking
Labile emotions	Labile emotions
Incontinence	Incontinence
May ignore things on affected side (more common in left hemiplegics)	May ignore things on affected side
May have difficulty following directions due to poor comprehension or poor retention; more consistent in remembering after he or she has mastered a skill	Poor short-term memory
Behavioral style is slow and cautious; may be disorganized when encountering a new or unfamiliar situation	Poor judgment; behavioral style is quick and impulsive; may tend to overestimate abilities or appear unaware of deficits, resident is a high safety risk
Poor balance	Poor balance
Fatigues easily	Fatigues easily
	Spatial-perceptual deficits
	May have difficulty reading or adding a column of numbers because the resident cannot keep his/her place on a piece of paper

with this condition cry or laugh for no apparent reason. Emotional lability may also cause involuntary outbursts of anger. This is very embarrassing for the resident. He or she is aware of the behavior but cannot control it.

Aphasia is the loss of ability to speak or understand what is spoken. **Expressive aphasia** occurs when the resident cannot form or express thoughts. A resident with **receptive aphasia** does not understand the spoken word. Residents with **global aphasia** have lost all speech and language abilities.

Treatment

The resident is usually hospitalized for aggressive treatment as soon as the signs and symptoms of CVA are recognized **(Figure 7–3).** Some treatments will reverse the damage done by the CVA. However, the treatment must be given within the first 4 hours. Recognizing the condition and getting the resident to the hospital quickly is very important.

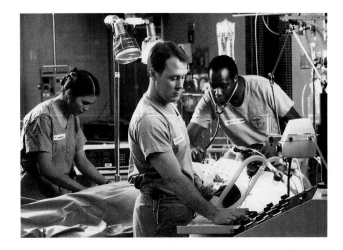

Figure 7–3 For the best outcome, the resident with a brain attack should be transported to the emergency department as soon as possible after the signs and symptoms are observed. Drugs to treat a stroke related to a blood clot must be administered within the first 4 hours to be effective. ("Be All You Can Be." Courtesy United States Government, as represented by the Secretary of the Army.)

Ⓢ︎ⒶRehabilitation and restorative nursing are started soon after admission or readmission to the facility. The resident will usually require the services of physical, occupational, and speech therapists. The goals of treatment are to:

- Maintain or improve the resident's condition
- Prevent deformities
- Restore as much self-care ability as possible

The goals of your care will be to prevent complications related to immobility and to restore self-care activities, such as ADLs and bowel and bladder control.Ⓢ︎Ⓐ Restoration of residents with CVA takes a long time. It is a great deal of work for the resident. **Table 7–2** lists approaches to use with residents who have hemiparesis.

Management of Specific Problems

Residents who have had a CVA on either side of the brain may have memory and behavior problems. These problems may interfere with the restorative program. Remember that these problems are beyond the resident's control. **Table 7–3** lists approaches to use with residents who are forgetful or who have behavior problems from a CVA.

Unilateral Neglect

When working with residents who show unilateral neglect, approach the resident from the affected side. Teach him or her to look at the affected side so he or she knows where it is. Periodically touch the extremity gently but firmly. Monitor the position of the affected extremities during transfers and ambulation to prevent injury.

Residents who have had a CVA often have an impaired sense of balance **(Figure 7–4).** Assist the resident to develop an awareness of good posture and balance. Use a transfer belt for transfers and ambulation. Position the resident in good alignment. Use pillows and props, if necessary.

Residents with hemiplegia may complain of pain in the affected arm and shoulder. This occurs because the force of gravity pulls it downward. Ⓢ︎ⒶAvoid pulling on the arm or shoulder during transfers.Ⓢ︎Ⓐ Pulling can cause **subluxation,** or dislocation. A sling may help support the arm. Other devices, such as a lap board or table, may also be used to provide support and relieve pressure on the shoulder joint.

Several restorative programs may be ordered for residents with CVA. Allow the resident to rest between treatments. Fatigue is a common problem. Increased **spasticity** in the affected extremities indicates that the resident is fatigued.

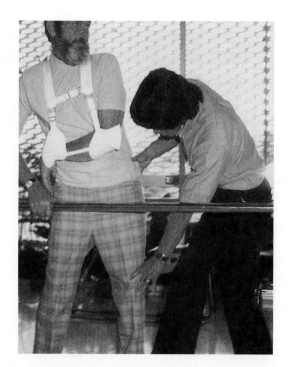

Figure 7–4 A stroke often causes a disturbance in balance. This resident with left hemiplegia is leaning to the right.

▇ PARKINSON'S DISEASE

Parkinson's disease (PD) is a neurological disease. Symptoms usually begin between the ages of 40 and 60. Occasionally they begin as early as the late teens or early twenties. About 1% of individuals over the age of 50 have the disease. Self-care in the home is difficult or impossible because the disease increases the risk of injury. Residents with Parkinson's disease have many restorative care needs.

Signs and Symptoms

In early stages of the disease, the individual is slow when completing ADLs. He or she has muscle stiffness, mild pain, tremors of the upper extremities, and difficulty walking. The disease is progressive and symptoms gradually worsen with age. As symptoms progress, voluntary movement becomes difficult. Pill-rolling develops in the fingers. In this condition, the fingers move involuntarily in a circular motion; it looks like the resident is rolling a pill between the thumb and fingers. The individual develops a stooped posture and shuffling gait. Falls are common. As the disease progresses, the resident develops a mask-like expression **(Figure 7–5, p. 107).** Speech becomes low-pitched and monotonous. The resident may have difficulty controlling oral secretions. Some individuals with Parkinson's disease develop dementia. The signs of the disease can be controlled to some degree with drug therapy. There is no known treatment for Parkinson's dementia.

Table 7–2 Approaches to Use in Restorative Care

Right Hemiparesis	Left Hemiparesis	Unilateral Neglect (More Common in Left Hemiplegia but Can Occur in Right)
Do not underestimate resident's ability to learn, despite the fact that he or she may have problems speaking and communicating.	Avoid overestimating resident's ability; spatial-perceptual deficits are easily overlooked.	Work on the unaffected side unless specifically directed to work with the neglected side.
Use pantomime and demonstrations if resident does not understand the spoken word; hand-over-hand technique may be effective.	Use demonstration and verbal cues.	Avoid making resident feel trapped or confined.
Avoid overloading resident with information. Keep messages and instructions brief, simple, and direct.	Break tasks into small segments.	Give frequent, orienting cues.
Avoid shouting; resident's ability to hear is not affected.	Give resident immediate feedback during each step of a task; do not wait until the entire task is completed.	Remind resident of the neglected side.
Divide tasks into many small . steps	Monitor resident for safety factors; know resident and avoid taking his or her word for what he or she can safely do.	Arrange environment so needed items are on the unaffected side.
Give resident immediate feedback during each step of a task; do not wait until the entire task is completed.	Avoid rapid body movements that startle resident.	
	Repeat procedures for learning often; use consistent methods for teaching resident.	
	Do not trust resident's yes and no answers; verify them.	
	Probably will need constant supervision and cuing when learning a new task.	
Keep comments positive; avoid giving negative feedback	Minimize clutter in the environment.	
Provide as much sensory stimulation as possible.	Use visual references to make your point.	

Table 7–3 Approaches to Use with Memory and Behavior Problems

Abusive language, inappropriate behavior	▦ Provide immediate feedback; waiting will dilute the effect. ▦ Remind the resident in a positive manner, that the behavior was inappropriate. ▦ Avoid angry, negative, punitive-sounding comments. ▦ Give prompt, positive feedback when the resident does something right or well. ▦ Work with the resident privately or in a small group; avoid large group settings.
Memory problems	▦ Establish a fixed schedule and routine and adhere to it as much as possible. ▦ Keep messages and directions brief and simple. ▦ Give directions one step at a time. ▦ Present new information one step at a time; get feedback from the resident before moving to the next step. ▦ Give frequent, positive feedback; the resident may have forgotten previous successes. ▦ Teach the resident new skills in the setting in which the information will be practiced. Although the resident may safely master a skill, he or she may be unable to perform it in a new location. ▦ Use memory aids such as written directions, memory cards, an appointment book, and pictures. ▦ Use familiar objects and old associations to teach new skills.
Emotional lability	▦ Interrupting inappropriate laughing or crying immediately may be very embarrassing; ignore inappropriate outbursts, change the subject, or leave the resident alone for a few minutes and return.

Treatment

Licensed nurses will administer medication to control the tremors. You will perform range of motion exercises several times each day. The muscular rigidity places the resident at high risk for contractures. The shuffling gait and stooped posture make walking difficult and unsafe. You may be assigned to ambulate the resident using a gait belt and walker. During ambulation, work with the resident to maintain good posture. Avoid flexion of the neck and shoulders by keeping the back straight and the head upright. Maintaining the ability to ambulate for as long as possible is important. Some therapists recommend that residents sleep on a firm mattress without a pillow. This decreases the risk of flexion contractures of the neck. Others recommend lying in the prone position several times a shift. This straightens the body as much as possible, reducing the risk of contractures.

The goal of restorative programs is to improve voluntary movement and decrease tremors that make ADLs difficult. The tremors are very embarrassing for some residents. You may work with residents on tasks such as grasping coins or other small objects in a pocket or sack, placing pegs in a board **(Figure 7–6),** or grasping the arms of a chair. These activities maintain range of motion. They help residents with functional tasks, while at the same time reducing tremors.

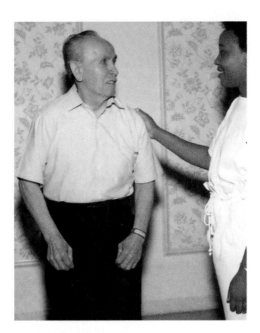

Figure 7–5 This resident with Parkinson's disease has a mask-like expression. His hands are flexed and are at risk of contractures.

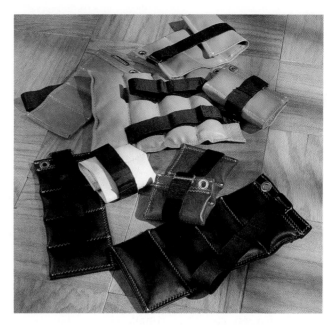

Figure 7–7A Many types of weights are available to encircle the arms and legs. (Courtesy of Sammons Preston)

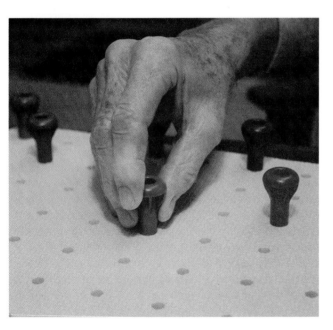

Figure 7–6 Inserting pegs into a board is an excellent activity for developing motor control of the small muscles in the hands.

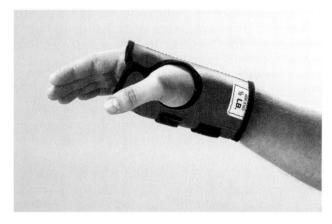

Figure 7–7B Special weights are available to conform to the shape of the hands. (Courtesy of Sammons Preston)

Some residents with Parkinson's disease have difficulty feeding themselves. The tremors may be so severe that the food spills before it gets to the mouth. In this situation, the therapist may evaluate the resident and establish a restorative program. Weights are often used to control the tremors **(Figure 7–7A).** Some therapists prescribe weights on the backs of the hands **(Figure 7–7B).** Others use weighted silverware. You will assist the resident to become proficient in eating using the weights or weighted utensils. Special cups with lids are also used to prevent spilling. Feeding the resident is not desirable, if it can be avoided. However, the resident's weight must be monitored closely. The tremors of Parkinson's consume extra calories. The resident is at very high risk for weight loss. This is because of the extra caloric need, combined with problems such as spilling. Residents are often given nutritional supplements or nourishing snacks to help maintain their weight.

Safety is a major consideration when caring for residents who have Parkinson's disease. The tremors cause them to be very slow with ADLs and movement. Some residents benefit from using assistive devices for ADLs. Allow adequate time for residents to complete tasks independently.

■■■ HUNTINGTON'S DISEASE

Huntington's disease (HD) is also called Huntington's chorea. This is a hereditary disease. In recent years, a genetic test has become available, to show if individuals with a family history of the disorder have the Huntington's gene. If the gene is present, development of the disease is inevitable. Some people with a family history choose not to be tested. They do not want to know if they will develop the condition.

Signs and Symptoms

Clinical signs of the disease usually begin when individuals are in their 40s or 50s. In some individuals, symptoms of the disease first appear in childhood or young adulthood. The disease is progressive and there is no cure. Disability and death occur within 15 to 20 years. Abnormal movements, called **chorea,** are the primary sign of Huntington's disease. The movements are subtle early in the course of the illness. The individual will appear anxious or restless. He or she appears to move frequently. Most people are aware of this movement. The resident may try to disguise the activity with voluntary movements, such as scratching the head or crossing the legs. As the disease progresses, rapid, jerking choreiform movements develop. These movements involve the entire body. The individual eventually loses voluntary control of all movement. He or she also loses control of the bowel and bladder. The involuntary movement increases with stress and attempts to control the choreiform motions.

Individuals who have Huntington's disease develop mental changes that progress to dementia. Early in the condition, the individual becomes nervous, suspicious of others, and irritable. Mood swings are common, as is depression. As the condition progresses, the individual develops dementia. He or she becomes totally dependent on others. The resident will develop difficulty swallowing and is at very high risk for choking.

Treatment

Residents who have Huntington's disease are commonly admitted to the long-term care facility because they cannot function safely at home. There is no known treatment or cure. Care is designed to keep the resident as independent as possible for as long as possible. The rapid movements consume many extra calories so the resident is at very high risk for weight loss. Extra nutrition and hydration will be ordered. Restorative nursing programs for residents with chorea usually involve ambulation with a gait belt. Some residents can walk independently by pushing an empty wheelchair.

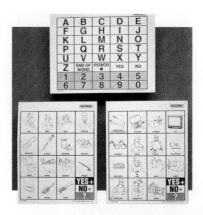

Figure 7–8   The Communicard trio is helpful for residents who are unable to speak. (Courtesy of Maddak, Inc.)

You may work with the resident on feeding, swallowing, and communication. These programs will be designed by licensed therapists. When residents with Huntington's disease are eating, they must sit completely upright to prevent choking. The speech therapist will teach you to remind the resident to tuck the chin. Keeping the chin down near the chest during swallowing prevents choking. Sometimes residents are taught to cough after each mouthful. This clears the throat of any remaining food. Mealtime should be stress-free. Allow extra time for the resident to eat. You may have to reheat the food. A mechanical soft or pureed diet or foods that are easy to swallow are served. Adaptive utensils may help the resident eat independently.

Poor muscular control makes communication difficult. The speech therapist will assess the resident and establish a communication program. The resident will be taught to use either hand signals, cards **(Figure 7–8),** or a communication board. Give the resident feedback when he or she speaks. Repeating what the resident says is a good way to show that the communication was successful.

■■■ MULTIPLE SCLEROSIS

Multiple sclerosis (MS) is another neurological disorder commonly seen in the long-term care facility **(Figure 7–9).** This progressive disease causes a degeneration of the nervous system that interferes with conduction of nerve impulses. The exact cause is not known. It is thought to be an **autoimmune disorder.** In this type of condition, the individual makes antibodies that work against his or her own body. Recent research suggests a virus may cause MS.

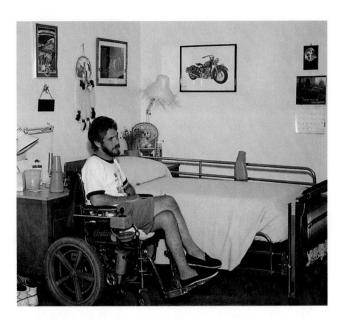

Figure 7–9 This young resident with multiple sclerosis has extensive paralysis and uses a motorized wheelchair to move about the facility. Using this chair allows the resident to move about freely.

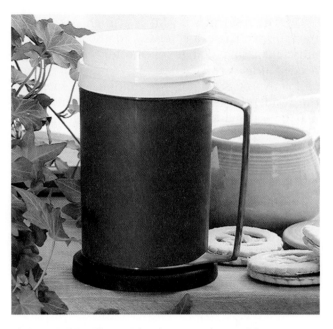

Figure 7–10 The weighted cup can be used for a number of conditions in which spilling is a problem. (Courtesy of Sammons Preston)

Signs and Symptoms

The signs and symptoms of MS vary widely. They include:

- Weakness
- Numbness and tingling in one or more extremities; eventual progression to complete loss of sensation
- Visual disturbances
- Poor coordination or incoordination
- Poor muscular control
- Paralysis
- Uncontrolled emotions
- Slow, scanning speech
- Short attention span
- Fatigue
- Incontinence
- Urinary retention

Residents who have MS often develop a **neurogenic bladder.** In this condition, the resident cannot feel the sensation of urine in the bladder. The bladder will become very full, retaining urine. The resident may have to be catheterized to relieve the problem. Some residents have seizures. Fatigue is common and often becomes worse as the day progresses. Involuntary muscle spasms and tremors occur. These interfere with motor control and self-care. Many individuals with MS also have symptoms of depression.

Multiple sclerosis is a condition in which there are exacerbations and remissions. During an exacerbation, signs and symptoms worsen. Stress, infection, and injury are risk factors for exacerbations. Some residents are relatively stable for long periods of time. Others deteriorate rapidly. They quickly become dependent on staff for care. Residents in remission appear stable and relatively symptom free.

Treatment

Preventive skin care is an important program for the resident with MS. Residents with this condition are at high risk for breakdown. MS causes impairment in the resident's sensation. He or she may not notice the discomfort of an early pressure ulcer. Pressure-relieving mattresses and other preventive devices are used routinely.

The restorative nurse will develop a bowel and bladder management program for the resident. Following the toileting schedule is very important. If the toileting program is not successful, the resident may be taught self-catheterization. If this is not possible, an indwelling catheter may be inserted. The goal of bowel and bladder management is to avoid the need for catheterization.

The restorative nurse or therapist will develop ADL programs for the resident. Consider the resident's fatigue when planning your schedule. Allow time for rest between activities. You may work with the resident with weights or weighted adaptive devices **(Figure 7–10).** This reduces tremors during feeding and self-care.

The resident with MS is at high risk of contractures. These are related to the involuntary muscle spasms. Range of motion exercises are needed at least twice a day. Active range of motion and active assistive range of motion will maintain the resident's strength. Splints and other devices may be ordered to keep the resident in good alignment and prevent contractures.

BRAIN DAMAGE

Some individuals are admitted to the long-term care facility because of head injuries. These usually result from trauma, falls, or automobile accidents. The injury often results in severe, permanent brain damage. Many young adults with this condition are admitted to long-term care facilities.

Signs and Symptoms

Signs and symptoms of brain damage vary widely. Most residents admitted to the nursing facility show signs and symptoms of severe damage. Residents are often dependent on staff for care. Although they may open their eyes, they seem unaware or are minimally aware of their surroundings. They are not able to follow commands, make decisions, or participate in their care. Loss of bowel and bladder control is common. The resident may be unable to speak or communicate. Paralysis of the extremities may be present. The resident is at high risk for injury. He or she may be unable to interpret dangers in the environment. The resident may also have impaired sensation. This increases the risk of skin breakdown.

Treatment

Treatment for the severely brain-injured resident involves preventive care. The goal of restorative care is to prevent complications. Skin breakdown and contractures are common. The restorative nurse will develop a skin care program. Pressure-relieving mattresses and other devices are used. Passive range of motion exercises are ordered at least twice a day to prevent deformities. Props, such as a footboard, are used to prevent contractures.

SPINAL CORD INJURIES

Some residents are admitted to the facility because of injuries or other conditions of the spinal cord that have resulted in **paralysis.** Paralysis affects sensation and voluntary movement below the level of injury **(Figure 7–11).** The most common cause is trauma. Conditions such as tumors, infection, cerebral palsy, **congenital disorders** (conditions present at birth), and neurological diseases can also cause paralysis. **Paraplegia** is paralysis of the lower half of the body, including both legs. **Quadriplegia** is paralysis affecting the arms and legs. **Flaccid** paralysis involves loss of muscle tone and absence of tendon reflexes. Some residents have **spastic** paralysis. These residents have no voluntary movement. The extremities move in an involuntary pattern, similar to muscle spasms. The resident is aware of the movements, but cannot stop them. The type of paralysis is determined by the level of injury. Residents with upper motor injuries are more likely to exhibit spastic paralysis.

Signs and Symptoms

Signs and symptoms of paralysis vary with the level of the injury. The resident will be paralyzed below the level of injury to the spinal cord. For example, an injury to the upper vertebrae in the neck will cause respiratory depression. The resident will be unable to move the arms and legs. He or she will lose bowel and bladder control. An injury near the waist will also cause loss of bowel and bladder control. The resident will be unable to move the legs.

Treatment

Treatment depends on the level of injury. Overall, treatment is directed at:

- Preventing complications of immobility
- Preventing deformities
- Restoring the resident to the highest degree of independence possible

Paralyzed residents will need range of motion exercises for the rest of their lives to prevent contractures.

When moving and positioning residents with paralysis, move the extremities slowly and gently. Rapid, rough movements will cause spasticity. If a resident's extremities move into a position of flexion, position them in extension. If the extremities move into a position of extension, position them in flexion. Positioning devices may be necessary to maintain position. However, attention to proper positioning is important. This is a major key to preventing contractures and deformities in these high-risk residents.

COMMUNICATION DISORDERS

Vision disorders have many causes. You learned the care of residents with vision and hearing impairment in your nursing assistant class. You will use these principles when giving restorative care, but they are not repeated here.

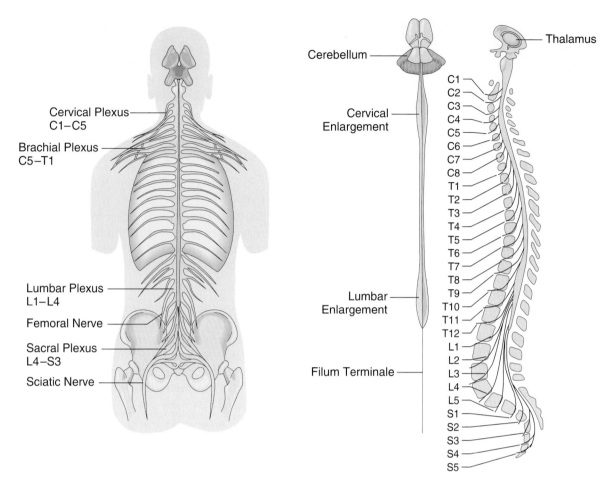

Figure 7–11   The type of paralysis is determined by the level of injury to the spinal cord.

Caring for Residents with an Artificial Eye

Some residents have had an eye removed. They may wear an artificial eye during the day. The eye is removed at night. You may be responsible for inserting and removing the eye. The socket is cleansed and irrigated. ⓈⒶIrrigation of the socket may be a licensed nursing procedure in your facility. Know and follow your facility policy.ⓈⒶ Apply the principles of standard precautions when caring for the artificial eye and mucous membranes in the eye socket.

Warm and Cold Eye Compresses

Many elderly residents have dry, itchy eyes. This may be caused by allergies, irritants, squinting, rubbing, or blinking the eyes. The eyes may appear red, with swollen eyelids. If residents rub or scratch their eyes, they may become infected. Residents with dry, itchy eyes may complain of:

▪ Burning
▪ Scratchy feeling
▪ Light sensitivity
▪ Difficulty moving eyes
▪ Excess mucus production
▪ Severe pain
▪ Blurred vision
▪ Seeing halos

Observe the resident for:

▪ Drainage from eyes
▪ Redness of eyelid rims
▪ Scaly, flaky skin around the eyes
▪ Edema of the eyelids

Report your observations to your supervisor. You may be instructed to apply warm or cool soaks to the eyelids. Apply the principles of standard precautions when performing this procedure. If an infection is suspected, use separate equipment for each eye. This will prevent the infection from spreading.

PROCEDURE

6 CARE OF AN ARTIFICIAL EYE

1. Perform your beginning procedure actions.
2. Assemble equipment:
   sterile gauze pads
   eye cup
   cotton balls
   small basin of warm water
   washcloth
   towel
   prescribed cleansing agent (if any)
   sterile water or normal saline
   disposable gloves
3. Position the resident for comfort. Cover the neck and shoulders with a bath towel.
4. Apply disposable gloves.
5. Instruct the resident to close his or her eyes and turn the side with the artificial eye toward you.
6. Dip a cotton ball in the water and cleanse the upper eyelid from the inner corner to the outer corner. Using a second cotton ball, cleanse the lower eyelid.
7. Remove the artificial eye:
   a. Press your thumb gently against the lower eye area to remove the eye. Simultaneously lift the upper lid with your finger. Cup your other hand to avoid dropping the eye.
   b. Some residents use a small suction cup to remove the eye. Gently hold the eye open with the fingers of one hand. Depress the suction cup between your thumb and index finger. Place the suction cup in the center of

the artificial eye. Release the pressure. Gently pull the eye from the socket.

8. Place the eye in the eyecup containing the prescribed solution.
9. Gently clean the eye socket in the same manner as you cleaned the outer eye. Avoid rubbing back and forth. Use a separate cotton ball for each stroke.
10. Pat the skin dry.
11. Cleanse the artificial eye, using only the prescribed solution. Never use alcohol, ether, or acetone to clean an artificial eye. These will damage the eye by dissolving or dulling the plastic. If not rinsed off well, they will injure the mucous membranes in the eye socket.
12. Store the artificial eye in sterile water or saline or the prescribed solution.
13. Perform your procedure completion actions.

To replace the artificial eye:

1. Perform your beginning procedure actions.
2. Apply disposable gloves.
3. Clean and rinse the artificial eye with the prescribed solution.
4. Gently open the upper eyelid while gently depressing the lower eyelid.
5. Slip the artificial eye under the upper lid.
6. Release the upper lid.
7. Draw the edge of the lower lid forward, covering the lower edge of the eye.
8. Perform your procedure completion actions.

Caring for Residents with Speech Disorders

Speech disorders have many causes. Residents who have had a CVA may have speech problems. The speech therapist will work with these residents initially. He or she will assist them to learn to speak or use other methods of communication. The therapist may develop a restorative program for the resident. A number of board games (**Figure 7–12**) are available for teaching communication, perception, reading, counting, color, and number recognition.

Playing the games is fun for the resident and serves many useful purposes.

The speech therapist or restorative nurse may suggest other methods of communication. If the resident can read, keep a notebook of simple words and phrases that the resident can point to. Make a notebook with pictures of common items that you have cut from magazines. Tell the resident to point to the item that he or she needs. For example, use a picture of a glass of water, a toilet, or pills. Sample pictures are shown in Appendix D.

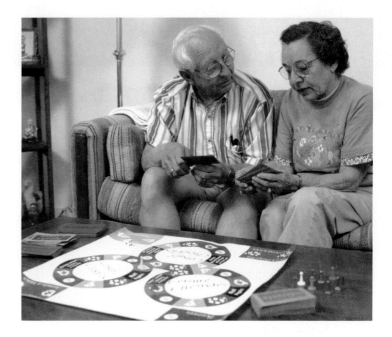

Figure 7–12 Board games are fun for the resident and help him learn communication, perception, reading, counting, color, and number recognition. As a bonus, the skills learned provide information the resident will need to return to living independently in the community. (Courtesy of Briggs Corporation, Des Moines, IA. (800) 247–2343)

PROCEDURE

7 WARM EYE COMPRESSES

1. Perform your beginning procedure actions.
2. Assemble equipment:
   towel
   small bottle of sterile saline solution
   small basin
   sterile gauze pads
   disposable gloves
   plastic bag
3. Position the resident for comfort. For warm compresses, assist the resident to a Fowler's or high Fowler's position, if possible. This position helps reduce edema. Cover the neck and shoulders with a bath towel.
4. Heat the bottle of sterile saline solution under hot running water, or place it in a second bowl of hot water. The solution should become warm, not hot. Check the temperature with a thermometer. It should be approximately 105°F.
5. Pour the heated solution into the small, sterile bowl.
6. Wash your hands.
7. Apply disposable gloves.
8. Place the gauze pads into the bowl.

9. Remove a gauze pad from the bowl, squeezing out the excess solution.
10. Instruct the resident to close his or her eyes.
11. Apply one compress to the affected eye.
12. Remove a second gauze pad from the bowl, squeezing out the excess solution.
13. Apply the second compress on top of the first.
14. Repeat with the other eye, as directed.
15. If the resident complains that the compress is too hot, remove it immediately.
16. Change the compresses every few minutes for the prescribed length of time. The treatment should not last longer than 15 to 20 minutes. Check the skin under the compress each time you change it for signs that the solution was too hot.
17. After 15 to 20 minutes, or as directed, remove the compresses. Discard in the plastic bag.
18. Use the remaining, clean gauze pads to dry the eye. Wipe from the inner corner to the outer corner. Use each gauze pad one time, then discard in bag.
19. Perform your procedure completion actions.

PROCEDURE

8   COOL EYE COMPRESSES

1. Perform your beginning procedure actions.
2. Assemble equipment:
   towel
   small bottle of sterile saline solution
   ice
   small basin
   sterile gauze pads
   disposable gloves
   plastic bag
3. Position the resident for comfort. The supine position is best for this procedure, as it reduces edema. Turn the resident's head slightly so the affected eye is up. Cover the neck and shoulders with a bath towel.
4. Place some ice chips into the small, sterile basin.
5. Pour the saline solution into the basin.
6. Wash your hands.
7. Apply disposable gloves.
8. Place the gauze pads into the bowl.
9. Remove a gauze pad from the bowl, squeezing out the excess solution.
10. Instruct the resident to close his or her eyes.
11. Apply one compress to the affected eye.
12. Remove a second gauze pad from the bowl, squeezing out the excess solution.
13. Apply the second compress on top of the first.
14. Repeat with the other eye, as directed.
15. If the resident complains that the compress is too cold, remove it immediately.
16. You may be directed to cover the compress with an ice pack. Make a small ice pack by placing ice chips in a sandwich bag or disposable glove. Squeeze the air out of the bag and tie the end. Keep the pack size small. Cover the cool compress with the ice pack, as directed. Remove it immediately if the resident complains of pain.
17. Change the compresses every few minutes for the prescribed length of time. The treatment should not last longer than 15 to 20 minutes. Check the skin under the compress each time you change it for signs that the solution was too cold. If an ice pack is used, it will be left in place for the duration of the treatment. Check the skin under the pack every 5 minutes for signs of injury.
18. After 15 to 20 minutes, or as directed, remove the compresses. Discard in the plastic bag.
19. Use the remaining, clean gauze pads to dry the eye. Wipe from the inner corner to the outer corner. Use each gauze pad once, then discard in bag.
20. Perform your procedure completion actions.

General Guidelines for Communicating with Residents with Aphasia and Other Speech Disorders

▪ Communicate in a quiet, relaxed, distraction-free environment. Residents with speech problems may speak very quietly and may be easily distracted.

▪ Treat the resident with intelligence. Show empathy and reinforce your understanding of the problem.

▪ Avoid treating or speaking to the resident like a child.

▪ Teach other staff members how to communicate with the resident during care.

▪ Try to learn if the resident understands what you are saying. Evaluate the resident's ability to respond by speaking, writing, or gestures. Some residents are taught to blink their eyes to communicate.

▪ Allow adequate time for the resident to process the information before responding.

(continues)

General Guidelines for Communicating with Residents with Aphasia and Other Speech Disorders, *continued*

- Listen carefully and concentrate on what the resident is saying.
- If you think you understand what the resident is saying, restate it in simple terms that the resident can acknowledge.
- Some speech problems are consistent. Look for patterns in speech that give clues to the meaning of words.
- Encourage the resident to use gestures.
- Provide paper and pen or magic slate if the resident can write.

- Ask simple, direct questions that do not require lengthy answers. Yes and no questions may be best.
- Encourage the resident to work on the communication problem. Avoid allowing the resident to become fatigued or frustrated.
- Be patient and persistent.
- Praise the resident. Express sincere approval for trying.

The speech therapist will design the restorative program. If the resident is in a skilled speech program, encourage him or her to use and practice new words. Remind the resident to use the tongue, lips, and facial movements he or she has learned. The resident may need frequent reminders. New movements and ways of forming words will not be automatic. Printed cards are used to remind the resident how to form words. The cards show mouth and facial movements. A mirror in the center of the card helps the resident practice **(Figure 7–13)**.

Speech therapy is directed toward helping the resident learn to communicate. Some residents will never be able to speak again. In this case, the therapist develops other methods of communication. Examples are communication cards, boards, or talking recording and electronic speaking devices. You will work with the resident to help him or her practice using these electronic methods of communication.

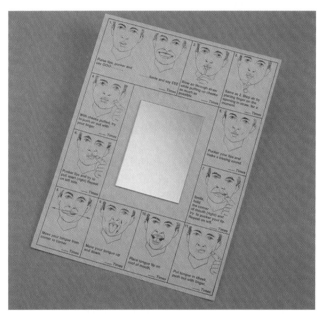

Figure 7–13 The facial images represent different mouth positions for speaking. Use the mirror in the center of the card when working with the resident. (Courtesy of Sammons Preston)

KEY POINTS IN CHAPTER

- *Cerebrovascular accident is caused by a sudden interruption of blood flow to the brain. This decreases blood supply and causes permanent damage. Most residents who have had a CVA will experience a recurrence some time later in life.*
- *Paralysis on one side of the body is called hemiplegia.*
- *Hemianopsia is loss of half of the visual field.*
- *Loss of ability to differentiate right from left, or up from down, is called spatial-perceptual deficit.*
- *Unilateral neglect is when the resident ignores the affected side of the body.*
- *Residents with CVA may have emotional lability, in which they cry or laugh for no apparent reason.*

(continues)

KEY POINTS IN CHAPTER *continued*

Aphasia is the loss of ability to speak or understand what is spoken.

Expressive aphasia occurs when the resident cannot form or express thoughts.

A resident with receptive aphasia does not understand what is spoken.

Residents with global aphasia have lost all speech and language abilities.

Parkinson's disease is a progressive neurological disease. It causes tremors, shuffling gait, stooped posture, and difficulty controlling secretions.

Huntington's disease is a genetic condition. Residents with this condition develop choreiform movements and dementia.

Residents with multiple sclerosis have remissions and exacerbations. The condition may remain stable for years, or the resident may deteriorate rapidly.

Paralysis affects sensation and voluntary movement of the area.

Paraplegia is paralysis of the lower half of the body, including both legs.

Quadriplegia is paralysis affecting the arms and legs.

Speech therapy is directed toward helping the resident learn to communicate. Some residents will never be able to speak, so other methods of communication will be used.

CLINICAL APPLICATIONS

1. Mr. Harvey is a 62-year-old resident who was admitted with a CVA and left hemiparesis. You will assist this resident with range of motion exercises. Mr. Harvey can move and use his right arm and leg. Does he need passive exercises on all four extremities? What do you think?

2. Mrs. Estes is a 34-year-old resident with multiple sclerosis. The condition began when she was in her early 20s. Her children are ages 7, 9, and 11. The resident misses and worries about her children. How can you assist Mrs. Estes?

3. Mr. Decicco is a resident with Huntington's disease. He is unable to participate in ADLs and requires total care. Is this resident a candidate for a restorative program? Why or why not?

4. Miss Stonaar was recently admitted with Parkinson's disease. She never married. She lived in her own home with a home health aide before admission. She has a strong desire to maintain her independence. The resident ambulates with assistance. She cannot bathe herself. She feeds herself, but spills much of her food. Is this resident a candidate for a restorative program? Why or why not? What do you suggest?

5. Mr. Davies is a paraplegic. You perform passive range of motion exercises on his legs twice each day. Each shift is assigned to perform passive range of motion as well. This week you notice that Mr. Davies's feet are showing signs of foot drop. Should you report this observation? Why or why not? If you think the condition should be reported, describe what you will say. What activity will help prevent this early condition from developing into a severe deformity?

Restorative Care of Residents with Integumentary System Disorders

OBJECTIVES

After reading this chapter, you should be able to:

Spell and define key terms.

Describe the structure and function of the skin system.

List nine changes to the integumentary system caused by aging.

Describe nursing measures to prevent pressure ulcers.

List the risk factors for pressure ulcer development.

Describe pressure ulcer staging, measurements, and documentation.

Describe the similarities and differences between three types of leg ulcers.

Describe nursing measures to prevent leg and foot ulcers.

State the purpose of the semisupine and semiprone positions.

THE INTEGUMENTARY SYSTEM

The integumentary system **(Figure 8–1),** or skin system, covers the body. Functions of the skin are to:

▪ Protect against infection
▪ Maintain fluid balance
▪ Excrete waste products
▪ Maintain temperature
▪ Provide sensations of touch, heat, cold, and pain

The skin consists of the outer layer, or **epidermis,** and a thicker, inner layer called the **dermis.** Beneath the dermis is a layer of **subcutaneous tissue,** or fat. The hair and nails are also part of the integumentary system. The skin joins with mucous membranes that line openings into body cavities. Some of these areas are covered with hair. The hair is a natural body defense that traps invading microbes, preventing them from entering.

Aging Changes

Aging changes to the integumentary system are more apparent than those to any other system of the body. Residents of long-term care facilities have many problems related to the skin system; the most common in long-term care facilities is pressure

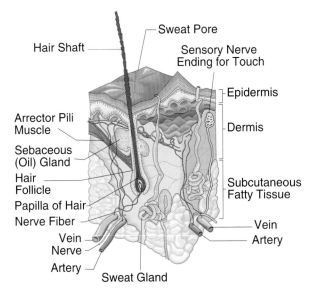

Figure 8–1 The skin protects against infection, maintains fluid balance, excretes waste products, maintains temperature, and provides sensations.

ulcers. Any condition that disrupts skin integrity increases the risk of infection. Complications of skin infections can be serious. You have many important responsibilities in caring for problems related to the skin system.

Several changes to the integumentary system occur with aging:

- The skin thins and loses elasticity. It becomes dry and wrinkles appear. Skin becomes irritated and breaks more easily.
- Blood vessels that nourish the skin become more fragile and break easily. This causes bruises, or **senile purpura (Figure 8–2),** and skin tears.
- Blood flow in vessels that nourish the skin is reduced, so injuries heal slowly.
- Oil glands that supply the skin secrete less, causing dry skin and itching.
- Perspiration decreases, reducing the ability to regulate temperature.
- Subcutaneous fat decreases. The loss of body fat may cause the resident to feel cold.
- Blood supply to the feet and legs is reduced. This increases the risk of ulcers.
- Fingernail and toenail growth slows. Nails become brittle.
- Hair thins and turns gray.

▬ PRESSURE ULCERS

You learned that one of the main purposes of moving and positioning residents is to prevent pressure ulcers. Pressure ulcers occur over bony

prominences. These are areas where the skin is close to an underlying bone **(Figure 8–3).** The pressure reduces the flow of blood and oxygen necessary to nourish the tissue. As the name implies, pressure ulcers are caused primarily by pressure. Moisture, powder, **friction, shearing,** chemicals, and other irritants also contribute to skin breakdown. Friction occurs when the skin rubs against another surface. Damage to the skin from friction is worsened by rapid movement. Shearing occurs when the skin is stretched. The skin moves in one direction while the underlying bone moves in the opposite direction. Friction and shearing may occur when staff pull the resident up in a bed or chair.

Pressure ulcers can develop on any area of the body if tubing or clothing constricts, presses, or rubs on the skin. They can develop rapidly, causing severe tissue destruction. Residents can develop pressure ulcers while lying in bed or sitting in a chair. Pressure ulcers are painful and heal slowly.

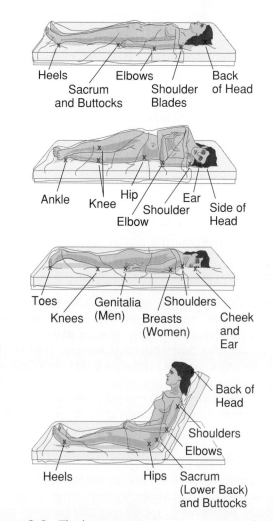

Figure 8–3 The bony prominences are areas in which skin is close to the underlying bone. These areas are at greatest risk of pressure ulcers.

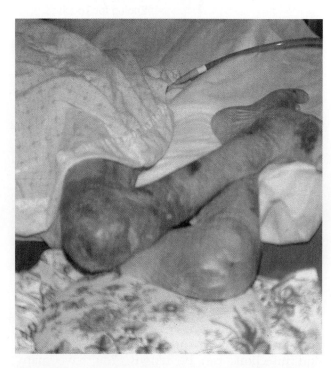

Figure 8–2 The skin in the elderly is fragile and breaks easily. This resident has arthritic deformities, contractures peripheral vascular disease, and senile purpura.

They are much easier to prevent than they are to treat. Ulcers may become infected, causing serious complications.

Ⓢ Detecting and treating a pressure ulcer in the early stages can prevent the ulcer from worsening. Residents with a history of healed ulcers are also at higher risk of developing additional ulcers. Residents with conditions such as incontinence, and certain diagnoses, are at high risk of developing pressure ulcers. Residents with CVA and neurologic conditions are in this category. If a resident is being treated for a pressure ulcer, assume that he or she is at very high risk. Residents with existing ulcers often develop additional ulcers at different sites on the body. The care plan will specify preventive care. Other conditions that increase the risk of pressure ulcers are listed in **Table 8–1**.Ⓢ Many facilities use a written risk assessment tool **(Figure 8–4)** to determine the degree of risk. You may be asked to help do the risk assessment. The care plan will reflect the resident's risk and preventive measures.

Stages of Pressure Ulcers

The Health Care Financing Administration (HCFA) defines **pressure ulcer** as an **ischemic** ulceration and/or **necrosis** of tissues overlying a bony prominence that has been subjected to pressure, friction, or shear. An *ischemic area* is one that has been deprived of blood flow and oxygen. *Necrosis* is tissue death. Necrotic tissue is black and leathery in appearance. Another name for necrotic tissue is **eschar.** A pressure ulcer cannot be staged if it is covered with eschar. Staging should be done after the eschar has been removed. Pressure ulcers are staged according to their severity.

■ Stage I pressure ulcers **(Figure 8–5A, p. 121)** begin as red areas. The redness does not go away within 30 minutes after pressure has been relieved. In a dark-skinned person, a stage I pressure sore begins as a dark blue or black area on the skin. The skin is not broken in a stage 1 area.

Table 8–1	**Clinical Conditions That Increase the Risk of Pressure Ulcer Development**	
Resident is **moribund,** or terminally ill, semicomatose, or comatose.	■ Life-sustaining measures have been withdrawn or discouraged	
Resident immobility and two or more of the following diagnoses:	■ Urinary incontinence ■ Chronic bowel incontinence ■ Severe peripheral vascular disease ■ Diabetes ■ Severe COPD ■ Hemiplegia ■ Paraplegia ■ Quadriplegia ■ Sepsis ■ Terminal cancer ■ Chronic or end-stage renal, liver, and/or heart disease ■ Disease or drug-related immunosuppression ■ Full body cast	
The resident receives two or more of the following treatments:	■ Steroid therapy ■ Radiation therapy ■ Chemotherapy ■ Renal dialysis ■ Head of bed elevated the majority of the day	

Malnutrition and dehydration, whether secondary to poor appetite or another disease process, place the resident at risk for poor healing. Clinical signs of malnutrition or dehydration are evident in the resident's laboratory values. Additionally, the resident's risk is increased if he or she has had a weight loss of 10% or more in the previous month.Ⓢ

BRADEN SCALE—For Predicting Pressure Sore Risk

HIGH RISK: Total Score ≤ 12 MODERATE RISK: Total score 13 - 14 LOW RISK: Total score 15 - 16 if under 75 years old OR 15 - 18 if over 75 years old.				DATE OF ASSESS. ➡	1	2	3	4
RISK FACTOR	**SCORE/DESCRIPTION**							
SENSORY PERCEPTION Ability to respond meaningfully to pressure-related discomfort	**1. COMPLETELY LIMITED**—Unresponsive (does not moan, flinch, or grasp) to painful stimuli, due to diminished level of consciousness or sedation, **OR** limited ability to feel pain over most of body surface.	**2. VERY LIMITED**—Responds only to painful stimuli. Cannot communicate discomfort except by moaning or restlessness, **OR** has a sensory impairment which limits the ability to feel pain or discomfort over ½ of body.	**3. SLIGHTLY LIMITED**—Responds to verbal commands but cannot always communicate discomfort or need to be turned, **OR** has some sensory impairment which limits ability to feel pain or discomfort in 1 or 2 extremities.	**4. NO IMPAIRMENT**—Responds to verbal commands. Has no sensory deficit which would limit ability to feel or voice pain or discomfort.				
MOISTURE Degree to which skin is exposed to moisture	**1. CONSTANTLY MOIST**—Skin is kept moist almost constantly by perspiration, urine, etc. Dampness is detected every time patient is moved or turned.	**2. OFTEN MOIST**—Skin is often but not always moist. Linen must be changed at least once a shift.	**3. OCCASIONALLY MOIST**—Skin is occasionally moist, requiring an extra linen change approximately once a day.	**4. RARELY MOIST**—Skin is usually dry; linen only requires changing at routine intervals.				
ACTIVITY Degree of physical activity	**1. BEDFAST**—Confined to bed.	**2. CHAIRFAST**—Ability to walk severely limited or nonexistent. Cannot bear own weight and/or must be assisted into chair or wheelchair.	**3. WALKS OCCASIONALLY**—Walks occasionally during day but for very short distances, with or without assistance. Spends majority of each shift in bed or chair.	**4. WALKS FREQUENTLY**—Walks outside the room at least twice a day and inside room at least once every 2 hours during waking hours.				
MOBILITY Ability to change and control body position	**1. COMPLETELY IMMOBILE**—Does not make even slight changes in body or extremity position without assistance.	**2. VERY LIMITED**—Makes occasional slight changes in body or extremity position but unable to make frequent or significant changes independently.	**3. SLIGHTLY LIMITED**—Makes frequent though slight changes in body or extremity position independently.	**4. NO LIMITATIONS**—Makes major and frequent changes in position without assistance.				
NUTRITION Usual food intake pattern ¹NPO: Nothing by mouth. ²IV: Intravenously. ³TPN: Total parenteral nutrition.	**1. VERY POOR**—Never eats a complete meal. Rarely eats more than 1/3 of any food offered. Eats 2 servings or less of protein (meat or dairy products) per day. Takes fluids poorly. Does not take a liquid dietary supplement, **OR** is NPO¹ and/or maintained on clear liquids or IV² for more than 5 days.	**2. PROBABLY INADEQUATE**—Rarely eats a complete meal and generally eats only about ½ of any food offered. Protein intake includes only 3 servings of meat or dairy products per day. Occasionally will take a dietary supplement, **OR** receives less than optimum amount of liquid diet or tube feeding.	**3. ADEQUATE**—Eats over half of most meals. Eats a total of 4 servings of protein (meat, dairy products) each day. Occasionally will refuse a meal, but will usually take a supplement if offered, **OR** is on a tube feeding or TPN³ regimen, which probably meets most of nutritional needs.	**4. EXCELLENT**—Eats most of every meal. Never refuses a meal. Usually eats a total of 4 or more servings of meat and dairy products. Occasionally eats between meals. Does not require supplementation.				
FRICTION AND SHEAR	**1. PROBLEM**—Requires moderate to maximum assistance in moving. Complete lifting without sliding against sheets is impossible. Frequently slides down in bed or chair, requiring frequent repositioning with maximum assistance. Spasticity, contractures, or agitation leads to almost constant friction.	**2. POTENTIAL PROBLEM**—Moves feebly or requires minimum assistance. During a move, skin probably slides to some extent against sheets, chair, restraints, or other devices. Maintains relatively good position in chair or bed most of the time but occasionally slides down.	**3. NO APPARENT PROBLEM**—Moves in bed and in chair independently and has sufficient muscle strength to lift up completely during move. Maintains good position in bed or chair at all times.					
TOTAL SCORE	Total score of 12 or less represents **HIGH RISK**							

ASSESS.	DATE	EVALUATOR SIGNATURE/TITLE	ASSESS.	DATE	EVALUATOR SIGNATURE/TITLE
1	/ /		3	/ /	
2	/ /		4	/ /	

NAME—Last, First, Middle   ATTENDING PHYSICIAN   ID NUMBER

BRIGGS, Des Moines, IA 50306 (800) 247-2343 PRINTED IN U.S.A.
Form 3166P

Source: Barbara Braden and Nancy Bergstrom
Copyright, 1988. Reprinted with permission.

BRADEN SCALE

Figure 8–4 The Braden scale is a research-based tool that is commonly used to predict the development of pressure ulcers. (Courtesy of Briggs Corporation, Des Moines, IA. (800) 247-2343)

- Stage II pressure ulcers **(Figure 8–5B)** are blistered or open areas. They may look like **abrasions,** or scrapes. Stage II ulcers are shallow. They involve part of the top layer of skin.
- Stage III pressure ulcers **(Figure 8–5C)** are areas in which the entire layer of skin is lost. The subcutaneous fat and muscle are exposed. These ulcers look like a deep crater.
- Stage IV pressure ulcers **(Figure 8–5D)** involve destruction of the entire top layer of skin. Damage extends through the fat into the muscle, tendon, and bone.

Tunneling or **undermining** may be present in stage III or stage IV ulcers. Some experts consider tunneling and undermining to be the same thing. They are similar, but not identical. Tunneling involves deep areas, or tunnels, that extend far back from the wound crater into the subcutaneous tissue. Undermining is also called *rimming.* It refers to

a loose area of skin forming a lip, rim, or edge surrounding the wound. In both cases, the skin overlying the area is intact. The tunnels or rim cannot be seen from the ulcer bed or skin surface.

Prevention of Pressure Ulcers

Ⓢ Keeping pressure off the skin over bony prominences is the most important way to prevent pressure sores. This is done by proper positioning, good padding, and frequent moving of residents. Some facilities use turn schedules **(Figure 8–6)** for residents who cannot reposition themselves. Good nutrition and hydration are important for keeping the body healthy and preventing breakdown. Ⓢ

Pressure ulcers are a leading cause of lawsuits against long-term care facilities. Prevention of pressure ulcers was part of your nursing assistant program. As a review, guidelines for prevention are listed in **Table 8–2.** You may have been taught to massage reddened skin areas and skin over bony prominences. This practice is outdated and is no

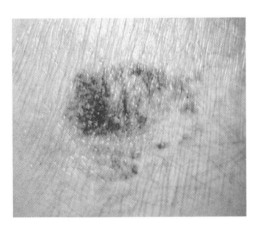

Figure 8–5A The stage I pressure ulcer is a red area that does not fade within 30 minutes after pressure is relieved. (Permission to reproduce this copyrighted material has been granted by the owner, Hollister Incorporated.)

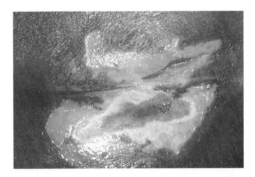

Figure 8–5C The stage III pressure ulcer has eroded through the subcutaneous fat and involves the underlying muscles and tendons. (Permission to reproduce this copyrighted material has been granted by the owner, Hollister Incorporated.)

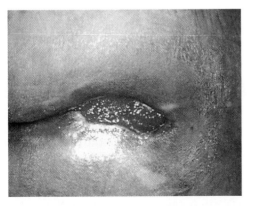

Figure 8–5B The stage II pressure ulcer presents as a blister, abrasion, or shallow crater. (Permission to reproduce this copyrighted material has been granted by the owner, Hollister Incorporated.)

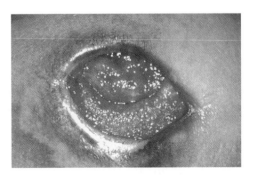

Figure 8–5D The stage IV pressure ulcer has eroded through the subcutaneous fat and involves the deeper structures of muscle, tendon, and bone. This extensive tissue damage is difficult to heal. (Permission to reproduce this copyrighted material has been granted by the owner, Hollister Incorporated.)

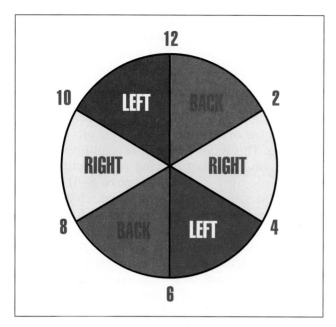

Figure 8–6 The turning clock is posted at the bedside to remind staff that the resident must be repositioned every 2 hours. (Courtesy of Briggs Corporation, Des Moines, IA. (800) 247-2343)

longer used. Research has shown that massage worsens damage to underlying tissue. Avoid massaging reddened areas and the skin over bony prominences!

You will be positioning residents with contractures, traction, fractures, and other complicated positioning needs. A ring that looks like a doughnut was a common positioning device at one time. Research has shown that doughnut-type devices increase pressure on the skin. They are no longer recommended. Licensed therapists may make recommendations for special positions and props to use for high-risk residents. Special devices **(Figure 8–7)** may be used for turning residents.

⑤ⓐPressure ulcers are declines under the OBRA regulations. The long-term care facility must prevent them. The facility is expected to provide care and treatment to heal the ulcers and prevent new areas from developing. If residents develop pressure sores while in the facility, surveyors will look for evidence that the ulcers were medically unavoidable. They will ask for proof that the facility provided aggressive preventive care. This is difficult to prove, even if the resident is at high risk. Surveyors view the high-risk conditions in Table 8–1 as "red flags" for the staff. If residents are at risk, staff are expected to take measures to prevent ulcers. Surveyors will review the MDS, care plan, flow sheets, and documentation of pressure ulcers. During a survey, they will observe staff caring for the ulcers.⑤ⓐ

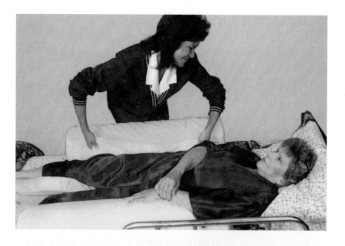

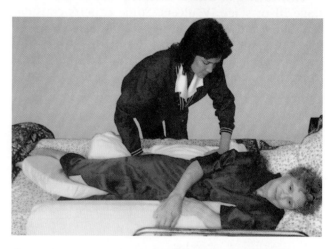

Figure 8–7 The turn aid system makes moving residents easier for the restorative nursing assistant and the resident. (Courtesy of Briggs Corporation, Des Moines, IA. (800) 247-2343)

Pressure Ulcer Documentation

The nursing assistant should check the skin daily for signs of red or open areas. ⑤ⓐHe or she must report problems to the charge nurse immediately.⑤ⓐ Licensed nurses in many facilities conduct weekly skin checks of all residents and document their findings. If a pressure ulcer develops, the nurse will document it and notify the physician immediately. The diameter and depth of the ulcer are measured with a disposable metric ruler **(Figure 8–8, p. 124)**. If the area is irregular in shape, the nurse will measure the length and width. He or she will stage the area and record information about the surrounding skin, skin temperature, odor, drainage, and necrosis. Thereafter, weekly measurements are taken. Many facilities also take photographs of pressure ulcers upon occurrence and periodically thereafter.⑤ⓐWhen taking pictures, staff must protect the resident's privacy. The wound is draped so that it is the only thing showing in the picture. Other areas of the anatomy must not be exposed and pho-

Table 8–2 Measures for Preventing Pressure Ulcers

■ Turn the resident at least every 2 hours, and more often if necessary. Follow the care plan and the resident's individual turning schedule.

■ Avoid positioning residents directly on the trochanter.

■ Encourage residents who are able to move to reposition themselves frequently in bed to relieve pressure.

■ Teach residents who are seated in chairs to shift their weight every 15 minutes, if physically able, to relieve pressure.

■ Residents who are sitting in chairs should also be moved and repositioned every hour.

■ Avoid elevating the head of the bed more than 45 degrees, to prevent shearing. If the head of the bed is elevated for any reason, assist the resident to change positions frequently to prevent pressure on the buttocks and hip area. A good rule to follow is to elevate the head of the bed as little and for as short a time as possible.

■ Place high-risk residents on pressure-relieving mattresses. Use pressure-relieving pads in the chair. Most of these devices are made of foam. Previously sheepskin mattresses were thought to relieve pressure. Research has shown that sheepskin prevents friction and shearing, but does not relieve pressure.

■ Avoid pressure on the heels by keeping them elevated or extending them over the end of the mattress.

■ Keep the skin clean and dry. Excessive moisture promotes skin breakdown.

■ Avoid massaging the skin over bony prominences.

■ Avoid massaging reddened areas.

■ Avoid using very hot water to bathe residents.

■ Use nonirritating soap to bathe residents.

■ Rinse the skin well after using soap. Soap residue promotes irritation and skin breakdown.

■ Avoid using powder and corn starch, which can be irritating to the skin.

■ If the resident is incontinent, wash the resident well with soap and water or a facility-approved cleansing agent after each incontinent episode. Rinse the skin well. Urine and feces are very irritating to the skin.

■ Use facility-approved moisturizing lotions on residents who have dry skin. Skin that is supple and well hydrated will not break as easily as dry skin.

■ Keep bed linens crumb- and wrinkle-free. The pressure from wrinkles and crumbs can cause skin breakdown.

■ Use lifting sheets to move residents in bed, whenever possible, to avoid friction and shearing.

■ Pad areas of the resident's body where the skin or bones rub together.

■ Use pillows, pads, and other props to maintain the resident's position.

■ Inspect the resident's skin daily for red or open areas. Report abnormal findings to the charge nurse.

■ Check the skin folds under the breasts, abdomen, and groin for signs of redness or irritation. Dry these areas well after bathing.

■ Follow the directions on the care plan for preventive skin care.

■ Provide adequate nutrition to meet the resident's calorie and protein needs. Provide adequate fluids. Provide oral nourishments, supplements, and snacks as ordered. Report to the charge nurse if the resident does not eat.

■ If the potential for improving a resident's mobility and activity exists, rehabilitation and restorative programs should be implemented. Maintaining mobility and activity should be the minimum goal for all residents.

■ All interventions and outcomes should be monitored and documented.

■ Wear gloves and apply the principles of standard precautions if contact with blood, body fluids (except sweat), secretions, excretions, mucous membranes, or nonintact skin is likely.

tographed. In fact, surveyors will note a resident rights deficiency if certain parts of the anatomy are exposed in photographs. They will also write deficiencies if an employee's ungloved hands are in the photograph next to the wound.

Measurements and photographs of wounds are objective. Information is not based on an individ-ual's opinion. Measurements are recorded on a flow sheet **(Figure 8–9, p. 125)** so progress can be tracked. Without this objective information, each nurse might describe the wound differently. One nurse will state that it is healing; another believes it is unchanged; yet another will say the wound is worsening. Measurements and photographs are

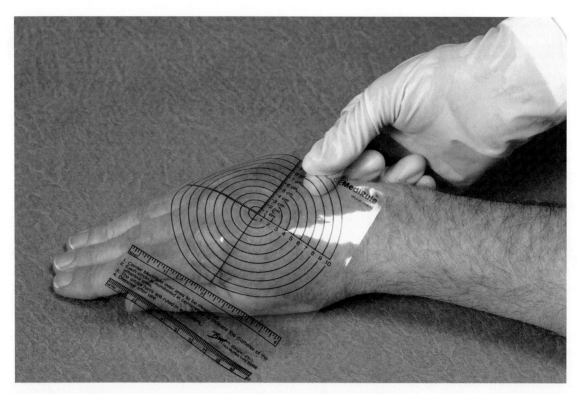

Figure 8–8 The flexible metric ruler is an accurate method of measuring pressure ulcers and skin wounds. The ruler is discarded in a biohazardous waste container after use. (Courtesy of Briggs Corporation, Des Moines, IA. (800) 247-2343)

essential to the wound management process. Measurements must be accurate. A camera that provides an instant photograph **(Figure 8–10, p. 126)** is used. By using this camera, you will know immediately if the quality of the picture is acceptable. The photograph supports written documentation and validates its accuracy. Some films have a grid covering the photograph area **(Figure 8–11, p. 126)**. Each square on the grid represents 1 centimeter (cm). The size of the wound is easily determined from the photograph. Sometimes the photos and measurements are used to support reimbursement. Measuring the wound and documenting weekly shows that the facility is monitoring the wound and taking appropriate action.

Pressure Ulcer Treatment

The nurse will contact the physician for a treatment order when a pressure ulcer is discovered. Because a pressure ulcer is a change in condition, the resident's responsible party is also notified. Many different treatments are used for healing pressure ulcers. If the ulcer is infected, the infection must be eliminated before the wound will heal. Treatment is selected by matching the properties of the product to the characteristics of the wound. Wounds heal best if a moist environment is maintained in the wound bed. The treatments should keep the edges of the wound dry while keeping the ulcer bed

moist. Some treatments are done several times each day. Others are done two or three times a week. The nurse evaluates the wound at each dressing change. If the wound is healing, the original treatment continues. If the wound does not heal, or worsens, the physician is contacted for a new treatment order.

Debridement. Wounds covered with eschar will not heal properly. To heal the ulcer, the eschar must be **debrided.** Debridement is a process of removing eschar. One way to do this is by using medications. These treatment products are very powerful. The debriding medication will be discontinued when the eschar is removed. A new treatment will be started. Continuing to treat the wound with the debriding agent will damage the skin further. Most superficial ulcers are treated using clean technique and standard precautions. Mechanical debridement is performed by removing the eschar with sterile instruments. Deep and infected wounds are also treated using sterile technique. You will be asked to set up the sterile dressing tray **(Figure 8–12, p. 126)** and assist with the procedure. Apply the principles of sterile technique as you learned them in Chapter 4.

Hydrotherapy. Pressure ulcers covered with eschar may also be treated by **hydrotherapy**, or whirlpool **(Figure 8–13, p. 126)**. The warm, circulating water loosens the tough, leathery tissue. Many types of whirlpool tubs are used in long-term

PRESSURE ULCER RECORD
(Reference tags: F157, F309, F311, F314, F441)

IDENTIFY SITE(S) BELOW BY DESIGNATING ALPHA CHARACTER A, B, C OR D	RISK FACTORS/CAUSE

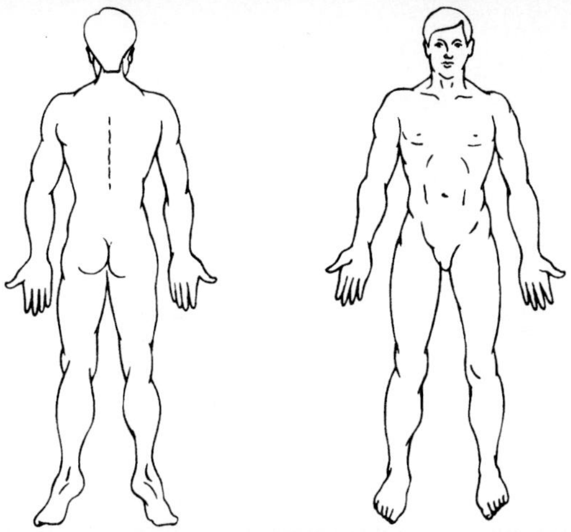

RISK FACTORS/CAUSE

☐ Diabetes ☐ Incontinence ☐ Paralysis ☐ Sepsis

☐ Peripheral vascular disease ☐ End stage disease

☐ Other_____

DESCRIPTION OF STAGES

STAGE 1: A persistent area of skin redness (without a break in the skin) that does not disappear when pressure is relieved.

STAGE 2: A partial thickness loss of skin layers that presents clinically as an abrasion, blister, or shallow crater.

STAGE 3: A full thickness of skin is lost, exposing the subcutaneous tissues—presents as a deep crater with or without undermining adjacent tissue.

STAGE 4: A full thickness of skin and subcutaneous tissue is lost, exposing muscle or bone.

SITE A	SITE B	SITE C	SITE D
Date First Observed _____	Date First Observed _____	Date First Observed _____	Date First Observed _____
Stage _____	Stage _____	Stage _____	Stage _____
Size _____ CM	Size _____ CM	Size _____ CM	Size _____ CM
Granulation _____	Granulation _____	Granulation _____	Granulation _____
Drainage _____	Drainage _____	Drainage _____	Drainage _____
Odor _____	Odor _____	Odor _____	Odor _____

If not a pressure ulcer, identify site(s) and describe: _____

DATE	SITE	STAGE	SIZE IN CM (WIDTH x LENGTH)	DEPTH	DRAINAGE	ODOR	COLOR	CULTURE SENT Yes/Date	No	RESPONSE TO TREATMENT	DATE NOTIFIED Dietary	Physician	NURSE'S SIGNATURE

NAME—Last _____ First _____ Middle _____ Attending Physician _____ Chart No. _____

CFS 6-5HH © 1992, 1995 Briggs Corporation, Des Moines, IA 50306 (800) 247-2343
R298 Printed in U.S.A.

PRESSURE ULCER RECORD
☐ Continued on Reverse

Figure 8–9 The pressure ulcer is staged and measured as soon as it is observed. After the initial measurements are taken, the area is measured weekly, or any time there is a significant change. The metric system is always used for measuring pressure ulcers. (Courtesy of Briggs Corporation, Des Moines, IA (800) 247-2343)

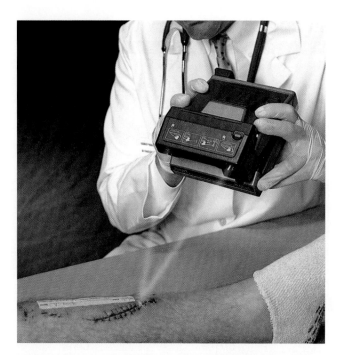

Figure 8–10 Most facilities use instant photographs for pressure ulcer pictures. The quality of the picture is known immediately. The picture becomes a part of the permanent legal record of the resident's care. (Courtesy of Briggs Corporation, Des Moines, IA. (800) 247-2343)

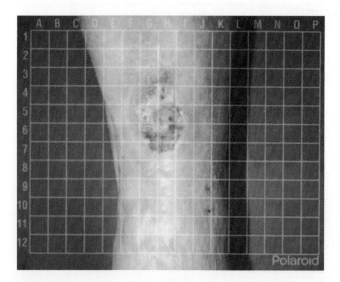

Figure 8–11 Each square in the grid is 1 cm., so one can look at the picture and determine the size of the ulcer. (Courtesy of Briggs Corporation, Des Moines, IA. (800) 247-2343)

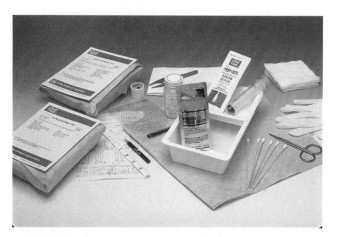

Figure 8–12 You may be responsible for setting up the wound tray and assisting with the dressing change. Apply the principles of standard precautions during this procedure. Bring a separate plastic trash bag to the room, for discarding dressings and other items that are disposed of as biohazardous waste. (Courtesy of Acme United Corporation (800) 243-9852)

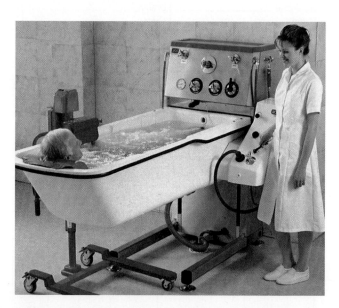

Figure 8–13 Previously, the whirlpool was used for treating most pressure ulcers. Research has shown that this can damage healing tissue, so whirlpool use is now reserved for ulcers with eschar that must be removed.

care facilities. Some facilities have more than one type. The procedure for giving a whirlpool varies with the type of tub being used. An overview of this procedure is given in Appendix E. Following the whirlpool, chemical or manual debridement may be done to remove more tissue.

Pressure ulcers are usually treated by nurses. However, therapists may treat complicated wounds. They perform mechanical debridement and some types of hydrotherapy. An overview of assisting with hydrotherapy and mechanical debridement was given in Chapter 4.

Measuring, photographing, and treating pressure ulcers often requires two caregivers. The restorative nurse completes the staging and treatment. You will assist by positioning the resident or photographing the wound. The nurse wears gloves to measure the wound. He or she cannot write down the measure-

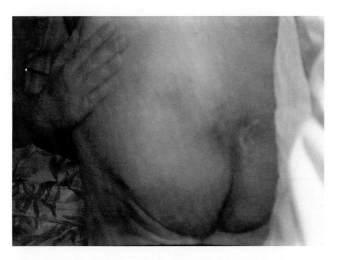

Figure 8–14 The crater of a pressure ulcer does not heal normally. The area becomes scar tissue, which is fragile, and subject to additional breakdown.

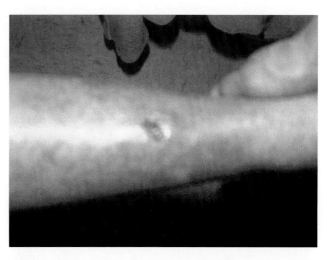

Figure 8–15 This resident has peripheral vascular disease, with a venous ulcer. The brown, rash-like skin and location of the ulcer are clues to the underlying cause.

ments while wearing gloves. You will record the measurements as the nurse calls them out. Apply the principles of standard precautions when assisting with wound care. Follow the principles of sterile technique in Chapter 4, and the nurse's or therapist's instructions.

Backstaging Pressure Ulcers

You have learned that nurses track wound healing and measure ulcers weekly. As the ulcer begins to heal, it decreases in size and depth. A properly healing wound heals from the bottom up. It seems logical for wounds to heal from a stage IV to a stage III, then to a stage II, and so forth, but this is not what happens. After an ulcer has developed, the underlying tissues and structures are permanently damaged. Although the surface of the ulcer eventually heals, the deep tissue damage persists. A healed pressure ulcer **(Figure 8–14)** consists of scar tissue. The tissue is fragile and is always at risk of further or renewed breakdown. Pressure ulcers do not heal like cuts. Healing pressure ulcers should be described as "healing stage IV, healing stage III," and so forth. Technically, they cannot be reverse-staged.

The inability to reverse-stage or backstage pressure ulcers presents an interesting dilemma for long-term care facilities, because of the reimbursement mechanisms and survey process. Some facilities backstage healing ulcers because they are required to do so by third-party payers and state surveyors. Although these facilities know better, they feel they have no other options. Some document each ulcer both ways. For example, they will chart a "healing stage III," and also "stage II" to describe the same ulcer. Know and follow your facility policies.

The National Pressure Ulcer Advisory Panel (NPUAP) is a group that studies pressure ulcers and

makes recommendations. This group has developed a tool to solve the problem of reverse-staging. The tool is called the Pressure Ulcer Scale for Healing (PUSH). The objective of PUSH is to assess the ulcer, then rate it with a score describing it. PUSH is an outcome tool that has been clinically tested. It is available through NPUAP.

■■■ LEG ULCERS

Ulcers of the lower legs **(Figure 8–15)** are often seen in long-term care facility residents. These leg ulcers are called *stasis ulcers*. They are common in residents with diabetes. **Neuropathy** is a painful condition of the nervous system. It affects the lower legs and predisposes residents to ulcers. Decreased blood flow to the area is also a common cause. Lower leg ulcers are not usually caused by pressure. They can be venous, arterial, or diabetic; 70% of all leg ulcers are venous. **Table 8–3** compares the three high-risk conditions and appearance of leg ulcers. The treatment is determined by the type of ulcer. Leg ulcers are difficult to treat. They heal very slowly because of reduced blood supply to the area. The same conditions that originally contributed to the formation of the ulcer also interfere with healing.

Caring for Residents with Leg Ulcers

You may be responsible for range of motion or ambulation programs for residents with leg ulcers or who are at risk of developing them. The resident's legs will be wrapped in Ace bandages or anti-embolism stockings **(Figure 8–16, p. 129).** These will be worn daily to improve circulation. The stockings keep the blood from pooling in the legs. You may perform range-of-motion exercises on residents with leg ulcers. Ankle flexion and calf muscle

Table 8–3 Leg Ulcer Comparison

Arterial Leg Ulcers	Diabetic Leg Ulcers	Venous Leg Ulcers
Causative or Predisposing Factors		
■ Diabetes mellitus ■ Advanced age ■ Peripheral vascular disease	■ Diabetes mellitus with peripheral neuropathy ■ Hyperglycemia	■ Inefficient valves in leg veins ■ Pooling of blood in ankle and foot ■ History of blood clots ■ History of leg ulcers ■ Obesity ■ Advanced age
Common Location of Ulcers		
■ Between toes or on tips of toes ■ Over the knuckle area of toes ■ Tip of heel ■ Ankle area ■ Over bony prominences ■ Any area subject to rubbing by clothing or shoes ■ Any area subjected to trauma	■ Under the heel ■ Over the knuckle area of toes ■ On the tips of toes ■ Between the toes ■ On the bottom (ball) of the foot	■ Ankle ■ Can occur anywhere on lower extremity, but pressure is greatest on the middle of the lower leg, so this is the most common location
Appearance and Characteristics of Lower Legs and Feet		
■ Skin dry, shiny, thin ■ Skin appears "tight" ■ Loss of hair on foot and ankle ■ Thick toenails ■ Lower legs pale when elevated ■ Lower legs red when down ■ Atrophy and loss of subcutaneous fat ■ Cyanosis ■ Coolness, decreased skin temperature ■ Absent or decreased pulses ■ Pain on walking; in later stages, pain at rest	■ Diminished or absent sensation in feet ■ Diminished or absent ability to feel temperature changes ■ Deformities of feet ■ Palpable pulses present ■ Skin warm to touch ■ Atrophy and loss of fatty tissue ■ Resident complains of "pins and needles" sensation ■ Pain may be relieved by ambulation	■ Edema, firm to touch ■ Pitting edema ■ Palpable pulses ■ Dilated veins visible on surface of skin ■ Dry, thin skin ■ History of healed ulcers ■ Area around wound highly colored or brown color in Caucasians ■ Rashes
Appearance of Ulcerated Area		
■ Wound margins regular and even ■ Necrotic tissue present ■ Gangrene possible; high risk ■ Wound bed pale in color ■ Skin surrounding wound purple or blanched ■ Severe pain, particularly when legs are elevated ■ Cellulitis, infection ■ Minimal drainage ■ Heals slowly	■ Wound margins regular and even ■ Wound bed deep ■ Cellulitis, infection ■ Resident may have **osteomyelitis,** a severe inflammation and infection of the bone ■ Small to moderate amount of drainage ■ Diminished or absent sensation in foot ■ Skin may be brown in color	■ Wound margins irregular ■ Ulcer is superficial ■ May be covered with yellow, moist tissue ■ Red-brown color skin surrounding the wound ■ Usually not painful ■ Moderate to heavy drainage ■ Dry, scaly, rash-like area surrounding wound ■ Resident may complain of intense itching

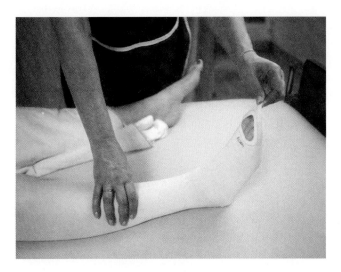

Figure 8–16 Anti-embolism hosiery may be ordered by the physician. Apply the hose before the resident gets out of bed in the morning. Make sure the seams are smooth and that the hose do not twist or bind. Check the resident's circulation in the toes frequently. Remove the hose every 8 hours for 20 minutes, or according to facility policy.

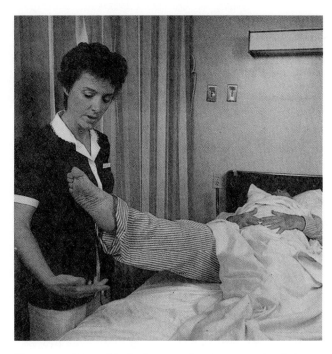

Figure 8–17 Ankle flexion exercises improve circulation.

contraction exercises **(Figure 8–17)** are particularly helpful. These exercises prevent blood clots and improve circulation. Apply the principles of standard precautions. You will be given specific directions for these exercises. Consult your supervisor if the resident complains of pain or if you feel that your treatment is causing the ulcer to worsen.

Preventive Care

Residents who are at risk for leg ulcers can be identified by the appearance of their lower legs. The legs may appear edematous, brown, red or blue, dry, and scaly (see Figure 8–15). Scar tissue from healed ulcers may be present. Keeping the feet and legs clean, dry, and free from injury is the most effective means of preventing ulcers. Drying well between the toes after bathing promotes good skin integrity. It also reduces the risk of infection. You may not be permitted to clip residents' toenails. This is because of the risk of clipping the skin. A small cut in the skin of the feet, or a crack between the toes, can easily become infected or ulcerate. Lower extremity injuries are difficult to heal. The rate of complications, including amputation, is great, particularly in residents with diabetes. The physician may order support hosiery or Ace bandages if the legs are edematous. Routine leg and foot care for residents at risk of leg ulcers includes:

▪ Applying a bed cradle to keep pressure from the linen off the feet and legs.

▪ Elevating the feet on pillows when in bed, or using heel protectors.

▪ Inspecting the feet and area between the toes daily. Report redness, irritation, open areas, injuries, or other problems.

▪ Washing and drying the feet well, particularly between the toes. Make sure no moisture remains. Moisture promotes fungal growth.

▪ Using moisturizer after bathing the feet to reduce cracking. Never put lotion between the toes. Pat moisturizer on the legs. Avoid massage, which can cause complications. If a blood clot is present, massage may dislodge it.

▪ Checking the inside of the resident's shoes daily before putting them on. Look for ridges, nails, torn, or irregular leather or fabric.

▪ Making certain that socks are clean, fit correctly, and are free from seams, holes, or mended holes. Pressure from seams and holes can cause ulceration.

▪ If the resident's risk is very high, change socks every two hours during the day. Change the shoes every five hours. Changing socks eliminates moisture. Changing shoes changes pressure patterns on the feet.

Teach the resident to:

▪ Wear socks if the feet are cold. Avoid placing the feet in hot water, or using hot water bottles or heating pads. Instruct residents to keep feet away from electric heaters.

▪ Avoid wearing roll garters or hosiery with elastic across the top of the leg.

- Buy shoes that fit comfortably and break them in gradually.
- Avoid wearing shoes without socks or stockings.
- Avoid adding insoles to shoes; they can cause complications.
- Avoid going barefoot.
- Avoid wearing sandals with thongs between the toes.
- Avoid using over-the-counter remedies for corns and calluses.
- Remind the resident to avoid standing for long periods and to rest frequently.
- Remind the resident not to sit or rest in bed with legs crossed; this inhibits circulation.
- Elevate the legs periodically; a footstool can be used, but elevating them above the level of the heart is best.
- The podiatrist will clip toenails and care for corns and calluses. Discourage residents from treating these areas themselves.

BASIC BODY POSITIONS

Four basic body positions are used for positioning residents in bed. These are the **supine** (face up) **(Figure 8–18A)**, **lateral** (side-lying) **(Figure 8–18B)**, **Fowler's** (semi-sitting) **(Figure 8–18C)**, and **prone** (lying on the abdomen) **(Figure 8–18D)** positions. ⓢⒶThe semiprone and semi-supine positions are variations of these positions. They are excellent for relieving pressure and preventing ulcers.ⓢⒶ The Fowler's position also has several variations, which are determined by the height of the head of the bed. Special positions may be used if the resident has special medical needs.

You learned basic resident positioning and how to use props for pressure relief in your nursing assistant class. That information is not repeated in this text. You have an important role in preventive skin care programs. Review your nursing assistant textbook for information on basic bed positions, moving residents in bed, props, and preventive skin care.

You may be teaching moving and positioning techniques to other nursing assistants. In the past few years, the semiprone and semisupine positions have been introduced. Encourage others to use these positions. They provide excellent pressure relief and are very comfortable. Because use of these positions is relatively new, the information may not have been presented in your class. Therefore, the procedures are described here.

The Semisupine Position

The **semisupine position (Figure 8–19A)** is also called the *tilt position*. Do not confuse it with the lat-

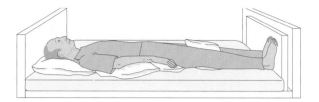

Figure 8–18A   The supine position

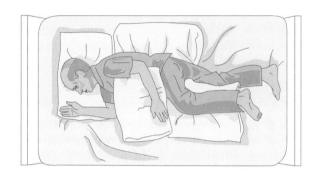

Figure 8–18B   The lateral position.

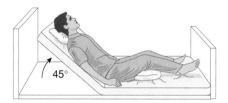

Figure 8–18C   Fowler's position is used for eating. Residents should not remain in this position for prolonged periods because the position increases the pressure on the hips, coccyx, and buttocks.

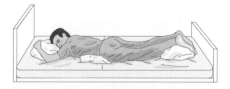

Figure 8–18D   The prone position

eral position. The resident in the lateral position is lying on the side. This increases pressure on the bony prominences of the ear, shoulder, elbow, hip, and ankle. The resident in the semisupine position is on his or her side, but is tilted at an angle. When used correctly, this position relieves pressure from all bony prominences. The spine is straight. The resident leans against a pillow for support. The legs are straight, with the top leg slightly behind the bottom leg. A pillow is placed under the top leg to keep it even with the hip joint. The lower shoulder is pulled forward. This causes pressure to be distributed across the back, not the shoulder joint. The arms can be at the sides or folded across the abdomen.

The Semiprone Position

The **semiprone position (Figure 8–19B)** is the opposite of the semisupine position. It is a very comfortable position for the resident. Like the semisupine position, it eliminates pressure on the bony prominences, reducing the risk of pressure ulcers. To place the resident in this position, begin by turning the resident prone. Lift the shoulder and chest on the side closest to you. Support them with a pillow. Position the opposite arm behind the resident. The legs and spine are straight. Fold a second pillow in half and place it under the top leg. Turn the resident's head to either side. Use a small pillow for comfort.

Follow your facility policy for using the semiprone position. Some facilities do not use the prone position without a physician's order. Check with your supervisor to see if this also applies to the semiprone position. Monitor a resident who is in the semiprone position every 15 minutes. Make sure that he or she is tolerating the position well and is not having difficulty breathing.

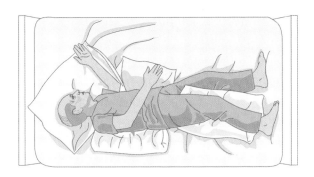

Figure 8–19A The semisupine position is a comfortable position that relieves pressure from the main bony prominences.

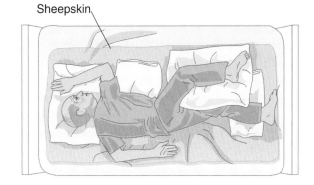

Sheepskin

Figure 8–19B The semiprone position is very comfortable. Check your facility policy to ensure that use of this position is permitted.

KEY POINTS IN CHAPTER

- *The skin protects against infection, maintains fluid balance, excretes waste products, maintains temperature, and provides sensations.*
- *The skin consists of three layers: the epidermis, dermis, and subcutaneous tissue or fat.*
- *The hair and nails are also part of the integumentary system.*
- *The most common skin problem in long-term care facilities is pressure ulcers.*
- *Pressure ulcers can develop on any area of the body, but are most common on skin over bony prominences.*
- *Pressure ulcers can develop when the resident is seated in a chair.*
- *Residents with existing or healed pressure ulcers are at high risk for new pressure ulcer development.*
- *Pressure ulcers are easier to prevent than they are to treat.*
- *Stage I pressure ulcers are red, intact areas. The redness does not go away within 30 minutes after pressure has been relieved.*
- *In a dark-skinned person, a stage I pressure ulcer begins as a dark blue or black area on the skin.*
- *Stage II pressure ulcers are blistered areas or shallow craters. They involve only the top layer of skin.*
- *Stage III pressure ulcers look like deep craters. They involve the entire skin surface. Subcutaneous fat and muscle are exposed.*
- *Stage IV pressure ulcers involve destruction of the entire top layer of skin. They extend through the fat into the muscle, tendon, and bone.*

(continues)

KEY POINTS IN CHAPTER *continued*

- *Tunneling or undermining are conditions that occur in stage III or stage IV ulcers. Tunnels extend far back from the wound crater into the subcutaneous tissue. Undermining is a loose area of skin forming a lip, rim, or edge surrounding the ulcer. The skin overlying both areas is intact. The tunnels or rim cannot be seen from the skin surface.*

- *Pressure sores are a leading cause of lawsuits against long-term care facilities.*

- *Massaging red areas and bony prominences destroys tissue under the surface.*

- *Pressure ulcers are declines in condition.*

- *Pressure ulcers are staged and measured each week. Photographs are taken at discovery and periodically thereafter.*

- *Pressure ulcers cannot be backstaged, because the skin fills with scar tissue. It does not return to its original condition.*

- *Three types of leg ulcers are venous ulcers, arterial ulcers, and diabetic ulcers.*

- *Foot and leg ulcers cause serious complications, including amputation.*

- *The most effective method of preventing lower extremity ulcers is preventing injury.*

- *The semisupine and semiprone positions are excellent for pressure relief.*

CLINICAL APPLICATIONS

1. Mrs. Perinello is a diabetic resident who was recently admitted to your facility. The resident tells you that she previously had an ulcer on her lower leg that took two years to heal. Should you report this information? Is this resident at risk of developing additional leg ulcers? List the general preventive measures for leg and foot ulcers.

2. Mr. Jones is a diabetic resident who had two toes amputated because of gangrene. Is he at risk of developing foot ulcers? List measures to take for residents who are at high risk of developing foot ulcers.

3. Mrs. Lieu is a 68–year-old resident in the late stage of Alzheimer's disease. She is incontinent and totally dependent on staff for care. Is Mrs. Lieu at risk for skin breakdown? List general nursing measures to prevent pressure ulcers.

4. Miss Rodriguez is a 33-year-old resident admitted to your facility with multiple sclerosis. She is within her ideal body weight range. She consumes an adequate amount of food and fluids. Her skin is in good condition, and she has never had a pressure ulcer. This resident has a neurogenic bladder. She cannot walk, and has muscle spasms in her legs. Is this resident at risk of skin breakdown? Why or why not? What measures will you take when caring for the resident's skin?

5. You are assisting the restorative nurse with the measurements and photographs of Mr. Swain's pressure ulcers. Mr. Swain has a large stage IV ulcer on the coccyx. He has a large stage III ulcer on the left hip. Explain how to drape the resident and take the pictures of the ulcers.

Consideration of Special Needs

After reading this chapter, you should be able to:

Spell and define key terms.

Demonstrate the use of restorative equipment used for contracture prevention and treatment.

Define adaptive device.

Explain how adaptive devices are used to promote independence and positive self-esteem.

Demonstrate the use of positioning aids to prevent skin breakdown, deformities, and complications.

Demonstrate correct application of an elasticized bandage.

Describe the restorative nursing assistant's responsibilities for the restraint reduction program.

▬ RESTORATIVE EQUIPMENT AND SUPPLIES

Providing restorative care requires very few special articles. Most of the equipment and supplies are found in the long-term care facility. If not, they can be easily obtained from suppliers. This chapter reviews some of the basic items that you will use when providing restorative care.

Restorative Equipment Used for Prevention and Treatment of Contractures

Restorative equipment is used for many residents to prevent contractures and deformities. These conditions can develop very quickly as a result of immobility. Immobility has a negative effect on the resident's quality of life. Follow the care plan. Use common sense in selecting, applying, and using restorative equipment. ⓢⒶYou will be responsible for placing and applying the equipment. Some items, such as splints, are worn according to a schedule. Other equipment, such as handrolls, is used at all times. Placing a device on a resident before a contracture develops will keep the muscles and tendons from shortening. A contracture will not occur. If the equipment is fastened to the resident's body, keep the skin clean and dry under the device. Restorative equipment is removed to perform range-of-motion exercises, then replaced. Follow the care plan and your facility policy.ⓈⒶ

Handrolls and Cones

Handrolls and cones are used to keep the fingers from contracting into a tight fist **(Figure 9–1).** Some devices can be fashioned from common items in the facility. However, using commercially manufactured handrolls is best. ⓈⒶFor many years health care workers used rolled washcloths in place of handrolls. Research has shown that the softness and texture of a rolled washcloth promotes squeezing. This

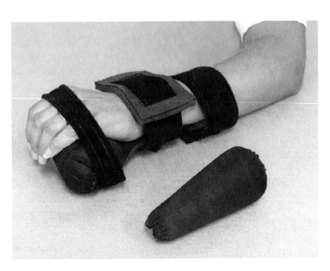

Figure 9–1 The NeuroFlex splint is an advanced form of contracture management that incorporates the new flex concept into contracture correction. (Courtesy of Restorative Medical, Inc. (800) 793-5544)

encourages contracture development. Handrolls should be used routinely in all dependent residents. A doctor's order is not necessary unless the resident has severe deformities or contractures of the hands. After the handroll is placed, support the wrist. The wrist should be in a neutral position to prevent wrist drop. This condition is another type of contracture.⑤

When selecting handrolls, check the size. The diameter should not be smaller than the surface area over which the hand can be stretched. The handroll should stretch the hand very slightly toward normal alignment.

Soft handrolls **(Figure 9–2A)** are very comfortable. They are commonly used in long-term care facilities. Most commercial varieties have a Velcro® strap attached that fastens across the back of the hand. Semirigid, cone-shaped handrolls **(Figure 9–2B)** are also used. Therapists recommend these

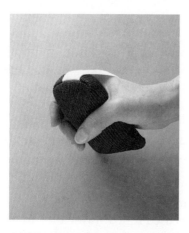

Figure 9–2A   The soft handroll is secured to the hand with a Velcro® fastener. (Courtesy of Skil-Care Corporation, Yonkers, NY (800) 431-2972)

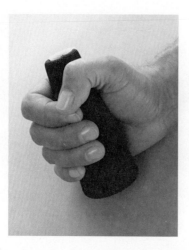

Figure 9–2B   The large part of the cone is positioned by the little finger. The cover is removable for washing. Avoid drying it in the dryer. (Courtesy of Skil-Care Corporation, Yonkers, NY (800) 431-2972)

for residents who have early contractures. They may also be used for residents whose fingers are very rigid. The cones are fastened to the hand with the large end by the little finger.

Keep the residents' fingernails short and clean. Residents with rigidity and contractures often keep the hand closed in a tight fist. ⑤Long, soiled fingernails increase the risk of injury and infection.⑤ Sometimes, two assistants must clip and clean the fingernails because the fingers are so rigid. One assistant positions the hand, while the other clips the nails. After the nails are clipped, file them with an emery board to remove sharp edges. Remove the handroll at least once each shift and wash the hand. Dry well before reapplying the splint. If the splint becomes soiled, follow manufacturers' directions for cleaning it. Most handrolls (or the removable covers) can be washed in the washing machine. Air drying prevents shrinkage in the dryer.

Avoid prying open a hand to clip fingernails. Massage the fingers and palms. Insert your index fingers on either side of the hand. Gently massage each joint. After massaging the inside and outside of the hand, gently extend the fingers. Stop at the point of resistance.

Splints

An *orthosis* is a device that maintains an extremity in a fixed position. Splints are orthoses used on the hands, arms, legs, and feet. Splints are sometimes used to stabilize fractures before casting. They may also be used in place of a cast. If a fractured extremity is very edematous, a splint may be applied. When the edema decreases, a cast will be applied. Some extremities, such as fractured **digits** (fingers and toes), cannot be casted. Splints are used to immobilize them during healing.

Many long-term care facility residents have orders for splints. Splints maintain good alignment and prevent and reverse early contractures. They maintain an extremity in a fixed position. The physical or occupational therapist may fabricate splints. He or she may also order splints from a medical supplier. The therapist orders or fashions the splint to meet a resident's specific medical needs. A variety of splints are available.

Static splints are stiff. They increase the risk of injury and are not used for residents with increased spasticity. **Dynamic splints** are flexible. They enable the resident to move the joint in flexion and extension. Dynamic splints are recommended for most immobility contractures. The care plan will describe the reason for the splint. It lists the instructions for applying and removing it. The care plan will also describe when the splint is to be worn. Do not remove splints used to immobilize broken bones.

Splints used to prevent or reverse contractures are worn according to a schedule. For example, the splint is usually worn during the day. It may be removed at mealtime and for ADLs. Removing the splint allows the resident to perform self-care. Keeping the extremity under the splint clean and dry is very important. The splint must be removed at least once each 24 hours for bathing. Check the skin under the splint for signs of redness, irritation, and breakdown. Report your observations to your supervisor. Splints may be padded to prevent irritation.

Footboards

SAFootboards are used to prevent foot drop.**SA** Foot drop **(Figure 9–3)** is a severe contracture. Once developed, is difficult or impossible to reverse without surgery. It occurs quickly in residents who are confined to bed. Foot drop is also common in residents with spinal cord and head injuries. The muscles in the foot point downward. They become stiff, rigid, and fixed in a position called **plantar flexion.** The resident with this contracture will be unable to stand normally on the foot because he or she is unable to place the heel flat on the floor. The position of the foot is similar to that of a woman in high heels. Residents with contractures of the feet and ankles are unable to walk.

Footboards **(Figure 9–4)** are positioned at the end of the mattress. The heels hang over the end of the mattress. This prevents pressure ulcers on the heels. The ball and sole of the foot are positioned flat against the footboard. This keeps the toes from pointing downward. Other commercial devices that fasten to the foot may be used instead of a footboard **(Figure 9–5).** Preventing contractures of the feet is an important responsibility. Bedfast, dependent residents should always have a footboard or other means of foot support to prevent deformities.

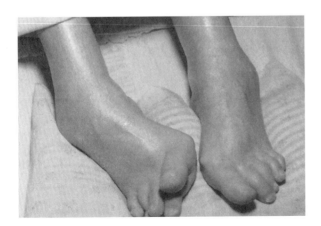

Figure 9–3 Foot drop is a severe contracture of the feet. This resident is unable to walk because of the deformities.

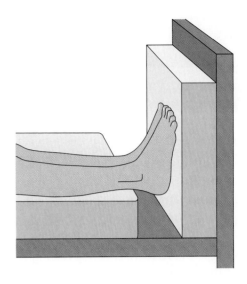

Figure 9–4 Bedfast residents are positioned so the heels hang over the end of the bed. The foot rests against the footboard to prevent flexion contractures. Some facilities apply high-top tennis shoes as an alternative to footboards.

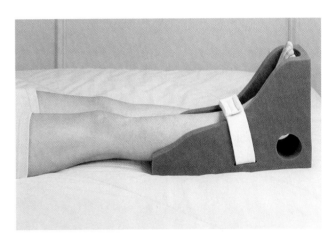

Figure 9–5 The foot drop orthosis may be used instead of the footboard. The heel area is padded to decrease pressure. (Courtesy of Sammons Preston)

Adaptive Devices

Adaptive devices are pieces of equipment used to assist residents to perform everyday tasks **(Figure 9–6A and 9–6B).** The devices change the way the task is done. This enables the resident to perform ADLs independently. Using adaptive devices improves self-esteem. The resident can complete the task according to his or her own schedule, not someone else's.

Sometimes adaptive devices are simple things that can be made by staff. For example, a resident with right-side hemiparesis cannot use a remote control with his right hand. Fasten a strip of Velcro® to the remote control. Fasten an opposite-side strip to the left side rail and the left arm of the chair. Place the remote control on the Velcro so it is close

PROCEDURE

9 APPLYING A FOOTBOARD

1. Perform your beginning procedure actions.
2. Gather equipment:
   footboard
   linen as necessary
   padding for footboard (bath blanket, sheepskin, foam), if necessary
3. Expose the resident's feet by folding the linen at the foot of the bed back.
4. Pad the footboard, if necessary, so the resident's feet are not touching a wooden surface.

5. Place the footboard at the foot of the bed, securing it according to the type of board you are using.
6. Position the resident so the feet are flat against the board.
7. Elevate the resident's heels from the surface of the bed by elevating them on a pillow, or hang them over the end of the mattress, depending on the type of footboard used.
8. Cover the footboard with the bed linen.
9. Perform your procedure completion actions.

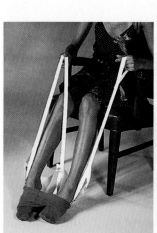
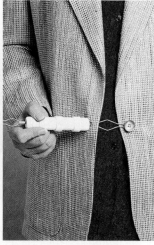

Figure 9–6A and 9–6B Adaptive devices give the resident the ability to perform tasks independently by changing the way that they are done. (Courtesy of Maddak, Inc.)

to the resident. This enables him or her to use the control without calling for help.

Adaptive devices are ordered by the occupational therapist or restorative nurse. The device ordered is based on an evaluation of the resident's needs. The resident is taught how to use the device for everyday tasks. Your role as a restorative assistant is to make sure the device is clean, available, and used by the resident. When the resident is learning to use it, provide support and encouragement.

When an adaptive device is first introduced, licensed personnel may work with the resident to teach him or her how to use the device correctly.

However, learning to use a device correctly takes time. You will continue working with the resident until he or she masters the task. The care plan will provide instructions. Report to your supervisor if a resident experiences a problem. If you feel that a modification or change to another device is appropriate, report this information to your supervisor.

Adaptive Devices for Eating

The adaptive devices most commonly used are those that enable residents to feed themselves. Feeding oneself promotes dignity and self-esteem. Residents who feed themselves usually eat better than when they are spoon-fed. Independent eating helps prevent weight loss, which is a common problem in long-term care facility residents.

Many types of adaptive devices are available to meet residents' needs. Adaptive silverware is commonly used **(Figure 9–7A).** Utensils that swivel are useful for residents whose food falls off the utensil because of tremors or weakness. Resting the resident's elbow on a piece of gripper, foam, or the table helps decrease tremors.

Residents who have difficulty grasping silverware will benefit from utensils with built-up handles. These can be commercially purchased or made with common materials. Bicycle handle grips or foam pipe wrapping can be used to enlarge the handle. ⑤ If you will be making a device, make sure it can be washed and sanitized.⑤ Some residents are unable to grasp silverware at all. These individuals will benefit from utensils with a Velcro® cuff that wraps around the hand. Use hand-over-hand technique to assist the resident to learn to use the utensils.

Some residents push food off the plate when trying to scoop the food onto a utensil. Plates with built-up edges **(Figure 9–7B)** and plate guards are useful. The resident can also use one hand to hold a piece of bread on the plate. He or she will be taught to push the food against it. Adaptive cups **(Figure 9–7C)** are used for residents who cannot hold a cup without dropping it. They can also be used for residents who drip or spill when drinking from a regular cup. Other items, such as a straw holder **(Figure 9–7D),** may also be used. If a commercial straw holder is not available, taping the straw to the inside of the glass may work. Residents who have had a CVA may scoop their food away from their bodies. This causes the plate to slide toward the center of the table. Placing a piece of gripper, Dycem **(Figure 9–7E),** or a damp washcloth, paper towel, or napkin under the plate solves the sliding problem.

You will help residents learn to use adaptive devices at each meal. Prompting, verbal cues, and hand-over-hand technique may be necessary to help residents learn to use adaptive devices. Over time, the resident will learn to use the device independently. Learning takes patience and practice.

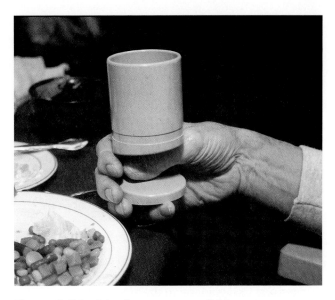

Figure 9–7C Adaptive cups are available to meet many individual needs.

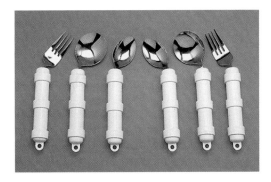

Figure 9–7A Many types of adaptive silverware are available to meet the individual needs of the resident. (Courtesy of Maddak, Inc.)

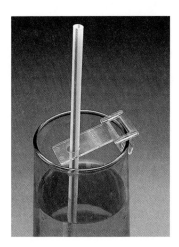

Figure 9–7D This device positions the straw securely. (Courtesy of Maddak, Inc.)

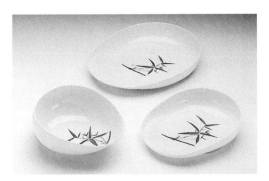

Figure 9–7B The resident scoops the food against the edge of the plate without spilling. (Courtesy of Maddak, Inc.)

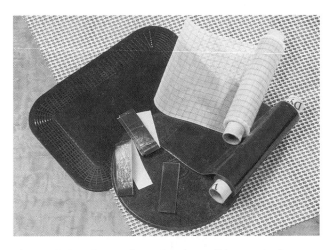

Figure 9–7E Dycem is used to keep dishes and other items from sliding. (Courtesy of Sammons Preston)

Adaptive Devices for Grooming and Hygiene

Being able to bathe and groom oneself are important skills. Everyone has a personal hygienic routine. Grooming and hygiene are very private activities. Adaptive devices enable residents to perform these skills independently. This increases self-esteem and personal comfort. You will work with residents during ADLs to help them become comfortable using the devices. Verbal cues, encouragement, demonstrations, and hand-over-hand technique may be used to help residents learn to use the items correctly.

Adaptive Devices for Dressing

Dressing aids **(Figure 9–8)** are also commonly used. These devices make it easier for residents to dress themselves. Using adaptive dressing aids may appear awkward to you. For the resident, being able to dress independently is important. Like personal hygiene, dressing is a private and personal activity for most people. Learning to use dressing devices may take considerable practice. At first they may seem unnatural to the resident. Over time, however, the resident will appreciate the devices because they allow him or her to dress independently. You will work with the residents daily while they are learning to use the devices. Verbal cues and demonstrations may be necessary. Avoid providing more assistance than the resident needs, even if the procedure is time-consuming.

▧ POSITIONING AIDS

Positioning aids are used for residents with many conditions. Keeping the body in good alignment:

- ▧ Improves oxygenation
- ▧ Prevents deformities

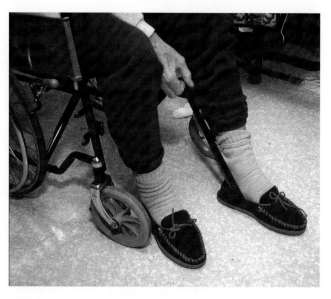

Figure 9–8 Dressing can be a difficult task for some residents. Adaptive dressing devices allow them to dress independently.

- ▧ Improves overall body function
- ▧ Improves appearance
- ▧ Promotes healthy self-esteem

Trochanter Rolls

The trochanter roll **(Figure 9–9)** is used to prevent external rotation of the hips. ⓢ Trochanter rolls should be used routinely for bedfast residents, to prevent deformities. ⓢ Unless a specific medical condition such as a hip fracture is present, no special order is necessary. To hold the trochanter roll in place, roll it away from the resident's body. Rolling the trochanter roll toward the body will cause it to slip, making it ineffective.

PROCEDURE

10 MAKING A TROCHANTER ROLL

1. Perform your beginning procedure actions.
2. Gather equipment:
   bath blanket
   disposable gloves if contact with blood or body fluids is likely
3. Place the bath blanket on a flat surface. Fold it in thirds lengthwise.
4. Place the blanket on the bed, extending from the waist to the mid-thigh area.
5. Position the resident in the center of the blanket.
6. Roll the center of the blanket outward (away from the resident) until it is firmly against the femur area.
7. Tuck the roll inward to maintain position.
8. Perform your procedure completion actions.

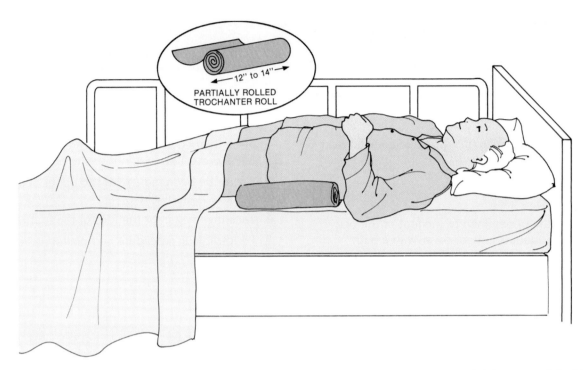

Figure 9–9 Trochanter rolls should be used for all bedfast residents to prevent contractures and deformities of the hip.

Bed Cradle

The bed cradle **(Figure 9–10)** keeps the weight of the upper bedding away from the resident's body. This may be necessary for several reasons. Some residents have serious skin conditions. Contact with the bedding causes irritation. In some residents, the weight of the bedding irritates a painful condition. Bed cradles are used to prevent foot drop for some residents. The weight of the bedding pushes the resident's feet into a position of plantar flexion, causing foot drop. A bed cradle may be used over a wet cast, allowing it to dry, while the bedding keeps the resident warm.

The bed cradle is a frame that attaches to the sides of the bed. The upper bedding is placed over the cradle. This keeps the weight of the covers off the resident's skin. Bed cradles are not used frequently, and some facilities may not have them. If a commercially made cradle is not available, a clean cardboard box can be substituted. First, pad the inside of a box with a sheepskin, bath blanket, or other material. Insert the resident's feet into the open end of the box and cover the box with the upper bed linen. If a bed cradle is needed higher up on the legs or arms, both ends can be cut from the box. A very heavy, stiff box is needed, to keep it from collapsing under the weight of the bedding. Cutting both ends from the box reduces its stability, but it can be done as a temporary measure until a cradle becomes available. Pad the box, then position the extremity inside. Cover the box with the bed linen. Use this method only until a commercially made bed cradle is available.

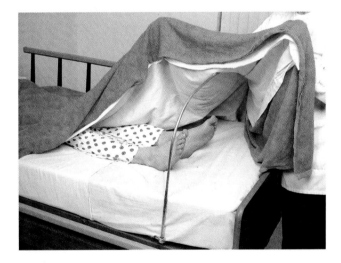

Figure 9–10 The bed cradle is fastened to the foot of the bed, then covered, keeping the weight of the upper bedding off the resident's legs.

Bridging

Bridging is a technique used to elevate an area off the surface of the bed. This method elevates an injured area, relieving pressure on the skin. It is useful for residents with healing pressure ulcers. Bridging is commonly used for the sacrum, hips, heels, and ankles. No special equipment is necessary. Facilities may use a combination of pillows, foam props, and bath blankets to support an area. The semiprone or semisupine positions are excellent alternatives to bridging. **Table 9–1** lists methods of bridging specific areas.

PROCEDURE

11 APPLYING A BED CRADLE TO THE BED

1. Perform your beginning procedure actions.
2. Gather equipment:
   bed cradle
   linen as needed
3. Fold the upper linen to the foot of the bed. If the resident is in bed, cover with a bath blanket before removing linen.
4. Place the bed cradle over the area of the bed to be protected. Fasten it to the bed frame.
5. Cover the bed cradle with the upper bedding. Remove bath blanket.
6. Tuck the linen in at the foot of the mattress.
7. Perform your procedure completion actions.

Table 9–1 Bridging Specific Pressure Areas

Location	Method
Sacrum	Place a pillow or folded bath blanket under both hips; place a pillow or folded bath blanket above and below the sacral area.
Trochanter	Position the resident in the lateral position; place a pillow under the trunk, place a second pillow under the upper leg. A pillow may also be needed to support and elevate the lower leg for comfort.
Ankle	Use a foam ring heel elevator which encircles the ankle, elevating the foot. An alternative when the resident is in the lateral position is to place a folded bath blanket or small pillow above and below the ankle.
Heel	Use foam ring heel elevators to elevate the heels off the surface of the bed, or elevate the length of the lower legs on pillows.

ELASTICIZED BANDAGES

Elasticized bandages are used to reduce edema from musculoskeletal injuries. They may also be used instead of anti-embolism stockings. The bandages will support a weakened joint or hold a splint in place. You may be directed to apply an elasticized bandage to an extremity. Select a bandage of the proper size and width. Before beginning the procedure, position the extremity in good alignment. Face the resident when wrapping the bandage. If the bandage is applied to a hand or foot, keep the fingers or toes exposed. This is necessary so the circulation can be monitored. Apply the bandage in a circular motion, using firm, even pressure (**Figure 9–11**). Always wrap distal to proximal (from bottom to top). Wrap in the direction of the heart.

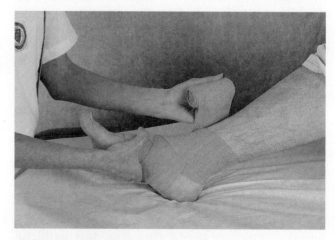

Figure 9–11 Always wrap the elastic bandage from distal to proximal, using overlapping turns.

PROCEDURE

12 APPLYING AN ELASTICIZED BANDAGE

1. Perform your beginning procedure actions.
2. Gather supplies:
   elasticized bandage of the proper length and width
3. Assist the resident to a comfortable position. Elevate the extremity you will be wrapping on the bed or table. Clean and dry the area, if necessary, before bandaging.
4. Hold the roll of the bandage facing up. Apply the bandage to the smallest part, distal to the joint you are wrapping.
5. Wrap the bandage around the extremity using two circular turns.
6. Wrap upward, using firm, even pressure in overlapping spiral turns. Each turn should overlap about two thirds of the previous turn.
7. Tape, pin, or clip the bandage in place.
8. Check the color and temperature of the fingers or toes distal to the bandage.
9. Perform your procedure completion actions.

Never apply an elasticized bandage from proximal to distal (from the top to bottom). Avoid wrapping it tightly. The bandage should maintain firm pressure on the extremity. It should not cut off or reduce blood flow. Check the circulation every hour. Remove the bandage immediately if changes in color or temperature are noted. Report your observations and action to your supervisor immediately. Remove and rewrap the bandage if it becomes loose or wrinkled. Wrinkles in the bandage can cause pressure ulcers.

■ RESTRAINT REDUCTION

You learned about using restraints in your nursing assistant program. In the past decade, a great deal of research has been done on the use of restraints. This research has shown that residents in restraints require more care than residents who are not restrained. Another interesting finding involves injuries. Incidents involving residents in restraints resulted in more serious injuries than incidents involving residents who were not restrained. Although restraints may be used to keep some residents safe, they also have many negative side effects.

Health care regulatory and accrediting organizations have specific rules regarding restraints. ⓢⒶHospitals and long-term care facilities must reduce restraints as much as possible.ⓈⒶ Though many health care workers in the United States oppose restraint reduction, nurses in other countries, particularly in Europe, rarely use restraints. ⓈⒶSome states are considering eliminating the use of vest restraints in long-term care facilities.ⓈⒶ This may occur as early as 1999 or 2000.

ⓈⒶThe intent of the OBRA '87 requirements is for each resident to reach his or her highest state of well-being. The law prohibits the use of restraints for discipline or convenience. Facilities must limit restraint use to circumstances in which the resident has medical symptoms that cannot be treated in any other manner. If restraints are used, the least restrictive device to keep the resident safe is used for the least amount of time possible.ⓈⒶ

Differentiating Restraints from Other Devices

Physical restraints are defined as any manual method or physical or mechanical device, material, or equipment attached to or adjacent to the resident's body. The resident cannot remove the device easily. It restricts freedom of movement or normal access to one's body. Examples of physical restraints are vests, belts, and geriatric chairs. Vest restraints are associated with a high risk of injury and death. ⓈⒶVisually observe residents in restraints every 15 to 30 minutes. Release the restraint every 2 hours for 10 full minutes. Reposition, ambulate, or take the resident to the bathroom during this time. If the resident is bedfast or chairfast, provide range-of-motion exercises. Reposition him or her to relieve pressure.ⓈⒶ

Enablers are devices that empower residents. They help residents function at their highest level. For example, a resident in a wheelchair is unable to sit up straight to feed herself. She is fed by staff. A support that corrects her posture, allowing her to feed herself, is an enabler. Enablers that maintain body position and alignment are called **postural supports.** Used correctly, they give residents a higher degree of independence. The device enables the resident to perform tasks that he or she was previously unable to do. In this case, using the device improves the resident's self-esteem.

Differentiating a restraint from an enabler or postural support may be difficult. Generally, devices that assist or enable residents to perform a task are enablers. (SA)The device is not a restraint if the resident has the physical and mental ability to remove it.(SA) If the resident can remove the device, it is a restraint alternative. If he or she cannot remove the device, it is a restraint. For example, many facilities use geriatric chairs. If the resident cannot remove the tray on the chair, it is a restraint. Some trays fasten to the chair with Velcro® straps. If the resident has the physical and mental ability to release the Velcro®, the chair is a restraint alternative. Some facilities do not use Velcro® to fasten the tray to the chair, because the trays are heavy. If a resident pushes the tray onto the legs, it may cause injury.

Role of the Restorative Nursing Assistant in Restraint Reduction

Restraint reduction is restorative care. Restorative nurses are responsible for the restraint reduction program in many facilities. Assisting with the restraint reduction and elimination program may be one of your responsibilities.

You have learned that a device is a restraint if the resident does not have the physical or mental ability to remove it. For example, many soft belt restraints are fastened with Velcro®. The belt is simple to unfasten. However, if the resident does not have the mental ability to remove it, it is a restraint. The restorative nurse may develop a restorative program to teach the resident to remove the restraint. You will work with him or her using verbal cues and hand-over-hand technique. You will also teach the resident basic safety, such as locking the wheelchair brakes. Carefully document the resident's progress and understanding. Over a period of time, cognitively impaired residents can learn to release safety devices.

Factors to Consider and Risk Factors to Eliminate

You will have a great deal of direct contact with the residents. You may know what does or does not work in managing the problem that is causing the need for the restraint. Important information to consider and report to your supervisor is:

- Does the resident see and hear well? Does he or she normally wear glasses? Is the resident wearing them now? Are they clean? Does the resident's hearing aid work? Are the resident's ears plugged with wax? Sometimes behavior

problems, balance problems, and other safety factors are caused because the resident is out of touch with the environment. He or she may misinterpret environmental clues. Applying eyeglasses and hearing aids may eliminate the need for a restraint.

- Is the resident able to make his or her needs known? Unsafe behavior may be caused by an unmet need. Discovering the unmet need and meeting it may help you avoid using a restraint. Pain, hunger, thirst, need to use the bathroom, and boredom are all unmet needs. Use trial and error to see if you can discover the problem.

- Does noise or confusion in the environment agitate the resident? Noise can be caused by other residents or staff, the intercom, radios, or television. Eliminating the noise may stop the behavior.

- Does the behavior occur during a certain time of day, during a certain activity, when the resident is in a specific location, or when a certain person is providing care?

- Does the resident seem uncomfortable? Physical discomfort or uncomfortable environmental temperature can cause unsafe behavior.

- Does the resident seem lonely, isolated, or bored? Boredom, loneliness, or looking for a misplaced item can cause unsafe behavior.

- Does the resident try to get out of the bed or chair without help? Is the resident unsteady on his or her feet? Does he or she normally use a cane or walker? Is the resident using it now? Is the call signal available, and does the resident know how to use it? Would the resident benefit from use of an alarm that sounds when he or she stands up? Would using an alarm remind the resident to sit down, alert the staff, and eliminate the need for a restraint?

Remember that behavior problems requiring restraints are often the result of unmet needs. (SA)Identifying these needs and meeting them is the first step in successfully eliminating restraints.(SA)

If the resident is a wanderer, he or she may be looking for a state of mind, not a physical location. Attempt to provide the state of mind the resident is seeking. If the resident says that he must go to work, talk to him about his job. If a resident says she must go make dinner for her children, discuss her cooking. This helps restore the state of mind and decreases wandering behavior.

Restraint Alternatives

Differentiating positioning devices from restraint alternatives may be difficult. Many devices are used for both purposes. When trying to decide how to meet the resident's positioning needs, consider restraint alternatives. Some alternatives provide support and keep residents in good alignment. Familiarize yourself with the restraint alternatives used in your facility. Review the medical supply and restraint manufacturers' catalogs so you know what type of devices are available. You may see something in a catalog that will benefit one of your residents. You may see something that you can make easily. The following are other suggestions that may be helpful to eliminate the need for restraints:

▪ Use magnetic sensor bracelets **(Figure 9–12)** that set off alarms if the resident enters a dangerous area or tries to leave. These work on the same principle as the magnetic detectors placed in stores to prevent shoplifting. They are applied to the dominant hand, making them difficult to remove. Follow facility policy and manufacturers' directions.

▪ Alarm cushions are available that signal when the resident stands up or tries to get out of bed. Some facilities attach the signal cord to the resident's gown or clothing. If the cord is too short to reach the resident, tie a string to it. If the resident stands, or moves too far forward, the cord will pull from the wall, sounding an alarm.

▪ Beds that are low and close to the floor are available. The risk of injury is reduced if the resident falls out of bed. Using this type of bed eliminates the need for side rails.

▪ Self-releasing seat belts **(Figure 9–13)** are similar to the lap belts used in cars. Some belts have buckles. Some have Velcro® fasteners.

▪ Lap buddies **(Figure 9–14)** are foam cushions placed on the lap. They are lightweight, provide a support surface, and are easy to remove. Trays that fasten to the chair with Velcro® can be used for the same purpose.

▪ Some chairs are designed to make standing more difficult. Many chairs are available for residents with special positioning needs **(Figure 9–15).** Use caution, however. A common restraint alternative is a commercial reclining chair. This type of recliner is designed for health care facilities. Although some residents benefit from this device, it causes serious complications in others. Residents who use a reclining chair for prolonged periods develop weakness in the neck muscles and lose the ability to hold the head up. They cannot feed themselves in the reclining position, and must be fed by staff. Eventually, they lose the ability to feed themselves. Residents in recliners look at the ceiling all day. They lose touch with the environment because they cannot see it. This creates or increases confusion. The resident cannot participate in activities because he or she cannot see well enough in the reclined position. If recliners are used, head rests are available to position the head forward and promote eye contact. Using these chairs as a restraint alternative must be seriously considered. Although they solve one problem, they have the potential to create many others.

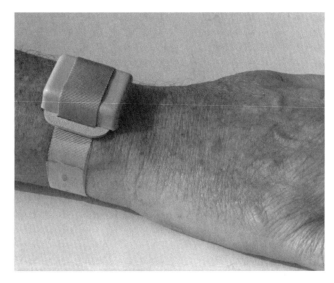

Figure 9–12 The magnetic sensor bracelet sounds an alarm if the resident attempts to go out an exit door. (© 1996 R.F. Technologies, Inc. Used by permission.)

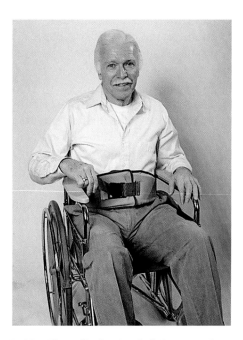

Figure 9–13 The self-releasing belt is a restraint alternative if the resident can remove it. It is a restraint if the resident is physically or cognitively impaired and unable to release it. (Courtesy of Skil-Care Corporation, Yonkers, NY (800) 431-2972)

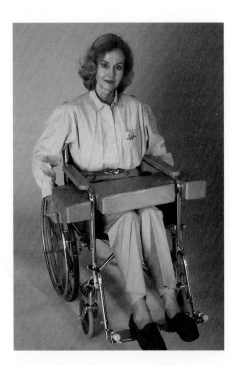

Figure 9–14   The lap buddy is foam covered with vinyl. It is lightweight and comfortable, and may be used for an arm support instead of the heavier lap tray. It is a restraint if the resident is physically or cognitively impaired and unable to remove it. (Courtesy of Skil-Care Corporation, Yonkers, NY (800) 431-2972)

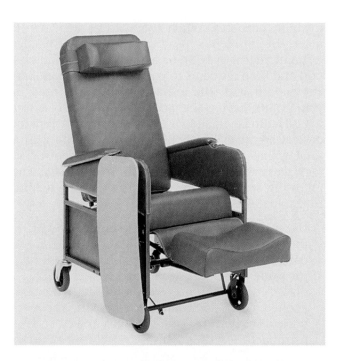

Figure 9–15   Potential candidates for the reclining geriatric chair should be evaluated carefully. The chair is useful for many residents, but can cause complications in others. It is a restraint if the resident is physically or cognitively impaired and unable to remove the tray. (Photo courtesy of Hill-Rom® Long Term Care Division)

- For residents who remove tubes or dressings on the arms, chest, and abdomen, consider applying a turtleneck shirt or other tight-fitting shirt. An alternative to a shirt is using a fabric cover, such as stockinette, or an abdominal binder.

- Nonslip matting, called "gripper" or Dycem, is available in the housewares department of most department stores. Most medical suppliers also sell this inexpensive product. When placed under a resident's body, movement, particularly sliding forward in a chair, is difficult.

- Inverted wedge cushions **(Figure 9–16)** prevent the resident from sliding the hips forward in the chair. Gripper can be placed over and under the seat cushion for extra security. Avoid using gripper if it is wet. Wash it in the sink and hang it up to dry before using it again.

- Beanbag chairs are comfortable to sit in. They make it very difficult for residents to get up. Wanderers with Alzheimer's disease often wear themselves out. They use many extra calories pacing about the facility all day. The beanbag keeps the wanderer safe and comfortable, allowing him or her to rest.

- Physical and diversionary activities promote empowerment and self-esteem, reducing

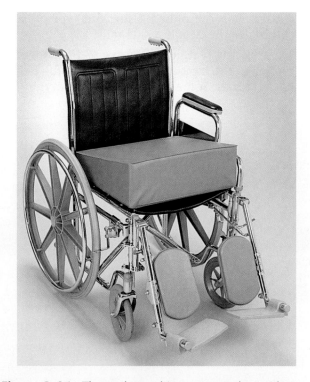

Figure 9–16   The wedge cushion prevents the resident from sliding the hips forward in the chair. Dycem can be used over and under the seat for extra security. Make sure the resident's feet and legs are supported. (Courtesy of Skil-Care Corporation, Yonkers, NY (800) 431-2972)

behavior problems. Ask your activity director for suggestions and assistance.

▪ Ribbons or streamers across doorways may prevent wanderers from entering. Signs, such as "stop," "do not enter," or "construction zone," may be attached to the streamer.

▪ A small personal stereo with earphones, playing the resident's favorite music, is very effective for calming agitated residents.

▪ Minimizing environmental noise, confusion, and activity reduces agitation.

▪ Place soft sponges or other objects in the resident's hands to keep them busy.

▪ Regularly remind and reassure residents that they are safe and in the right place.

▪ Provide distraction. Smile and talk to residents when you pass by. Spend a few minutes talking whenever possible.

▪ Avoid telling a wanderer, "Don't go outside." Telling the resident not to leave makes the resident think about going outside. If someone tells you not to think of a purple dog, you will think of it. Then you must unthink it. Saying "Stay inside" is more effective. In cognitively impaired residents, this approach requires a less complicated thought process.

▪ Leave the bathroom light on or use night lights at bedtime.

▪ Taping dark construction paper to the floor, or painting an area of the floor (such as in front of an exit door) black may be helpful. Cognitively impaired persons perceive this as a hole and will not try to cross it.

▪ Provide adequate lighting at all times. This enables residents to interpret environmental objects, equipment, and individuals correctly.

▪ Make sure the environmental temperature is comfortable.

▪ A warm bath or shower may calm an agitated resident.

KEY POINTS IN CHAPTER

Restorative care requires very little special equipment.

Handrolls are used for dependent residents to prevent contractures.

Splints are used to prevent deformity and stabilize fractures.

Keep the skin clean and dry under handrolls and splints.

Do not remove splints that are stabilizing fractures.

Footboards are used to prevent plantar flexion of the feet.

The bed cradle is used to keep the weight of bed linen away from the resident's body.

Adaptive devices are used to assist residents to perform everyday tasks.

Bridging is used to relieve pressure from the bony prominences of the sacrum, trochanters, heels, and ankles.

An elasticized bandage is used to prevent or relieve edema and provide support.

An elasticized bandage is always wrapped from distal to proximal.

Residents in restraints require more care than residents who are not restrained.

Restraints can have serious side effects.

An enabler is a device that allows a resident to perform an activity that he or she could not perform without the device.

A restraint is attached to or adjacent to the resident's body, restricts movement and access to the body, and cannot be removed by the resident.

A postural support maintains the resident in good body alignment.

A restraint alternative is any item or device that is used instead of a restraint. To qualify, the resident must have the physical and mental ability to remove the device.

The OBRA '87 legislation requires long-term care facilities to reduce restraint use.

If restraining a resident is necessary, the device selected should be the least restrictive to keep the resident safe. It should be used for the least amount of time possible.

CLINICAL APPLICATIONS

1. Mrs. Neale is a 77-year-old resident who was recently admitted to your facility because of a massive CVA. The resident is not responsive. She is bedfast and requires total nursing care. She is fed through a gastrostomy tube. Mrs. Neale has a large stage I pressure ulcer on her coccyx. Her paralyzed arm is flaccid. She keeps her unaffected hand in a tight fist. What restorative nursing measures and adaptive devices do you recommend for this resident?

2. Mr. Horst has contractures of both hands. He uses splints daily. When the splints are removed, it is very difficult to open his hands to replace them. Bathing his hands and clipping his nails are also difficult. What measures do you suggest for making this task easier for both the resident and staff?

3. Miss Paluay has a fractured hip. She is a poor surgical candidate, so her fracture is being managed with traction. The resident will be on bed rest for at least 4 weeks. What restorative nursing measures do you suggest for preventing skin breakdown and deformities?

4. Mrs. Halstrom is a dependent resident. She is 5'1" tall, and weighs 82 pounds. Her extremities are very rigid. She is transferred to the chair by two assistants. After she sits for an hour, she begins to slump forward. Sometimes she leans over the side of the chair. Presently, Mrs. Halstrom is restrained with a vest to keep her upright and prevent falls. Suggest restorative nursing measures and restraint alternatives that may be helpful to this resident.

5. Mr. James has Alzheimer's disease. He has lost 8 pounds in the past month. He wanders about the facility most of the day. Mr. James does not sit in one place long enough to finish a meal. If he leaves the dining room, he refuses to return. In the late afternoon, he takes a long nap. When he awakens, he begins wandering again. He often wanders into the early morning hours. Mr. James has never left the facility, but several times recently he has set off alarms on the exit doors. Describe some nursing measures to use to assist this resident.

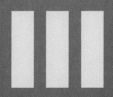

Preventing Personal Injury

CHAPTER 10

Preventing Musculoskeletal Injuries

OBJECTIVES

After reading this chapter, you should be able to:

Spell and define key terms.

Describe common causes of injuries in health care workers.

Describe how musculoskeletal injuries can be prevented in health care workers.

Demonstrate proper body mechanics for lifting and moving residents and heavy objects.

Define ergonomics.

Identify ergonomic hazards in the long-term care facility.

List the components of an ergonomics program.

BACK INJURIES IN HEALTH CARE WORKERS

Lifting and moving residents is an important part of restorative care. Many procedures also involve bending. A review of how to protect your musculoskeletal system is presented in this chapter.

Back injuries are the most common injury in health care workers. Some have been disabled for life because of work-related back injuries. Most of these were caused by lifting and moving residents. The most common causes of back injuries are:

- Poor posture
- Being in poor physical condition
- Using improper body mechanics
- Incorrect lifting
- Jobs that require high energy
- Transferring residents in confined spaces, such as bathrooms or cluttered bedrooms

Pay attention to how your body feels. Become aware of aches, pains, and feeling stressed. Discomfort, pain, and stress suggest that something is wrong! Pay attention to how you perform certain tasks. Pay attention to your working conditions. Paying careful attention will show you where the hidden dangers are. Tasks that involve awkward posture, force, repetition, and insufficient rest periods are risk factors for injuries. Take shorter, more frequent breaks, before becoming fatigued. If possi-

ble, take a 5-minute break every hour instead of one 15-minute break after 3 hours. Use common sense when doing your job. You have learned many methods of lifting and moving residents. No single technique will work in all circumstances. Use good judgment. Select the technique that will make the job the easiest for both you and the resident. One way to do this is to use a transfer belt. ⓢⒶWhen in doubt about your ability to move a resident, always ask for help.ⓢⒶ Do not let someone tell you that you can lift a resident alone. If you think you need help, you probably do. Get it before moving the resident. Remember that working safely means:

- Using common sense
- Using ergonomics
- Staying healthy and physically fit
- Getting enough rest at night
- Making injury prevention a top priority

Causes of Musculoskeletal System Injuries

Your posture determines which joints and muscles are used to perform certain tasks. Posture also determines the amount of force or stress that your body can tolerate. For example, twisting or bending while you lift, lower, or handle objects increases stress on the spine. These tasks cause less stress when the back is straight. Tasks that require repeated or sustained bending or twisting of the wrists, knees, hips, or shoulders also increase the stress on your joints. Tasks that involve frequent or prolonged work at or above shoulder height are very stressful.

Exertion.   Performing duties that require forceful exertion intensify the stress on your body. The stress increases the risk of injury. Lifting, pushing, and pulling are tasks you do many times each day. These require forceful exertion. Increasing the force with which a job is done increases the demand on your body. Prolonged or recurrent tasks such as these cause fatigue. This leads directly to musculoskeletal problems if you do not get enough rest. The force necessary for a task increases as the weight of the resident or object you are moving increases. Other factors that affect the force used are:

■ Moving a bulky object

■ Standing in an awkward position

■ Moving quickly or abruptly

■ Lifting or moving a wet object or resident

Repetitive Motions.   **Repetitive motions** are those that are done often for prolonged periods. Repetitive motions increase fatigue. Over time, they cause muscle and tendon strain. Tendons and muscles will usually recover from the effects of stretching or forceful exertion. However, the body needs rest before performing the activity again. The effects of repetitive motions are increased if you stand in an awkward position. Using forceful exertion for the task also increases the negative effects on your body.

Duration.   The length of time a person is continually exposed to a risk factor is called **duration.** Job duties that require you to use the same muscles or movements for long periods of time increase fatigue. If a task requires sustained muscle contraction, a recovery or rest time is required to prevent injury.

Environmental Conditions.   Prolonged contact with hard or sharp objects or objects that vibrate increases the risk of injury. Contact with these items inhibits nerve function and blood flow. The risk of injury increases with cold temperature, insufficient breaks, and performing unfamiliar tasks. Studies are being done to see if mental stress also has a negative effect on the musculoskeletal system. One theory is that the stress caused by very close supervision and feelings of lack of control may also have a negative effect on the body.

   You can also prevent injuries by:

■ Following facility safety and health rules

■ Following policies and procedures related to your job

■ Reporting early signs and symptoms of work-related stress or injury

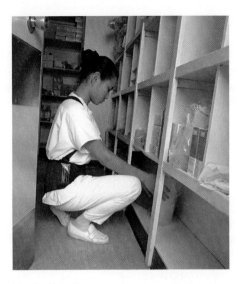

Figure 10–1   Wearing a back support belt encourages good body mechanics.

Back Support Belts

Use a back support belt if your physician recommends it, if this is your preference, or if this is facility policy. Many assistants feel better if they are wearing the belt for support. Use of the back belt is controversial. Some studies have shown that workers using back support have fewer back injuries. Other studies have shown that there is no difference in the rate of injuries. The belt reminds you to keep your back straight and to use good body mechanics. Using improper body mechanics when wearing the belt is difficult **(Figure 10–1).** For this reason alone, the belt is beneficial. You are less likely to become injured if you are using good body mechanics.

   Some workers believe they can lift heavier loads when wearing a back support. This is not true. Believing that the belt protects you increases your risk of injury. Avoid lifting more weight than you would without a belt. To date, there is no proof that wearing a back support increases the weight that you can lift or carry. Follow your facility policy and manufacturer's directions for wearing the back support belt.

■ BODY MECHANICS

Lifting, moving, and positioning residents and heavy objects is a major part of your job. You learned about body mechanics in your nursing assistant program. However, the subject is so important that it is summarized here. Using good body mechanics is important any time you:

■ Perform lifting or moving procedures

■ Transfer residents

■ Pick up items from the floor

■ Bend or lift

Using good body mechanics involves using the largest, strongest muscles to do the job. Your strongest muscles are in your legs and arms. Your weakest muscles are in your back and abdomen. Using good body mechanics makes work easier and prevents fatigue. Using your body correctly also helps prevent injury to you and residents.

Posture

The foundation of proper body mechanics is good posture. Good posture is the same whether you are standing, sitting, or lying down. Good standing posture involves:

▨ Keeping your back in good alignment with its natural curves

▨ Standing straight

▨ Keeping your feet flat on the floor

▨ Propping one foot on a stool if you will be standing in one place for a long time

▨ Distributing your weight evenly on both feet

▨ Standing with your feet at least 12 inches apart

▨ Bending your knees slightly

▨ Keeping your arms at your sides **(Figure 10–2)**

While practicing good posture, you should:

▨ Change your position often

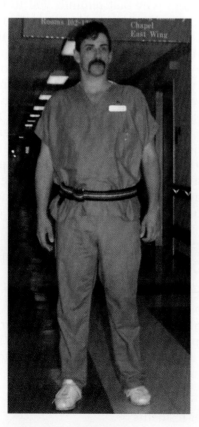

Figure 10–2 Good standing posture.

▨ Stretch frequently during your shift

▨ Keep your body flexible and as relaxed as possible

▨ Avoid forcing your body into a small or confined space

Body Mechanics for Residents

Teach residents the principles of good body mechanics. ⓢⒶPosition residents in good alignment in bed. Use supports and props if necessary. To position residents **(Figure 10–4, p. 152)** in chairs, make sure that the spine is straight and the:

▨ Ankles, knees, thighs, and elbows are at right angles

▨ Head is balanced naturally over the shoulders

▨ Shoulders are relaxed, not hunched forward or slumped to the side

▨ Hips are at a 90° angle at the back of the seatⓢⒶ

▨▨▨ ERGONOMICS

Ergonomics is a method of fitting or matching the job to the worker. Injuries commonly occur if the job and the worker do not match. **Ergonomic hazards** are work place conditions that create stress on the worker's body. Examples of ergonomic hazards are:

▨ Improper work methods

▨ Improper equipment

▨ Poor posture

▨ Force

▨ Repetition

▨ Inadequate rest periods

Two types of injuries commonly affect health care workers. **Instantaneous injuries** occur suddenly and without warning. Accidents, such as falls, are examples of this type of injury. **Cumulative trauma disorders** are injuries to nerves, tissues, tendons, and joints. These occur from repeated stress and strain over months to years. Cumulative injuries are caused by:

▨ Performing repetitious tasks

▨ Using muscular force to do the job

▨ Heavy lifting without assistance

▨ Poor posture

▨ Standing in awkward positions

▨ Inadequate rest or break time

Avoid placing stress on your body whenever possible. Use a cart to transport heavy objects instead of carrying them. The **safe lifting zone** is the area

General Guidelines for Using Good Body Mechanics While Lifting and Moving

Refer to **Figure 10–3.**

- Keep your back straight.
- Stand upright, using good natural posture.
- Keep your feet flat on the floor.
- Stand with your feet at least 12 inches apart to maintain a wide base of support.
- Use the large muscles in your legs when lifting residents or heavy objects.
- Bend from the hips and knees, never from the waist.
- Face your work.
- Avoid twisting at the waist. If you must turn, pivot.
- Tighten your abdominal muscles to support your back.

- Squat when lifting heavy objects from the floor.
- Keep heavy objects as close to your body as possible when lifting, moving, and carrying.
- Use both hands to lift or move heavy objects.
- Push, pull, or slide heavy objects instead of lifting them.
- Use smooth, even movements instead of quick, jerking motions.
- Avoid unnecessary bending and reaching.
- Check the care plan for directions before moving residents.
- Always use a transfer belt for moving residents, unless contraindicated.
- Ask for help from others if you are unsure whether you can move a resident or object.

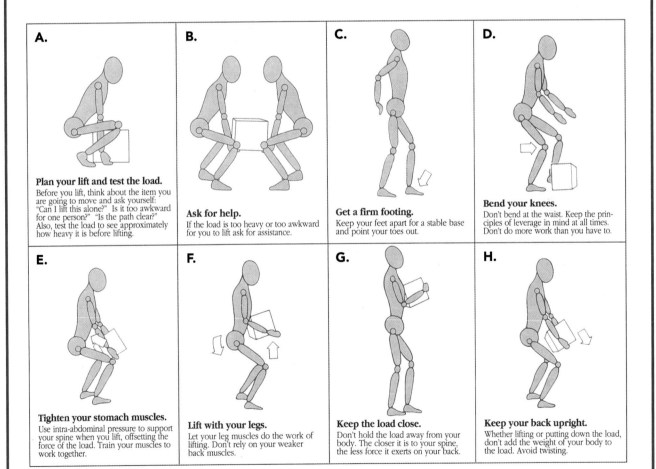

A. Plan your lift and test the load.
Before you lift, think about the item you are going to move and ask yourself: "Can I lift this alone?" Is it too awkward for one person?" "Is the path clear?" Also, test the load to see approximately how heavy it is before lifting.

B. Ask for help.
If the load is too heavy or too awkward for you to lift ask for assistance.

C. Get a firm footing.
Keep your feet apart for a stable base and point your toes out.

D. Bend your knees.
Don't bend at the waist. Keep the principles of leverage in mind at all times. Don't do more work than you have to.

E. Tighten your stomach muscles.
Use intra-abdominal pressure to support your spine when you lift, offsetting the force of the load. Train your muscles to work together.

F. Lift with your legs.
Let your leg muscles do the work of lifting. Don't rely on your weaker back muscles.

G. Keep the load close.
Don't hold the load away from your body. The closer it is to your spine, the less force it exerts on your back.

H. Keep your back upright.
Whether lifting or putting down the load, don't add the weight of your body to the load. Avoid twisting.

Figure 10–3   Eight rules for lifting and moving heavy objects. (Reprinted with permission from Ergodyne Corporation, St. Paul, MN)

(continues)

General Guidelines for Using Good Body Mechanics While Lifting and Moving, *continued*

- Use mechanical lifting devices for moving heavy residents.
- Elevate the bed to a comfortable height for your body when giving bedside care. Lower the bed to the lowest horizontal position after caring for the resident.
- Avoid bending at the waist when caring for residents in bed.
- When lifting a resident from the floor, use a mechanical lift, sheet, or other device. Always ask for help.
- Avoid:
  - twisting while lifting
  - bending in an awkward position to pick up an item from the floor
  - attempting to hold a falling resident up

- Never lift:
  - an object on the floor by bending at the waist
  - with one hand
  - over obstacles, such as the bed
  - while reaching or stretching
  - if you are in an uncomfortable or awkward posture
  - in a confined space
  - wet, slippery objects or residents
  - a resident who is grabbing at the arms of a chair, side rails, or your body
  - any resident or object if you are unsure of your ability to do it safely

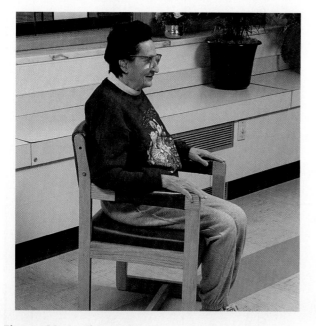

Figure 10–4 This resident is seated with her joints at right angles, head balanced, shoulders relaxed, and hips at a 90° angle to the back of the chair.

between your knees and shoulders. If you must lift an item below knee level, bend from your knees. Lift with your leg muscles. If you must lift from above shoulder height, stand on a stool or ladder. Rearrange shelves, if necessary. Place heavy and frequently used items on the middle shelves. If an item is heavy, ask for help. Work at waist height, whenever possible. Avoid bending or reaching up or down. Pivot to reach objects. Avoid twisting from the waist. Use good body mechanics when standing, lifting, moving, and turning.

Exercise

All people need exercise for health and life. Muscles normally contract and relax. During the contraction phase, the muscle forces blood out. Blood enters the muscle during the relaxation phase. Muscles receive nourishment from stored carbohydrates, fat, and protein. The human body depends on muscle function for survival. The heart is a muscle. Breathing, circulation of blood, and proper elimination all depend on muscular action.

Overexertion can cause injury. Anyone involved in an exercise program should be monitored by a physician. Consult your personal physician. Ask for an exercise program to meet your needs. Avoid doing too much too fast. Start slowly and gradually develop endurance. Monitor your pulse during exercise. Stop if the rate exceeds 100, or follow your physician's instructions.

Stretch at the beginning of your shift and before beginning a heavy task. This will loosen your muscles, making it easier to move. Stretching again when you finish will reduce stiffness. Stretch periodically during your shift. The exercises shown in **Figure 10–5** will help protect your back.

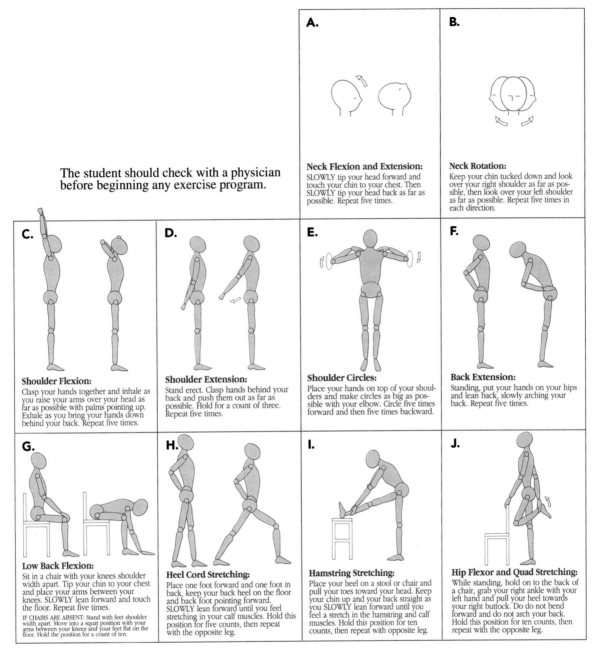

The student should check with a physician before beginning any exercise program.

A.

Neck Flexion and Extension:
SLOWLY tip your head forward and touch your chin to your chest. Then SLOWLY tip your head back as far as possible. Repeat five times.

B.

Neck Rotation:
Keep your chin tucked down and look over your right shoulder as far as possible, then look over your left shoulder as far as possible. Repeat five times in each direction.

C.

Shoulder Flexion:
Clasp your hands together and inhale as you raise your arms over your head as far as possible with palms pointing up. Exhale as you bring your hands down behind your back. Repeat five times.

D.

Shoulder Extension:
Stand erect. Clasp hands behind your back and push them out as far as possible. Hold for a count of three. Repeat five times.

E.

Shoulder Circles:
Place your hands on top of your shoulders and make circles as big as possible with your elbow. Circle five times forward and then five times backward.

F.

Back Extension:
Standing, put your hands on your hips and lean back, slowly arching your back. Repeat five times.

G.

Low Back Flexion:
Sit in a chair with your knees shoulder width apart. Tip your chin to your chest and place your arms between your knees. SLOWLY lean forward and touch the floor. Repeat five times.
IF CHAIRS ARE ABSENT: Stand with feet shoulder width apart. Move into a squat position with your arms between your knees and your feet flat on the floor. Hold the position for a count of ten.

H.

Heel Cord Stretching:
Place one foot forward and one foot in back, keep your back heel on the floor and back foot pointing forward. SLOWLY lean forward until you feel stretching in your calf muscles. Hold this position for five counts, then repeat with the opposite leg.

I.

Hamstring Stretching:
Place your heel on a stool or chair and pull your toes toward your head. Keep your chin up and your back straight as you SLOWLY lean forward until you feel a stretch in the hamstring and calf muscles. Hold this position for ten counts, then repeat with opposite leg.

J.

Hip Flexor and Quad Stretching:
While standing, hold on to the back of a chair, grab your right ankle with your left hand and pull your heel towards your right buttock. Do not bend forward and do not arch your back. Hold this position for ten counts, then repeat with the opposite leg.

Figure 10–5 Performing warm-up exercises before work will protect your back and prevent injury. (Reprinted with permission from Ergodyne Corporation, St. Paul, MN)

Using the Principles of Ergonomics When Moving Residents

To avoid back injuries, use common sense. Organize your work to save as many steps as possible. Think about the steps in the procedures you are performing. See if you can combine them. For example, before showering residents, you routinely toilet them. First, you take the resident to the bathroom. You transfer him or her from the wheelchair to the toilet and back. Next, you transfer the resident to the shower chair. Then you transport him or her to the shower room. Instead, transfer the resident to the shower chair first. Center the chair over the toilet. This eliminates two transfers. Cover the resident when finished, and transport him or her to the shower room. Good organization of supplies, equipment, and tasks reduces stress on your body. Modifying the way you do certain tasks also reduces stress. Before moving residents, evaluate the move. Ask yourself these questions:

- Is the resident larger than you are?
- Can the resident follow directions?
- Can the resident help with the transfer?

- Can you move the resident with a lifting sheet, mechanical lift, or other device?
- Can you use a sliding board to transfer the resident instead of lifting?
- Do you need help? Ask for help if residents exceed one-third to one-half of your body weight, or if the resident the resident cannot help with the transfer.
- Does the resident grab at persons or objects? If so, always get help.
- Is the resident within your safe lifting zone?
- Is it necessary to twist or stretch to move the resident?
- Do you need special equipment?
- Did you stretch your muscles before lifting?

- Are you wearing nonslip footwear?
- Have you moved any obstacles in your path?
- Are you in a confined space?

Developing an Ergonomics Program

An ergonomics program will be developed by your employer. Many long-term care facilities recognize that ergonomics saves money. More important, these programs prevent worker injuries. The Occupational Safety and Health Administration (OSHA) has developed guidelines for facilities to use in developing ergonomics programs. They recommend that employees participate in developing the program. As a restorative nursing assistant, you may be asked to assist. The components of an ergonomics program are listed in **Table 10–1.**

Table 10–1 Components of an Ergonomics Program

1. Look for signs of potential musculoskeletal problems, such as frequent worker reports of aches, pains, and injuries, or tasks that require repetitive, forceful exertions.

2. Show a commitment in addressing potential problems and encouraging worker participation and input into problem-solving activities.

3. Provide training to all employees to recognize and evaluate potential musculoskeletal problems.

4. Gather information to identify jobs, tasks, or working conditions that are most problematic, using information such as incident reports, injury and illness logs, medical records, and job analyses.

5. Identify effective controls for tasks that pose a risk of musculoskeletal injury. Evaluate these approaches to see if they reduce or eliminate the problem.

6. Emphasize the importance of early detection and treatment of musculoskeletal disorders for preventing permanent impairment and disability.

7. Minimize risk factors for musculoskeletal disorders when planning new work processes and operations. Doing this from the beginning is less costly than redesigning tasks later.

8. Assess all work activities to ensure that tasks can be accomplished without exceeding the physical capabilities of the worker.

9. Provide initial and periodic in services on body mechanics for all employees.

10. Provide a surveillance program to identify potential work-related musculoskeletal problems.

11. Include a medical management program.

KEY POINTS IN CHAPTER

You have many responsibilities that include lifting, moving, and bending. Protecting your back is very important.

Back injuries are the most common injury in health care workers.

Pay attention to how your body feels and take steps to prevent injury.

A short break every hour is better than a longer break after several hours of work.

Posture determines the amount of force or stress that your body can tolerate.

Your posture determines which joints and muscles are used to perform certain tasks. It also determines the amount of force or stress that your body can tolerate.

When lifting and moving residents, use good judgment. Select the technique that will make the job the easiest for both you and the resident. Using a transfer belt is one way of doing this.

Tasks that require repeated or sustained bending or twisting increase the stress on your joints.

Tasks involving prolonged work at or over shoulder height are particularly stressful.

Jobs that require forceful exertion increase stress on your muscles, tendons, ligaments, and joints. This increases the risk for injury.

The longer you perform a task requiring sustained muscle contraction, the longer the recovery or rest time required.

The back belt does not prevent injury, but reminds you to use good body mechanics.

The back belt does not increase your ability to lift more weight. Avoid lifting more than you would if you were not wearing the belt.

Using good body mechanics involves using the largest, strongest muscles to do the job.

The foundation of proper body mechanics is good posture.

Stretching at the beginning of your shift and before beginning a heavy task loosens your muscles and helps prevent injury.

Good organization and modification of the way tasks are done reduce stress on your body.

CLINICAL APPLICATIONS

1. Susan, CNA, confides in you that she has had problems with back pain in the past. She is worried that moving residents will cause a back injury. What advice will you give her?

2. David, CNA, tells you that he wears a back support belt because he can lift heavy residents by himself if he wears the belt. Without it, he must ask another assistant to help. What advice will you give him?

3. Your facility has formed a committee to develop an ergonomics program. You have been asked to participate. You have been short-staffed lately. Many of the nursing assistants are not taking their breaks because they cannot get their work done. What will you suggest? Explain why ergonomics is important in the long-term care facility.

4. The bathrooms in your facility are small. Most residents are transferred from the wheelchair to the toilet by nursing assistants. This is difficult in such a small space. During the ergonomics committee meeting, the administrator asks your opinion of how to solve this problem. He tells you that making structural changes in the facility is impossible. What do you suggest?

5. Karen, CNA, tells you that she is dieting. She has not seen her physician. She is not eating during the day. She tells you she is exercising at the gym after work. She confides that she becomes dizzy sometimes. You know that when she transfers residents, she bends from the waist. What advice will you give her?

Lifting, Moving, and Ambulation Procedures

CHAPTER 11

Restorative Exercise and Bed Mobility

OBJECTIVES

After reading this chapter, you should be able to:

- *Spell and define key terms.*
- *List 10 reasons for exercising residents.*
- *Demonstrate active group exercises.*
- *State the purpose of therapeutic exercises.*
- *Name five types of therapeutic exercises.*
- *Define passive range of motion, active range of motion, active assisted range of motion, and resistive range of motion.*
- *Describe the similarities and differences of each type of range of motion*
- *Describe how to teach residents to move independently in bed.*

EXERCISE

You have learned that exercise is essential to all individuals for health and life. Like you, residents in long-term care facilities need exercise for good health. The licensed therapist or restorative nurse develops the exercise programs for residents. The principles of beginning an exercise program for residents are the same as they are for employees. Residents must be under the supervision of a physician. Some exercises require a physician's order. Begin the program gradually. Avoid doing too much too fast. Start slowly and gradually develop endurance to exercise. Monitor the pulse during exercise. Stop if the rate exceeds 100. Your supervisor and the care plan will provide guidelines.

Reasons for Exercise

Exercises are done for many reasons. The most common reasons are to:

- Maintain normal range of motion for all residents
- Improve range of motion in certain residents
- Maintain muscle strength
- Increase or restore muscle strength
- Develop coordination and control
- Prevent deformities
- Improve circulation
- Improve sense of well-being
- Promote healthy self-esteem
- Provide beneficial sensory stimulation

Exercising a joint several times a day is better than exercising it once. For example, performing 5 range of motion exercises twice a day is better than performing 25 repetitions once a day. Some facilities have exercise groups and activities. These groups are fun for residents. They provide an excellent opportunity for physical movement. In most long-term care facilities, residents begin arriving in the dining room 30 minutes before mealtime. Many facilities assign a staff member to the dining room. This person can assist residents with group exercises while they wait for meals to be served. The residents may exercise to music, and look forward to participating **(Figure 11–1)**.

Exercising for Fun

Some facilities have separate exercise rooms for residents. These rooms usually have permanent exercise equipment. Pulleys, shoulder ladders **(Figure 11–2)**, and shoulder wheels **(Figure 11–3)** are mounted on the wall for residents to use. Residents can visit these rooms informally any time. You may conduct group activities in the room daily. Games such as Velcro® darts, horseshoes, and beanbag tosses are good exercise. They provide a sense of competition. These games also increase eye-hand

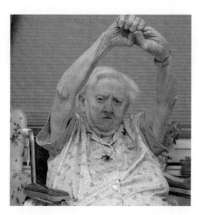

Figure 11–1   Active movement prevents deformity and strengthens the extremities. This resident is strengthening her unaffected arm while she exercises the affected arm to prevent deformity.

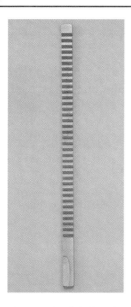

Figure 11–2   Residents "climb" the shoulder ladder with their fingers. (Courtesy of Briggs Corporation, Des Moines, IA. (800) 247-2343)

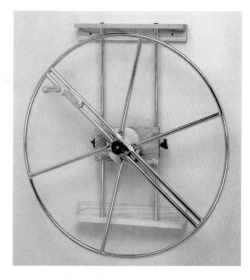

Figure 11–3   The range of motion on the shoulder wheel ranges from 10 inches to 30 inches. (Courtesy of Medline Industries, Inc. (800) MEDLINE)

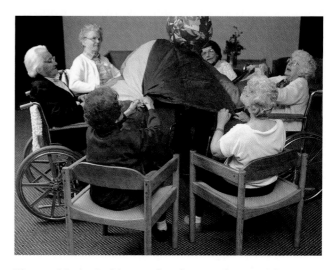

Figure 11–4   Residents enjoy the parachute activity, which improves gross motor skills. (Courtesy of Briggs Corporation, Des Moines, IA. (800) 247-2343)

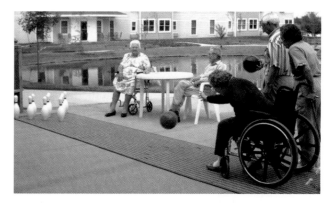

Figure 11–5   Bowling improves gross motor skills and coordination, as well as providing fun and enjoyment. (Courtesy of Briggs Corporation, Des Moines, IA. (800) 247-2343)

coordination, grip strength, and range of motion. A ball toss game is available that uses Velcro® mitts. A parachute activity **(Figure 11–4)** is fun and good exercise. The group holds a parachute and bounces a ball or balloon across it from one person to the next. This enjoyable activity is more difficult than it looks. Nevertheless, it strengthens the arms and hands and improves range of motion in the shoulders. Residents also enjoy bowling **(Figure 11–5).**

Gross Motor Exercises

Gross motor exercises are usually done with residents who have a limited response to the environment. Residents with mental confusion, short attention span, and inability to follow directions are good candidates. Gross motor exercises begin with activities such as catching a beach ball. The degree of difficulty is increased as the resident's attention span increases.

PROCEDURE

13 ACTIVE GROUP EXERCISES

These simple active range of motion exercises can be used for group or individual exercises. Performing these exercises daily improves activity tolerance. Performing them at least three times a week maintains activity tolerance. Repeat each exercise 10 times. Do not allow residents to become fatigued. Each person's activity tolerance is different. Some residents may not be able to do all of these steps. Encourage them to participate to the extent they are able. Some exercise is better than none. Playing music adds to resident motivation and fun.

1. Inhale normally through your nose, causing your abdomen to protrude. Hold your breath for several seconds. Take at least twice as long to exhale as you did to inhale. Purse your lips and pull your abdomen in. Exhale through your mouth. Relax.

2. Hold your arms at your sides. Keep your elbows straight. Shrug your shoulders and tighten your arm muscles. Hold for several seconds, then release. Relax.

3. Drop your chin to your chest. Curl your trunk forward. Do not bend your hips. Breathe out. Uncurl your trunk, lift your chin up, and breathe in. Relax.

4. Place your fingertips on your shoulders. Move your elbows in a circular motion (the movement originates in the shoulder joints).

Alternate a clockwise circle with a counterclockwise circle. Relax.

5. Place your arms at your sides. Raise them over your head. Keep your elbows straight. Tell residents to stretch and reach for the sky. Bring your arms back down to your sides. Relax.

6. Sit in a chair with both feet flat on the floor. Straighten your knee, lifting your right foot. Hold it for a few seconds, then return your foot to the floor. Relax. Repeat with your left leg. Relax.

7. Sit in a chair with both feet flat on the floor. Draw your right knee up toward your chest. Hold it for a few seconds. Return it to the floor. Relax. Repeat with left leg. Relax.

8. Sit in a chair with your heels resting on the floor. Extend your knees slightly. Pull your toes up toward your knees. Point your toes down, away from your body. Move your ankles clockwise in a circular motion. Move your ankles counterclockwise in a circular motion. Relax.

9. Sit in a chair with your hands resting on your knees. Raise your left arm up over your head. Keep your elbows straight. Inhale. Bring your left arm across your body. Exhale. Return to the starting position. Relax. Repeat with your right arm. Relax.

▦ THERAPEUTIC EXERCISES

Therapeutic exercises are planned for individual residents. These exercises maintain or improve joint function. Therapeutic exercises prevent and correct deformities, diseases, and injuries. Returning a joint to normal function depends on the strength of the muscles controlling the joint. Two types of range of motion exercises are used:

▦ Exercises that move the joints
▦ Exercises that stretch and lengthen the muscles that cross over the joint

The goals of therapeutic exercises are to:

▦ Retrain and strengthen muscles
▦ Restore normal movement
▦ Prevent deformity
▦ Stimulate the functions of various body systems

A therapist develops the therapeutic exercise program to meet the resident's needs. Sometimes the therapist performs the exercises on the resident. When the resident is stable, you will assist with the exercises. Active and passive range of motion exercises are a form of therapeutic exercises. Active exercise is always best. A summary of the various types of therapeutic exercises is found in **Table 11–1.**

Table 11–1 Types of Therapeutic Exercises

Type of Exercise	Description	Goals	Restorative Action
Passive	Performed by the restorative assistant	Maintain as much joint function as possible, prevent deformity	Support the proximal and distal joint. Gently and smoothly move the joint through its normal range of motion. Avoid pain; avoid forcing the joint farther than it will comfortably move.
Active Assisted	Performed by the resident with assistance from the restorative assistant	Promote normal muscle function, prevent deformity	Support the distal joint and encourage the resident to take the joint through its normal range of motion. Assist no more than necessary. Provide brief rest periods frequently throughout the activity.
Active	Performed by the resident without assistance during normal daily activities	Increase muscle strength, prevent deformity	Done during normal movement such as turning, moving, and performing ADLs. Monitor the resident in the early phases of the exercise program to make sure he or she does not substitute one joint movement for another. Remind the resident of each movement to use. Avoid physically assisting.
Resistive	Exercise performed by the resident against manual or mechanical resistance, such as sandbags or weights	Increase strength	A sandbag or weight is placed over the extremity. The resident moves the joint through the normal range of motion with the weight in place, against the slight resistance on the joint. Over time, the amount of weight is increased, which increases resistance. The hand may also be used to provide resistance instead of weights, but this procedure is usually performed by licensed personnel. Know and follow your facility policy.
Isometric	Exercises performed by a resident by contracting, then relaxing a muscle while maintaining a fixed position	Maintain strength in an immobilized joint	Contract the muscle without moving the joint. Hold the contraction for a few seconds, then relax. Practice deep breathing during the exercises.

PROCEDURE

14 SAMPLE ISOMETRIC EXERCISES

The exercises given here are samples only. The therapist or restorative nurse will develop a program for the resident. The resident will start gradually by performing each exercise two to three times, twice a day. This will be increased to ten times, three times daily.

1. Perform your beginning procedure actions.

2. Assist the resident to a position of comfort.

3. Instruct the resident not to hold his or her breath during exercise. Perform each exercise during exhalation.

4. Instruct the resident to contract the quadriceps (thigh muscles). Hold for 10 seconds and relax. Repeat as tolerated.

5. Tell the resident to contract the gluteal (buttocks) muscles. Hold for 10 seconds and relax. Repeat as tolerated.

6. Instruct the resident to contract the abdominal (stomach) muscles. Hold for 10 seconds and relax. Repeat as tolerated.

7. Perform your procedure completion actions.

Isometric Exercises

A therapist or nurse may teach residents **isometric exercises. Isometrics** is the science of exercise without movement. These exercises help maintain strength when a joint is immobilized. You may be assigned to remind and assist residents with isometric exercises by providing verbal cues. Isometrics involves alternately contracting and relaxing a muscle while maintaining it in a fixed position.

▄▄▄ RANGE OF MOTION EXERCISES

Maintaining a resident's range of motion is a very important part of restorative care. Range of motion is important for keeping residents active, healthy, and independent. Most restorative nursing programs and ADL skills are built upon the residents' ability to perform range of motion.

Range of motion is the normal movement of the joints. Ability to move the joints is affected by:

▄ Age

▄ Body size

▄ Genetics

▄ Activity

▄ Presence or absence of disease

▄ The effects of fractures, deformities, or injuries

We do range of motion many times each day in activities of daily living, and at work. Surveyors like to observe passive range of motion exercises during a survey **(Figure 11–6)**. The restorative nurse may observe the resident during morning care to evaluate range of motion. Most people go through the full range of motion when bathing. A summary of

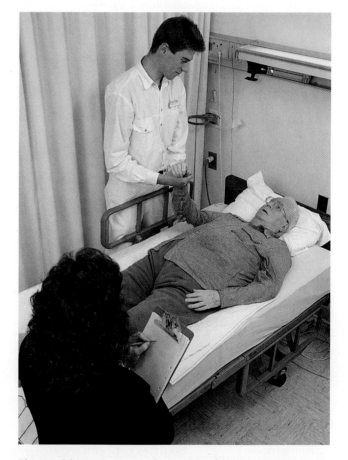

Figure 11–6 Surveyors frequently observe range of motion exercises during a survey.

motions used during a bed bath is found in **Table 11–2.** If you observe a resident having difficulty with these movements, notify your supervisor. He or she will assess the resident further.

Table 11–2 Observations of Range of Motion During Bathing

Activity	Range of Motion Movement or Body Alignment
Holds bath blanket while nursing or restorative assistant removes sheet	Pronation Finger flexion Elbow flexion
Washing resident's face, turning the head to the side	Neck rotation
Resident lying flat on back without pillow under head	Neck extension Dorsal spine extension
Resident or staff lift head for washing, toothbrushing, styling hair	Neck flexion
Washing shoulder, arm, **axilla** (underarm)	Elevation of shoulder External rotation of shoulder Flexion of shoulder Elbow flexion
Washing forearm	Internal rotation of shoulder Pronation and supination of forearm
Staff bathing hand or resident brushing own hair	Flexion and extension of wrist Finger flexion and extension Thumb abduction and adduction Thumb flexion and extension Thumb opposition
Washing chest and abdomen	Observe for symmetrical positioning of trunk
Placing foot in basin, drying leg and foot	Flexion and extension of hip and knee Dorsal flexion of foot Plantar flexion of foot
Washing inside and bottom of leg	Hip abduction
Moving leg in and out for washing and drying	Internal and external rotation of hip

In some facilities, the restorative nurse or therapists measure the residents' range of motion measurements. Measurements are recorded in degrees. This is done on admission and periodically thereafter. High-risk residents are measured quarterly, before the care conference. Having baseline measurements shows whether the resident is staying the same, improving, or declining. Many facilities take measurements at the time the range of motion program is ordered. An instrument called a **goniometer (Figure 11–7)** is used. The measurements are recorded in degrees. They are compared with a chart listing normal joint range of motion.

🆂🅰In some facilities, the restorative assistant screens residents' range of motion. This is done by marking the resident's range of motion on a picture. The nurse reviews the information. If the range of motion is limited, the nurse will assess the resident further. Surveyors in some states require facilities to take quarterly measurements of all residents.🆂🅰

Reasons for Range of Motion Exercises

Residents who have been ill or confined to bed are not as active, so joints do not move through the normal range of motion daily. Weakness and

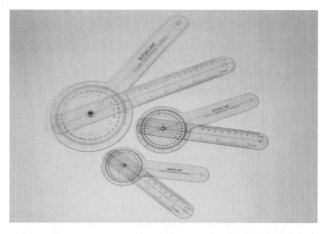

Figure 11–7 The goniometer is an instrument used to measure the degree of joint movement. Measuring joint function upon admission and periodically thereafter shows whether the resident's function is being maintained, improving, or declining. Surveyors in some states require that these measurements be taken quarterly. (Courtesy of Briggs Corporation, Des Moines, IA. (800) 247-2343)

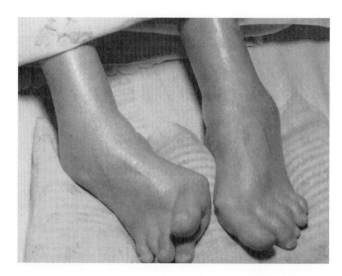

Figure 11–8 Contractures are difficult to reverse. This resident is unable to walk.

muscle wasting from lack of use is called **atrophy**. Over time, muscles become rigid. The joints do not move as freely as they once did. Joint movement may be painful because the muscles have shortened from lack of use. When the joint moves, the muscle stretches. This causes discomfort or pain. Contractures and deformities develop **(Figure 11–8).** *Contractures* are disfigurements caused by muscle shortening. They are serious, painful complications of inactivity. Contractures make caring for the resident more difficult. Residents with contractures of the feet and ankles cannot walk. Footboards should be used for all bedfast residents to prevent contractures. Placing residents in the prone position for 15 to 30 minutes daily stretches the muscles. This helps prevent contractures. Avoiding the sitting position for prolonged periods also helps prevent flexion contractures.

Residents' joints must be moved regularly to prevent complications. If residents cannot move independently, you may be responsible for exercising the joints. ⓢⒶAll residents should be exercised regularly to prevent deformities. This includes residents with no potential for rehabilitation. Like pressure sores, contractures and deformities are much easier to prevent than to reverse. However, they can be reversed, particularly in the early stages. If a resident has previously had a contracture in an extremity, he or she will be on a maintenance program. This will prevent the muscles from shortening again. Reversing contractures requires diligent effort by staff.ⓢⒶ

Frequency of Range of Motion Exercises

ⓢⒶIn most facilities, range of motion exercises are part of the routine care of all residents. Range of motion is a routine nursing measure.ⓢⒶ A physician's order is not required for most residents. Residents with contractures, arthritic deformities, chronic pain, injuries, or recent surgery must have an order. In many facilities, nursing assistants perform range of motion on residents without contractures. The restorative assistant performs range of motion on residents with contractures, arthritis, and other special problems. In some facilities, restorative assistants do range of motion exercises on all residents. Take your responsibilities for providing range of motion exercises very seriously. Sometimes the therapist or restorative nurse will prescribe a special routine. The care plan will describe the resident's individual program. Your facility will have a policy for how often to perform range of motion exercises. Most facilities exercise residents two or three times a day. Each joint is taken through its normal range of motion three to five times. Five repetitions for each joint is most common. In some circumstances, more repetitions are ordered. Know and follow your facility policy.

Types of Range of Motion Exercises

All range of motion exercises are based on the principles of passive range of motion. Knowing and understanding how to perform these exercises is important. Once you master passive exercises, other types of range of motion are simple. When assisting residents with active exercises, use verbal cues and demonstration as much as possible. Avoid giving hands-on assistance unless absolutely necessary.

Active Range of Motion

Active range of motion (AROM) exercises are done by most residents each day. Active range of motion maintains movement, prevents deformity, and strengthens muscles. AROMs are done during movement, ADLs, certain activities, and in exercise groups. Some residents do not remember to exercise. You will give verbal cues, talk, and demonstrate to help them with AROM exercises. Some residents cannot move all of their joints independently. However, they may be able to use a strong extremity to exercise a weaker extremity. For example, a resident who has had a stroke has a strong right arm and a weak left arm. Teach this resident to move the weak arm with the stronger arm.

Active Assisted Range of Motion

Active assisted range of motion (AAROM) may also be called active assistive range of motion. These exercises are either started or completed by the resident. The exercises are done when the resident needs assistance moving because of:

- Paralysis
- **Paresis** (slight paralysis)
- Weakness
- Pain
- Serious cardiopulmonary problems
- Increased spasticity

Limit your assistance to only what the resident needs. Sometimes, no hands-on assistance is necessary. You will provide verbal cues and demonstration. Supervise the resident to make sure that he or she exercises correctly. Sometimes pieces of equipment, such as pulleys, are used for exercising joints. This is another form of active assisted range of motion.

Passive Range of Motion

Passive range of motion (PROM) exercises are performed for residents when independent movement is impossible. Passive range of motion exercises maintain movement and prevent deformities. They do not strengthen the muscles. You will perform PROM for residents with conditions such as:

- Paralysis
- Contractures
- Orthopedic conditions
- Neurologic disorders
- Severe cognitive impairment

Passive range of motion exercises are also ordered when residents are unable to move joints safely or when active movement:

- Increases spasticity
- Causes pain
- Creates excessive stress on the heart

The resident must be comfortable and relaxed during the exercises. Each joint is taken through the normal range of movement.

If residents resist PROM, you can exercise them during a bath or in the whirlpool. The movements are easier and less painful in water. Some cognitively impaired residents may resist your attempts at exercise. However, they will do range of motion exercises with pulleys or a bicycle pedaler. If this is the case, allow them to do this each day. They will enjoy the activity and benefit from the exercise.

Resistive Range of Motion

Resistive range of motion exercises are prescribed to increase strength. Residents work against manual or mechanical resistance. At the beginning of the exercise program, the resistance is slight. The amount of resistance is increased as the resident develops strength and endurance.

Precautions and Special Situations

Residents with certain conditions require special care and handling. Avoid exercising extremities with fractures or dislocations. When assisting residents with healed hip or other joint replacements, avoid internal rotation. Also avoid adduction beyond the midline. Some residents have bones that break easily. Osteoporosis is a condition in which bone mass decreases. This leads to fractures with little or no trauma. You have learned that residents with this condition may develop spontaneous fractures. Check with your supervisor and the care plans for residents who have special situations or osteoporosis.

If the resident has a wound or pressure ulcer, check to see if exercise will harm the healing tissue. If a resident is combative or resists exercise, avoid forcing him or her. Gently explain and demonstrate the procedure. Try to coax the resident into participating. Sometimes singing an old song will distract the resident. Encourage the resident to sing along with you. If distracted, he or she may allow you to perform the exercises. The resident may even have fun! Notify your supervisor if the resident continues to refuse.

Some residents have muscle spasms and rigidity. When exercising residents with these conditions, move the joint slowly and smoothly. Stop at the point of resistance. Apply gentle, steady pressure until the muscle relaxes **(Figure 11–10)**. Avoid rapid, jerking movements. Avoid stretching the

PROCEDURE

15 RESISTIVE EXERCISES

The exercises listed here are for various parts of the body. The therapist or restorative nurse will provide information about the area(s) to exercise and the number of repetitions. The resident will begin gradually. Perform each exercise three times, two to three times daily. As the resident gains strength, the number of repetitions is increased. The goal is to perform 10 repetitions of each exercise, or as ordered.

1. Perform your beginning procedure actions.

2. Assist the resident to the supine position.

3. Using a rope attached to the foot of the bed, pull the body up to a sitting position (strengthens the shoulders and arms).

4. Assist the resident to the prone position, if able.

5. Instruct the resident to place the palms flat on the bed at shoulder height. Push down on the bed, elevating the upper part of the body (strengthens the arms).

6. Assist the resident to sit in a chair or dangle on the side of the bed.

7. Tell the resident to place the palms flat on the mattress or chair seat. Push up to lift the hips off the surface (strengthens the arms).

8. Assist the resident to the supine position.

9. Instruct the resident to bend the knees, then push the feet against the footboard (strengthens the legs).

10. Place the resident's leg through an elastic band and have the resident push against it while you hold the top **(Figure 11–9).**

11. Perform your procedure completion actions.

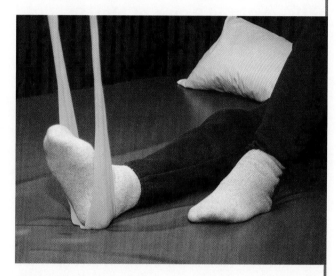

Figure 11–9 Use of this special elastic band is a form of resistive exercise. The resident pulls the leg down while the restorative nursing assistant holds the band.

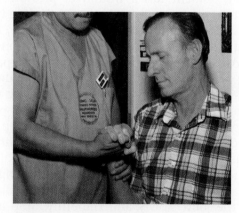

Figure 11–10 This resident's right arm is contracted. The restorative assistant is holding gentle, steady pressure on the forearm to relieve spasticity.

joint too far. These activities cause pain and worsen the condition. Suspect muscle spasms if resistance progressively increases during exercise. Rigidity presents as resistance to movement in any direction. Slow, continuous, sustained movements help prevent spasticity and rigidity. If rigidity and muscle spasms develop, hold steady, gentle pressure on the muscle. Avoid forcing the muscle past the point of resistance. This should enable you to complete the exercise. Report the problems to your supervisor. The restorative nurse or therapist will provide specific instructions.

Range of Motion Terminology

Some important terms used to describe common joint movements are listed in **Table 11–3.**

Table 11–3   Range of Motion Terminology

Term	Definition
Abduction	Moving an extremity *away from* the body.
Adduction	Moving an extremity *toward* the body.
Circumduction	A circular movement of a joint, such as the thumb or wrist.
Dorsal flexion or **dorsiflexion**	Pulling the toes and ball of the foot upward toward the head.
Eversion	Turning a joint outward.
Extension	Straightening a joint.
External rotation	Turning a joint outward away from the median line.
Flexion	Bending a joint.
Hyperextension	Gentle, excessive extension of a joint, slightly past the point of resistance.
Internal rotation	Turning a joint inward toward the median line.
Inversion	Turning a joint inward.
Medial	Pertains to or is situated toward the midline of the body.
Median	Situated in the median plane or in the midline of the body.
Opposition	Touching each of the fingers against the thumb.
Palmar flexion	Bending the hand down toward the palm.
Plantar flexion	Bending the foot downward, away from the body.
Pronation	Moving a joint to face downward.
Radial deviation	Turning the forearm toward the radius.
Retraction	Drawing back, away from the body.
Rotation	Moving a joint in, out, and around.
Supination	Moving a joint so it faces upward.
Ulnar deviation	Turning the forearm toward the ulna.

PROCEDURE

16 PASSIVE RANGE OF MOTION EXERCISES

1. Position the resident in good alignment in the supine position.

2. Exercise each extremity as indicated on the care plan. Support the extremity above and below the joint.

   a. Head and neck (if this is your facility policy or if you have a physician's order)

   1. Tip the head forward, bringing the chin to the chest (flexion) **(Figure 11–11A).**

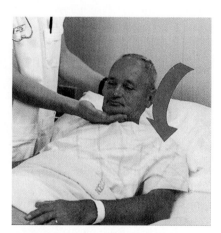

Figure 11–11A   Neck flexion

   2. Tip the head backward, with the chin up (extension).

   3. Move the head from side to side (rotation).

   4. Move the head back and forth in a circular motion (circumduction).

   b. Shoulders, arms, and elbows

   1. Raise the arm over the head, then return the arm to the side (flexion and extension).

   2. Move the arm from side to side, as far away from the body as possible, then return to the side (abduction and adduction) **(Figure 11–11B).**

   3. Move the arm across the chest until the fingers touch the opposite shoulder. Return the arm to the side (horizontal adduction and horizontal abduction).

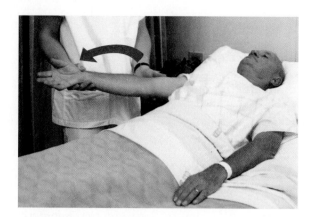

Figure 11–11B   Elbow extension

   4. With the arm straight out at the side, bend at the elbow and rotate the shoulder. Return the arm to the side (external and internal rotation).

   5. Bend at the elbow and bring the hand to the shoulder. Return the arm to the side (flexion and extension) **(Figure 11–11C).**

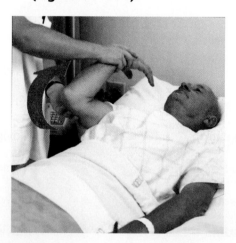

Figure 11–11C   Elbow flexion

   c. Wrists, fingers, and forearms

   1. Support the elbow.

   2. Grasp the hand as in a handshake. Turn the palm up, then down (supination and pronation).

   3. Bend the hand back gently at the wrist, then return to the neutral position (extension and hyperextension).

(continues)

PROCEDURE **16** *continued*

4. Bend the hand forward at the wrist, then return to the neutral position (flexion) **(Figure 11–11D).**

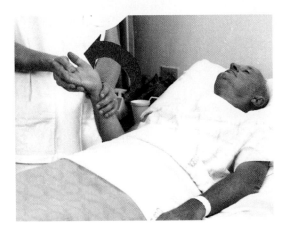

Figure 11–11D Wrist extension

5. Move the hand from side to side, first toward the thumb, then outward (radial deviation and ulnar deviation).

6. Move the hand in a circle (circumduction).

7. Clench the fingers and thumb as if making a fist (flexion).

8. Extend the fingers and thumb (extension) **(Figure 11–11E).**

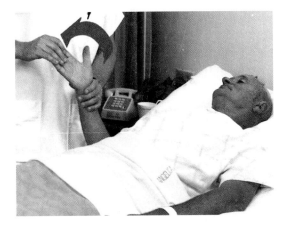

Figure 11–11E Finger extension

9. Spread the fingers and thumb together and then apart (adduction and abduction) **(Figure 11–11F).**

10. Flex and extend the joints in the thumb and fingers (flexion and extension).

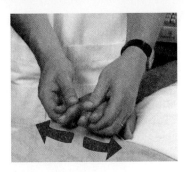

Figure 11–11F Finger abduction

11. Move the thumb in a circular motion (circumduction).

12. Touch each finger to the thumb (opposition) **(Figure 11–11G).**

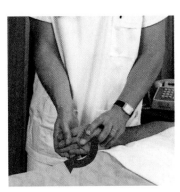

Figure 11–11G Thumb opposition

d. Legs, hips, and knees

1. Keeping the knee straight, raise the leg up and down (flexion and extension).

2. Bend and straighten the knee (flexion and extension) **(Figure 11–11H).**

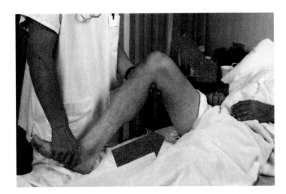

Figure 11–11H Hip and knee flexion

(continues)

3. With the leg resting on the bed, roll it inward and outward (internal rotation and external rotation).

4. Stretch the leg out from the body. Return the leg to touch the other leg (abduction and adduction) **(Figure 11–11I)**.

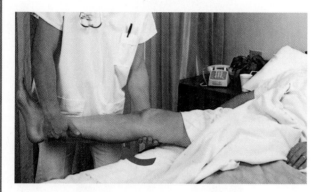

Figure 11–11I Hip abduction

e. Ankles, feet, and toes

1. With the leg straight on the bed, bend ankle toward the knee, then back down (dorsal flexion or dorsiflexion) **(Figure 11–11J)**.

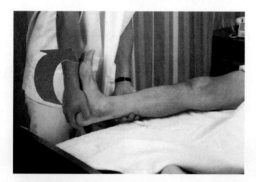

Figure 11–11J Dorsiflexion of the ankle

2. Push the foot and toes out gently downward, pointing toward the foot of the bed (plantar flexion) **(Figure 11–11K)**.

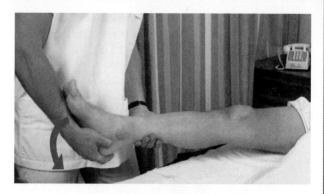

Figure 11–11K Plantar flexion of the ankle

3. With the leg straight, turn the foot and ankle from side to side (inversion and eversion) **(Figure 11–11L)**.

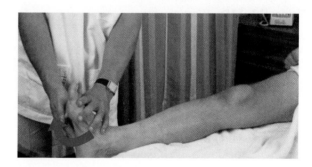

Figure 11–11L Foot eversion

4. Bend the toes downward and upward (flexion and extension).

5. Spread each toe apart, then back together again (abduction and adduction) **(Figure 11–11M)**.

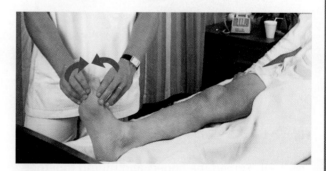

Figure 11–11M Toe adduction

General Guidelines for Assisting Residents with Range of Motion Exercises

- Check the care plan for specific guidelines and limitations.
- Explain the procedure to the resident.
- Before beginning, make sure the resident is comfortable.
- Position the resident in good body alignment, in the supine position, before beginning.
- Elevate the bed to a comfortable working height.
- Use good posture and apply the principles of good body mechanics.
- Encourage the resident to assist, if able, but keep your hands in position to provide support.
- Make sure you have enough space for full movement of the extremities.
- Expose only the part of the body you are exercising.
- Support each joint by placing one hand above and one hand below the joint.
- Move each joint slowly and consistently. Stop briefly at the end of each motion.
- Work systematically from the top of the body to the bottom.
- Never push the resident past the point of joint resistance. Move each joint as far as it will comfortably go.
- In many facilities, the neck is not exercised without a physician's order. Know and follow your facility policy.
- Perform each joint motion three to five times, or according to facility policy.
- Stop the exercise and report to your supervisor if the resident complains of pain. Watch the resident's body language and facial expression for signs of pain.
- Be alert for changes in the resident's condition during the activity. If you feel that the activity is harming the resident, stop. Notify your supervisor or a nurse. Changes that suggest a potential problem are pain, shortness of breath, sweating, and change in color.
- Help the resident relax during exercise.
- Use the exercise period as quality time to communicate with the resident.
- For residents who are stiff or combative, consider doing the exercise in the bathtub or whirlpool. Check with your supervisor.

ASSISTING THE RESIDENT WITH INDEPENDENT BED MOVEMENT

The progressive mobility program begins with independent movement in bed. Moving in bed:

- Provides exercise
- Prevents skin breakdown
- Permits the resident to reposition at will
- Prepares the resident to participate in transfer procedures

The directions here are for residents with hemiplegia or hemiparesis. They can be adapted for residents with many conditions.

PROCEDURE

17 ASSISTING THE RESIDENT TO MOVE INDEPENDENTLY IN BED

1. Perform your beginning procedure actions.

   ### a. Moving to the head or foot of the bed

   1. Instruct the resident to fold the affected arm across the abdomen. Grasp the leg with the strong hand.

   2. Instruct the resident to move the strong foot under the calf of the affected leg. Slide the foot down to the ankle.

   3. While maintaining this position, instruct the resident to flex the knee of the strong leg, placing the foot flat on the bed.

   4. Tell the resident to lift the head and hips, pushing up toward the head of the bed with the unaffected arm and leg.

   5. Repeat the procedure as necessary until proper positioning is achieved.

   6. Reverse the procedure to move to the foot of the bed.

   ### b. Moving to the head or foot of the bed using a trapeze

   A trapeze may be fastened over the head of the bed. The resident can use this device to move independently in bed. He or she moves by pulling on the trapeze, while simultaneously pushing with the feet.

   1. Instruct the resident to hold the trapeze with the strong hand.

   2. Tell the resident to move the strong foot under the calf of the affected leg. Slide the foot down to the ankle.

   3. While maintaining this position, instruct the resident to flex the knee of the strong leg, placing the foot flat on the bed.

   4. Tell the resident to lift the head, push down with the foot to lift the hips, and pull upward on the trapeze toward the head of the bed.

   5. Repeat the procedure as necessary until proper positioning is achieved.

   6. To move to the foot of the bed, reverse the procedure.

   ### c. Moving to the side of the bed

   The resident's body is moved in segments during this procedure.

   1. Tell the resident to fold the affected arm across the abdomen. Grasp the leg with the unaffected hand.

   2. Instruct the resident to move the strong foot under the calf of the affected leg. Slide the foot down to the ankle.

   3. Lift the strong foot and move the affected leg in the desired direction.

   4. Instruct the resident to remove the foot, flex the knee, and place the sole of the foot flat on the bed.

   5. Tell the resident to push the foot down, lift the hips, and move to the desired side of the bed.

   6. Tell the resident to place the strong arm on the leg or place the palm of the hand flat on the bed, depending on which direction he or she is moving. Lift the head and shoulders. If moving toward the strong side, have the resident pull on the leg. If moving toward the affected side, push the palm of the hand down on the mattress, lock the elbow, and slide the shoulders toward the affected side.

   ### d. Moving to the side of the bed using a trapeze

   1. Tell the resident to fold the affected arm across the abdomen. Grasp the trapeze with the unaffected hand.

   2. Instruct the resident to move the strong foot under the calf of the affected leg. Slide the foot down to the ankle.

   3. Lift the strong foot and move the affected leg in the desired direction.

   4. Instruct the resident to remove the foot, flex the knee, and place the sole of the foot flat on the bed.

   5. Tell the resident to grasp the trapeze with the strong hand.

(continues)

6. Instruct the resident to pull on the trapeze, while simultaneously pushing the foot down, lifting the hips over to the desired side of the bed.

e. Turning to the sides

1. Instruct the resident to move to the side of the bed opposite the direction in which he or she wishes to turn, following the directions in step c or d.

2. If the resident will be turning onto the affected side, have him or her grab the leg on that side with the strong hand and pull his or her body over. If the resident will be turning onto the strong side, instruct him or her to grasp the affected hand with the strong hand. Extend the arm and lock the elbow. Raise the arms in the air. Using the strong arm, swing the body over onto the strong side.

2. Perform your procedure completion actions.

KEY POINTS IN CHAPTER

Residents in the long-term care facility need exercise for their overall health and well-being.

Begin the exercise program gradually, increasing as the resident develops endurance.

Monitor the pulse during exercise, stopping if the rate exceeds 100.

Exercising a joint several times a day is better than exercising it once.

Therapeutic exercises are specifically planned for individual residents to maintain or improve joint function. The purpose of therapeutic exercises is to prevent and correct deformities, diseases, and injuries.

Range of motion is the normal movement of the joints. It is affected by age, body size, genetics, activity, and the presence or absence of disease.

Range of motion exercises prevent contractures and deformities, improve circulation, and enhance the resident's sense of well-being.

Active range of motion exercises are done by residents each day during movement, ADLs, certain activities, and in exercise groups.

Active assisted range of motion exercises are done when the resident needs assistance moving because of paralysis, paresis, weakness, pain, serious heart problems, or increased spasticity. The exercises are either started or completed by the resident.

Passive range of motion exercises are performed for residents with conditions such as paralysis, contractures, orthopedic and neurologic disorders, and severe cognitive impairment, or when independent movement is impossible.

Resistive range of motion exercises are prescribed by the licensed therapist to increase strength.

The progressive mobility program begins with teaching residents how to move independently in bed, providing exercise, preventing skin breakdown, and preparing the resident to participate in transfer procedures.

CLINICAL APPLICATIONS

1. Mrs. Springer has arthritic deformities of her elbows and knees. You are assigned to perform passive range of motion exercises on this resident. Are special instructions necessary? Where does the restorative nursing assistant find information about the resident's range of motion?

2. The residents in your facility begin arriving in the dining room 30 to 45 minutes before each meal. They sit and patiently wait for meals, and converse with each other occasionally. What restorative activities can you suggest while these residents are waiting for meals to be served? How would you go about convincing facility management that these activities would be beneficial to residents?

3. Mr. Li is receiving skilled physical therapy. He is doing well. The therapist is in the facility. She is running behind schedule in completing an assessment on a new resident. She asks you to perform range of motion exercises on Mr. Li. This resident had hip surgery two weeks ago. What will you do?

4. Mrs. Ianelli is an alert resident who had a CVA with right hemiparesis. She was previously right-handed. What type of range of motion exercises would you suggest for this resident?

5. Mr. Martinez is on a bed mobility program. He has a trapeze at the head of the bed. Explain how you will teach him to move to the head and foot of the bed using the trapeze.

CHAPTER 12

Progressive Mobility: Transfer Training and Wheelchair Mobility

After reading this chapter, you should be able to:

- *Spell and define key terms.*
- *List 10 preliminary activities the resident must complete before participating in a transfer or ambulation program.*
- *Identify the main parts of the wheelchair and explain the purpose of each.*
- *Describe how to measure a resident for a wheelchair.*
- *List at least five safety factors to consider when transferring residents.*
- *Describe two methods of relieving pressure for residents in wheelchairs.*

THE NURSING PROCESS AND RESTORATIVE MOBILITY PROGRAMS

You will have many responsibilities while working with residents in mobility programs. Mobility programs teach the residents to transfer and either propel a wheelchair or ambulate. Standing to transfer and ambulate keeps the resident healthy. If residents do not stand, calcium drains from their long bones, increasing the risk of injury.

Preliminary Activities

Residents must complete some initial goals before beginning a mobility program. Mobility programs also use the goal-oriented approach. Residents must meet several small goals first. This will enable them to put the pieces together to accomplish a larger goal. The preliminary activities are determined by the therapist or restorative nurse. The licensed person develops a program based on an assessment, including a task analysis. In the early stages of the program, the resident may receive skilled therapy. You may assist the resident with therapy. You may also reinforce what the resident has learned in the companion restorative program.

Progressive Mobility

Progressive mobility increases the resident's activity level gradually. A complete program is summarized in **Table 12–1**. Restorative care is individualized for each resident. Some residents learn to complete each step of the mobility program independently. Others will be able to complete only some of the steps without assistance. The resident may always need assistance with other tasks. Preliminary activities to transfer and ambulation programs include:

- Gradually increasing the length of time the resident is out of bed each day. You will assist the resident to be up for a short time twice a day. The time is increased according to the resident's tolerance.
- Teaching and assisting the resident to perform active range-of-motion exercises. This strengthens uninvolved muscles. The resident may use these muscles more to compensate for the illness or injury.
- Performing passive range-of-motion exercises on involved muscles.
- Teaching the resident to roll over in bed to both the involved and uninvolved side.
- Teaching the resident to dangle.
- Teaching the resident to balance and sit unsupported.
- Teaching the resident to stand.
- Teaching the resident to transfer.
- Teaching the resident to propel a wheelchair.
- Teaching the resident to ambulate, with or without an assistive device

Table 12-1 Progressive Mobility Program

Program Task	Purpose and Implementation of Task
Bed mobility	■ Increases ability to move independently in bed ■ Prevents skin breakdown, pneumonia, and other complications related to lack of movement ■ Teaches resident how to move and turn using side rails and overbed trapeze ■ Teaches resident principles of positioning and body alignment to prevent complications, deformity, and injury, as well as promote comfort
Transfer training	■ Teaches resident to transfer from bed to chair and back ■ Teaches resident how to transfer without weight bearing on affected leg ■ Teaches staff members how to assist resident using transfer belt and no weight bearing on affected leg
Strengthening	■ Increases arm strength in preparation for learning to walk with a walker ■ Increases strength in unaffected leg ■ Involves a series of exercises at the parallel bars and no weight bearing on affected leg; gait belt may be used to support resident during exercise
Ambulation with walker and no weight bearing	■ This step is not always used, but some programs teach the resident how to ambulate with a walker and no weight bearing on the affected leg, to improve independence and ambulate short distances
Ambulation with walker and weight bearing	■ Weight bearing on affected leg begins at parallel bars ■ Resident initially begins to stand and balance at parallel bars ■ When resident can safely stand and balance, he or she is taught to walk holding parallel bars ■ Resident progresses to using walker, gait belt, and one assistant to walk short distances; distance is gradually increased
Progressive independence	■ If the resident is able, he or she will be taught to use a cane or to walk without assistive devices

Assisting Residents to Sit on the Side of the Bed

Dangling is the first step to getting out of bed **(Figure 12–1)** Dangling means sitting on the side of the bed with the legs hanging over the edge of the mattress. This is an important procedure for residents who have been admitted from the hospital. The resident may be weak and unsteady. Sitting on the side of the bed will help him or her balance before getting up. Residents may become dizzy after lying down because of postural and blood pressure changes. Dangling helps the resident regain stability before transfers or ambulation. It prevents fainting and loss of balance. Stay with the resident while he or she is dangling. Monitor the skin for perspiration or pale color. If you observe these changes,

return the resident to the supine position. Notify your supervisor or a nurse.

■■ WHEELCHAIRS

The wheelchair is an important piece of restorative equipment. Many residents use wheelchairs for mobility. Some will progress to ambulation. Others will always use the wheelchair to move about. ⒮ⒶWhenever possible, the facility must restore the resident's ability to ambulate.ⓈⒶ

Because residents spend so much time in wheelchairs, careful attention to fitting the chair to the resident is very important **(Figure 12–2)**. Sometimes wheelchairs are ordered to meet special resident needs. For example, some residents with hemiplegia

PROCEDURE

18 ASSISTING THE RESIDENT TO DANGLE

1. Perform your beginning procedure actions.
2. Place the bed in the lowest horizontal position.
3. Elevate the head of the bed.
4. Assist the resident to move to the side of the bed closest to you.
5. Place your arm closest to the head under the resident's shoulders, palm side up.
6. Place your other arm under the resident's knees, palm side up.
7. Lift the back and knees, and support the shoulders. Pivot the resident so the legs are hanging over the side of the bed with the back straight.
8. Assist the resident to maintain balance, if necessary.
9. If the resident will be getting out of bed, assist him or her to dress or put on robe and nonslip footwear.
10. Stay with the resident. Monitor for changes in color and moisture of the skin.
11. To return the resident to bed, reverse the procedure. Pivot the resident back to the supine position.
12. Perform your procedure completion actions.

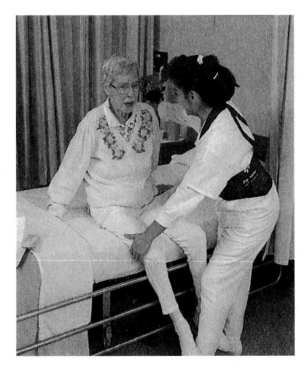

Figure 12–1 Dangling is the first step in getting out of bed. Return the resident to the supine position if she becomes weak or dizzy. When dangling, support the feet on the floor or a foot stool.

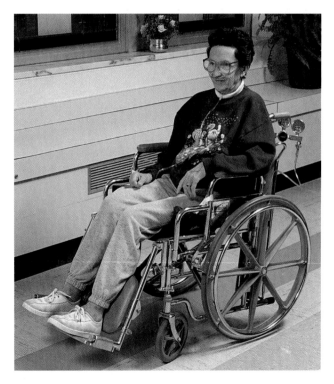

Figure 12–2 This resident is sitting in good body alignment and the chair fits her correctly. Attention to fitting the chair and proper positioning improves the resident's body function and ability to propel the chair.

can propel the wheelchair independently. They use their strong arm on the wheel and push the strong leg on the floor. The hemi wheelchair **(Figure 12–3)** has a seat that is four inches lower than a regular wheelchair. This makes foot propulsion easier.

Brakes

The brakes are an important feature of the wheelchair. Several types of brakes are available. The most common type uses a lever system to lock the chair. The brakes must be secure during transfers. Set them when the wheelchair is parked. ⑤If the chair slips even slightly, the brakes are not working properly.⑤ Notify your supervisor or the appropriate person in your facility if you believe the brakes are not working correctly.

Some residents do not lock the brakes on the wheelchair because they cannot reach them. For example, a resident with hemiparesis may not be able to reach the brake on the affected side. Extensions are available to lengthen the brake handle **(Figure 12–4)**. Some facilities create brake extensions by attaching PVC pipe. Some reclining wheelchairs have two brakes on each side. Both must be engaged to hold the chair securely. The first brake is the normal front wheelchair brake. When the back of the chair is reclined, the center of gravity changes. The single brake in front is not effective when the chair is tilted. A second brake in the back of the chair provides stability.

Caster Wheels

The small, front caster wheels of the chair provide the ability to move in all directions. The large part of the wheel faces back when the chair is moving. When the chair is parked, position the large part of the front wheel facing forward. This changes the center of gravity in the chair. Positioning the wheels to face forward prevents tipping if the resident leans forward. It helps stabilize the chair if the resident picks up an item from the floor. To reposition the wheels, back the chair up, then move it forward.

Drive Wheels

The large, rear wheels are the drive wheels. The most common type of wheel is made from solid rubber. An air-filled wheel may also be used. Air-filled tires are more comfortable and stable on soft or uneven surfaces. They must have enough air in them for the resident to propel the chair easily. If you believe a tire is low, notify the appropriate person.

The outer rim of the drive wheels is used for pushing the chair. Some residents have difficulty pushing because their hands slip. A nonslip surface can be applied to the outer rim. Special nonslip

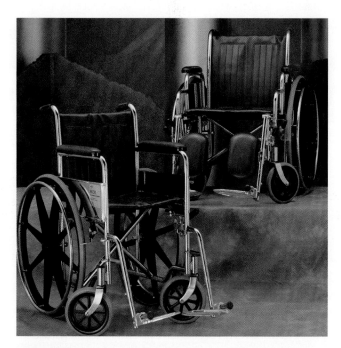

Figure 12–3 The seat on the hemiplegia wheelchair is lower than a regular wheelchair seat. (Courtesy of Medline Industries, Inc. (800) MEDLINE)

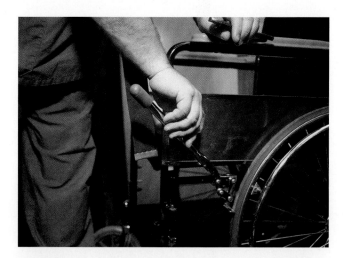

Figure 12–4 The brake extension is attached so the resident can reach it with the arm on the opposite side of the body, if necessary.

gloves will also correct the problem. Projections can be added to the outer rim for residents who cannot grasp the round wheel. The projections increase the width of the chair. However, they promote resident independence. Propelling the wheelchair independently is better for the residents. It provides exercise and permits them to move about the facility at will. This is much more satisfying than having to wait for someone to transport them.

Armrests

Armrests are available in two lengths. The desk-length armrest is lower in the front than in the back. This enables the resident to get close to tables. The chair works well for residents who sit in wheelchairs at mealtime. The full-length armrest is most common. The armrest is comfortable when the resident is seated. (SA)However, getting close to tables may be a problem. Elevating the table height does not solve the problem. Raising the table allows the resident to move closer. However, most residents are too short to benefit from the increased table height. They may end up eating with their elbows in the air because the table is too high.(SA) This is very uncomfortable and causes shoulder strain. It may cause some residents to have problems eating. Attaching a lap tray to the armrests corrects the problem.

Armrests can be removable or nonremovable. Removable armrests are necessary for sliding boards and some other transfers. The armrest height is adjustable in some chairs. (SA)Residents' shoulders should not be elevated when they are seated.(SA) This is more comfortable and prevents muscle strain.

Leg and Foot Rests

(SA)The resident's feet must be supported when the chair is being moved. They should never dangle in the air or drag the floor.(SA) The length for the legs can be adjusted in many chairs. This enables you to adjust the chair so the feet reach the footrests. If the leg length cannot be adjusted, a footrest elevator **(Figure 12–5)** can be used. Your maintenance department may make footrest elevators out of wood. (SA)When the wheelchair is parked, the resident's legs should be supported on the footrests or the floor. Allowing the legs to dangle is uncomfortable and increases the risk of blood clots.(SA) Advise residents to avoid leaning forward or picking up items from the floor. If the feet are on the footrests, the chair will tip. During the mobility program, you will teach residents how to pick up items safely.

You may teach residents with hemiparesis to propel the chair by moving the strong leg on the floor. Here, the footrest on the strong side is removed. One footrest is used to support the affected leg.

Many wheelchairs have removable legs. Remove the legs during transfers. However, make sure to replace them afterward. Facilities have many different types of wheelchairs. If the legs become separated from the chair, matching them up may be difficult.

Some wheelchairs have swing-away or pivoting legs. A lever on the side releases the leg. They are folded to the side during transfers. When using wheelchairs with fixed legs, raise the footrests during

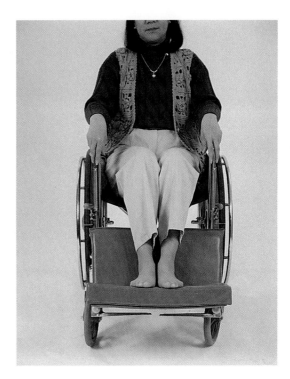

Figure 12–5 The feet must always be supported when the resident is sitting in a chair. Unsupported feet and legs are uncomfortable and increase the risk of blood clots. (Courtesy of Skil-Care Corporation, Yonkers, NY (800) 431-2972)

transfers. If they fall down, notify your supervisor or the proper person in your facility. The footrest is easily tightened. Heel loops may be used to keep the resident's feet from slipping off the back of the footrest. Pull the loop forward to raise the footrest.

Some residents with edema or fractures need chairs with elevating legs. This type of leg rest is also used for residents with contractures, or those who cannot flex the knees. Support the calf with a pad when the leg is elevated. A lock on the side holds the leg rest in place. For safety, support the leg with one hand while operating the lock with the other.

Reclining-Back Wheelchairs

Reclining-back wheelchairs **(Figure 12–6)** are used for residents who cannot sit upright. The chair back supports the head and neck. Adjust the back for comfort and maximum functional ability. Avoid reclining it farther than necessary. (The reasons for this are described in Chapter 9.) When adjusting the back, support the resident. Suddenly releasing the lock will cause him or her to fall back quickly. This causes pain and potential injury.

Amputee-Frame Wheelchairs

The center of gravity in the amputee-frame wheelchair is different from other chairs. The drive

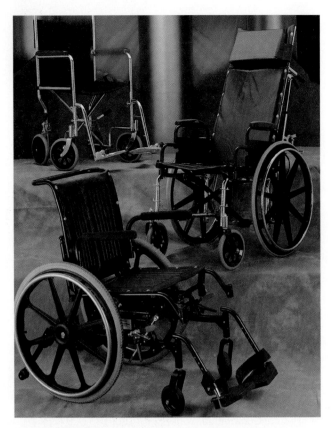

Figure 12–6 The reclining wheelchair is used for residents who do not have trunk, head, or neck control. Keep the back as upright as possible. Being upright helps the resident maintain orientation to the environment. (Courtesy of Medline Industries, Inc. (800) MEDLINE)

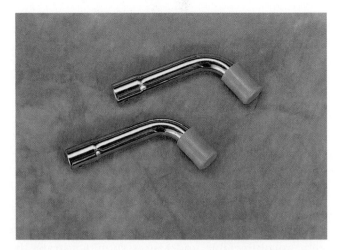

Figure 12–7 Anti-tipping devices are fastened to the back of the wheelchair to act as a counterbalance. (Courtesy of Medline Industries, Inc. (800) MEDLINE)

wheels are set behind the back support to prevent tipping. An amputation changes the resident's center of gravity. The chair compensates for this shift, keeping the resident stable.

Special Accessories

Some wheelchairs have small anti-tipping devices attached to the back. They are fastened to the bottom of the chair frame. These are optional accessories **(Figure 12–7)**. The extensions may have small wheels or weights that balance the chair. They stabilize the chair for residents who may tip over.

An extension piece can be fastened to the upper back rest of the chair to support the head. This accessory is usually used with reclining-back wheelchairs. However, some therapists recommend it for very tall residents or those with poor head and neck control.

Preventing Skin Tears

(SA) Torn armrests and seats on wheelchairs are a common cause of skin tears. Surveyors will write deficiencies if they observe worn wheelchairs. The armrests and seats should be replaced if they

become cracked or torn. Notify your supervisor if you observe a chair in disrepair.(SA)

Many health care workers fold wheelchairs by pulling the seat up quickly. This causes cracking and wear on the seat, making it unsafe. Fold the wheelchair by raising the footrests and gently pulling up on the seat. Some chairs have handles on either side of the seat. Pull the handles to fold the chair.

▉ WHEELCHAIR SIZE

There is no "one size fits all" wheelchair. Residents may not be able to propel a wheelchair that does not fit correctly. Fewer positioning aids are necessary if the chair fits the resident correctly. A wheelchair that is the wrong size contributes to skin breakdown. Reclining chairs used unnecessarily can cause serious physical and mental declines. Residents will not be comfortable if the wheelchair does not fit. As you can see, attention to chair size is very important.

The therapist or restorative nurse selects the size and type of wheelchair to meet the resident's needs. The distance between the seat and the floor of the standard adult chair is 36 inches. The distance between the seat and the floor of the hemiplegia chair is 32 inches. Standard measurements for wheelchairs are listed in **Table 12–2.** The type of chair selected is determined by:

▉ An assessment of the resident's physical condition

▉ The resident's special needs

▉ The needs of caregivers

▉ The environment in which the chair will be used

Table 12–2 Standard Wheelchair Sizes

Type of Chair	Seat Depth	Seat Width	Back Height
Standard adult	16″	18″	20″
Narrow adult	16″	16″	20″
Thin adult	16″	14″	20″
Tall adult	17″	18″	20″
Wide adult	16″	20″	20″
Extra-wide adult	16″	22″	20″
Heavy-duty adult	16″	24″	20″
Extra-heavy-duty adult	16″	26″	20″
Standard reclining back	17″	18″	23″
Hemiplegic adult	16″	18″	18″
Preschool	8″	10″	19-½″
Small child	11-½″	12″	19-½″
Standard child	11-½″	14″	18-¼″
Junior	16″	16″	18-½″

You may assist in measuring residents for wheelchair fit. Obtaining accurate measurements is very important. Always read the tape measure at eye level. The resident must sit on a flat, solid surface with a solid back while measurements are taken.

Seat Depth

The depth of the seat is very important to support the pelvis and thighs. The seat must be deep enough to support the thighs correctly. A short seat can be very uncomfortable for residents with long legs. If the seat is too long, the resident's weight is shifted toward the sacrum. This causes discomfort and increases the risk of skin breakdown. A long seat makes it more difficult for the resident to propel the chair. ⑤ⒶSome residents slide to the front edge of the wheelchair. A seat that is too long is often the problem. Facilities look for restraints and alternatives to keep residents from sliding. A different wheelchair may be all that is necessary!⑤Ⓐ Staff members may not be trained to recognize this problem. When the resident is seated properly in the chair, the hips should be near the back. The front edge of the seat should end two or three inches before the back of the knees.

To measure seat depth, position the resident in good alignment. Seat him or her on a flat surface with the buttocks and back supported. Measure from the bottom of the back support to behind the knee **(Figure 12–8).** Subtract three inches from this measurement.

Seat Width

Proper seat width is important for comfort. It also affects ease in moving the drive wheels and resting the arms on the armrests. A wheelchair that is too wide is difficult for residents to move. The resident may lean to one side. ⑤ⒶA seat that is too narrow increases pressure on the thighs, buttocks, and hips. This is uncomfortable and increases the risk of skin breakdown.⑤ When measuring seat width, an allowance of several inches is made. This provides extra space for prosthetic devices or bulky clothing.

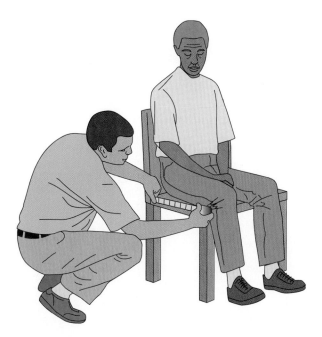

Figure 12–8 To determine seat depth, measure from the back of the chair to behind the resident's knee. Subtract two to three inches.

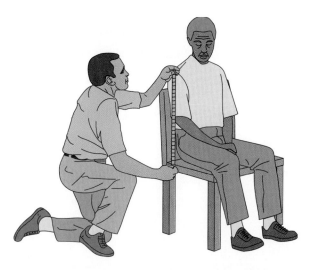

Figure 12–10 The back height is measured from the seat to the bottom of the shoulder blade.

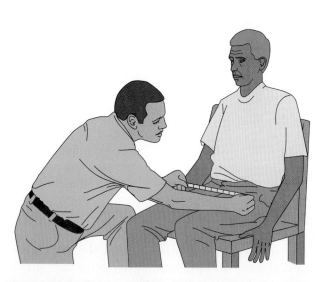

Figure 12–9 For seat width, measure the widest part of the resident's hips and thighs. You should be able to place a flat hand vertically between the resident and the armrest if the seat is the correct width.

To measure seat width, seat the resident on a flat surface. Measure the widest part of the hips and thighs. Add two inches **(Figure 12–9).**

Back Height

The height of the chair back is determined by the resident's need for back support. Measure from the top edge of the seat to the bottom of the shoulder blade **(Figure 12–10).** If the resident will be sitting on a foam cushion in the wheelchair, measure with the cushion in place.

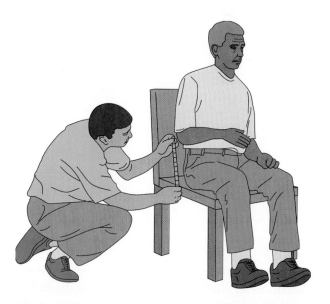

Figure 12–11 To measure the armrest height, fold the elbow across the abdomen, and measure the distance from the seat to the elbow.

Armrest Height

Armrest height is important for comfort and good sitting posture. If the armrests are too high, shorter residents will have problems propelling the chair. In short residents, the armrests will cause shoulder strain. In some residents, they cause bruising or other injuries to the arms. Sitting in a chair with high armrests is uncomfortable. Measure armrest height with the resident sitting on a flat surface. Flex the elbow so the hand rests against the abdomen. Measure from the seat of the chair to the elbow **(Figure 12–11).** If the resident will be sitting on a foam cushion, take the measurements with the cushion in place.

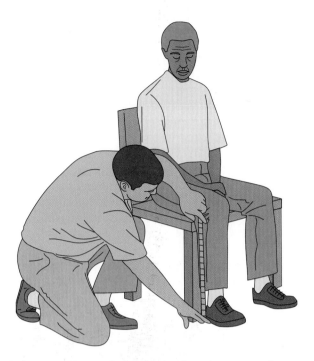

Figure 12–12 To determine leg length, measure from the back of the knee to the bottom of the foot.

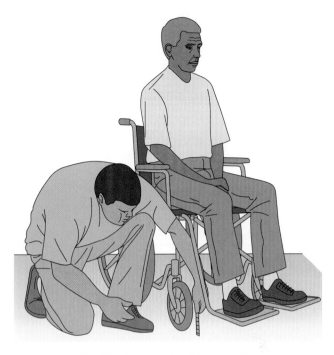

Figure 12–13 The footrest should never drag or scrape on the floor, particularly when going up inclines or over the threshold in a doorway. Measure from the lowest part of the footrest to the floor.

Leg Rest Length

The length of the wheelchair legs affects posture and body alignment. If the leg rests are too long, the resident's legs may dangle. He or she may slide forward in the chair to reach the footrests. This increases pressure on the buttocks and sacrum. It also increases the risk of tipping the chair. Measure the length of the leg rest from behind the knee to the foot **(Figure 12–12)**. Add the width of the foot. If the resident is sitting on a foam cushion, subtract the height of the cushion. The footrest should be at least two inches above the floor to prevent accidents. Transfer the resident to the wheelchair. After he or she is seated, measure from the lowest part of the footrest to the floor **(Figure 12–13)**.

Footrest Size

Some therapists also measure the footrest size. Foot support is important for preventing foot and ankle contractures. Long footrests may affect the resident's ability to move the chair. Support the foot from the heel to just below the toes. Measure the length of the resident's foot from the heel to the base of the toes.

▆▆▆ WHEELCHAIR MOBILITY

Propelling the wheelchair independently is good exercise. It promotes communication, independence, confidence, and self-esteem. Wheelchair mobility provides opportunities for residents to make choices and decisions. They can decide where

they will go and what activities to attend. A facility emphasis on efficiency may create problems with wheelchair mobility. Pushing the chairs is faster for staff than it is to cue and encourage residents to push them. *The wheelchair is a mobility device, not a transportation device.* Some residents do not propel their wheelchairs because of physical problems. However, adaptations may allow them to move independently. Some do not propel the chair because it does not fit correctly. Fitting wheelchairs and teaching residents to use them is best.

Wheelchair mobility is an activity that is individualized to the resident. After finding a chair that fits the resident, show him or her how to use it. Explain how to operate the brakes and footrests. Describe special features, such as removable arms. Show the resident how to propel the chair by using the arms and legs. Teach the resident how to transfer, if appropriate. After you have demonstrated, ask the resident to give you a return demonstration. Correct unsafe practices. The resident will not learn these skills immediately. It takes time to build the strength and endurance needed to propel a wheelchair. The restorative nurse will design a mobility program for the resident. The program may include exercises to strengthen the hands and arms. A wheelchair mobility program is similar to an ambulation program. However, the resident uses the wheelchair instead of walking. Follow the guidelines for ambulation programs in Chapter 13.

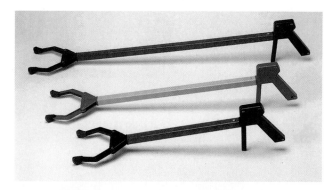

Figure 12–14 The pickstick or grabber is used to reach items on the floor. (Courtesy of Briggs Corporation, Des Moines, IA. (800) 247-2343)

WHEELCHAIR SAFETY

Remind residents about wheelchair safety, including:

- Locking the brakes when the chair is parked
- Parking the chair with the large part of the small front wheels facing forward
- Holding the armrests and feeling the chair with the back of the legs before sitting
- Not bending over to pick up items from the floor

Although residents should not pick up items from the floor while seated, many do anyway. Assistive devices are available to retrieve objects from the floor **(Figure 12–14)**. Residents with good balance and trunk control can be taught to pick up dropped items. Teach the resident to avoid shifting weight. He or she must avoid moving to the edge of the chair. To pick up items from the floor:

- Move the chair as close to the object as possible
- If necessary, move the chair forward beyond the object, then back up beside it so it is within reach
- Position the large part of the caster wheels facing forward
- Lock the brakes
- Lift the footrests and place the feet on the floor
- Avoid moving to the front of the seat; keep the hips near the backrest
- Reach to the side to pick up the item, instead of reaching between the knees

TRANSFER ACTIVITIES

You learned how to move a resident from bed to a wheelchair in your nursing assistant program. The transfers you learned were **dependent transfers.** The resident's participation is minimal in this type

of transfer. The transfers here are different, because they involve teaching the resident to be as independent as possible. The transfers described in this book are **assisted transfers,** in which the resident actively participates in the procedure. Your supervisor may teach you how to assist residents to sit in chairs without arms, soft chairs, and couches. The resident will be taught to sit slowly. He or she should avoid falling into the chair. Initially, the therapist or nurse will work with the resident. Your program will be designed to complement the skilled program. You will do this by giving demonstrations and verbal cues. Provide hands-on assistance, if necessary. Assist the resident only when necessary. Allow him or her to be as independent as possible. Knowing the resident's ability and specific mobility problem will help you provide exactly the amount of assistance needed.

Safe Transfers

Before beginning, explain the procedure to the resident. Tell him or her what is expected. Get feedback to make sure the resident understands. Use simple commands or counts to time your movements. For example, tell the resident, "We will move when I count to three," or, "We will move when I say lift." Moving simultaneously with the resident is important. This helps prevent injury to you and the resident.

SAThe care plan will list directions for the type of assistance to provide during moving procedures. The terms most commonly used are *standby, minimal, moderate,* and *maximum.* The Minimum Data Set lists different definitions (shown in **Table 12–3**). If you are in doubt about the level of assistance necessary, ask someone else to help. This will keep the resident and you safe during the transfer. Always use a transfer belt unless contraindicated. Stand close to the resident during the transfer.**SA** Never let the resident place his or her hands on your body. Never move the resident by lifting up under the arms. If the resident has hemiplegia, transfer toward the strong side. Use good body mechanics during moving and ambulation procedures **(Figure 12–15).**

The Transfer Belt

The transfer belt (also called a gait belt) is a heavy canvas belt. In some facilities, each resident is given a belt that is used only for that resident. Other facilities require the restorative assistant to wear the belt and use it for all transfers. Using the transfer belt:

- Prevents pulling on the resident's skin
- Makes it easier for you to move the resident
- Gives you control if the resident starts to fall
- Is safer for both you and the resident

Table 12–3 Definitions of Levels of Assistance

MDS Terminology	Definition
Independent	No help or staff oversight. Can also mean that staff help or oversight was provided only one or two times during the past seven days.
Setup	For bed mobility—handing the resident the trapeze. For transfers—giving the resident a sliding board or locking the wheels on the wheelchair. For walking—handing the resident a cane or walker. For wheeling—unlocking the brakes on the wheelchair or adjusting the foot pedals to facilitate foot motion while wheeling.
Supervision	Oversight, encouragement, or cueing provided three or more times during the past seven days. Can also mean that supervision (three or more times) plus physical assistance was provided only one or two times during the past seven days.
Limited assistance	The resident is highly involved in the activity. He or she received physical help in guided maneuvering of limbs or other nonweight-bearing assistance on three or more occasions. Can also mean limited assistance (three or more times) plus more help provided only one or two times during the last seven days.
Extensive assistance	Although the resident performed part of the activity over the last seven days, help of the following type(s) was provided three or more times: ■ Weight-bearing support provided three or more times ■ Full staff performance of activity three or more times during part, but not all, of the last seven days
Total dependence	Full staff performance of the activity during the entire seven-day period. Complete nonparticipation by the resident in all aspects of the activity.

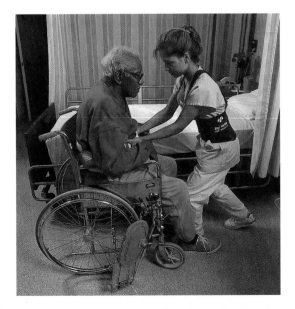

Figure 12–15 Always use good body mechanics when moving residents. The restorative nursing assistant is guarding the resident's leg with her foot and knee.

Never use the belt on a pair of pants in place of a transfer belt.

Contraindications for Use of the Transfer Belt. The transfer belt is contraindicated in some situations, for residents with certain conditions. Facilities have different policies for using the transfer belt. Know and follow your facility policy. Check with your supervisor or the resident's care plan. Residents may be afraid of the belt at first. Teach them why using it is safer. In general, avoid using the transfer belt for residents with:

■ An ostomy

■ A gastrostomy tube

■ Recent abdominal surgery or a fresh surgical incision

■ Severe cardiac or respiratory disease

■ Fractured ribs

■ Pregnancy

General Guidelines for Using the Transfer Belt

- The belt should never contact the skin. Dress the resident before applying the belt.
- The breasts of female residents should not be compressed under the belt.
- Encircle the waist with the belt, buckling it in front.
- Thread the belt through the teeth side. Then thread back through the opening on the other side. This double-locks the belt **(Figure 12–16)**.

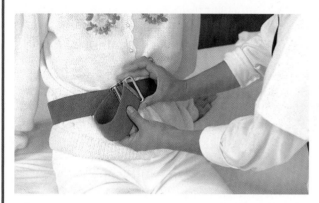

Figure 12–16 Thread the gait belt through the teeth and lock it securely.

- Check the fit of the belt with three fingers. It should be snug. There should be just enough space for your fingers to fit comfortably.
- Before you move the resident, his or her feet must be flat on the floor.
- When transferring a resident into or out of a wheelchair, move the footrests out of the way.

- After the resident is seated, support the feet on the floor or on the chair's footrests.
- Teach the resident to assist by pushing off the bed with the hands when you count to three.
- Always hold the belt with an underhand grasp. For transfers, position one hand on either side of the buckle in front **(Figure 12–17)**.

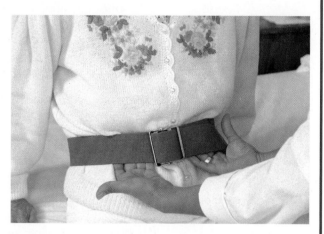

Figure 12–17 Insert your fingers under the belt, on either side of the buckle.

- When a dependent resident is standing, pivot him or her to transfer. More independent residents can take a few steps.
- Position the chair so the resident can feel the armrests with the hands before sitting.
- The resident should be able to feel the seat with the legs before sitting.
- Remove the belt after the resident is seated.

Preparing for Transfers and Ambulation by Using the Parallel Bars

For a resident to transfer and ambulate safely, he or she must be able to balance on one or both legs while standing. Parallel bars **(Figure 12–18)** may be used to teach residents these activities. The bars provide maximum stability. They require very little coordination on the part of the resident. Several activities help prepare the resident for progressive mobility. These are:

- Standing between the parallel bars and shifting weight from side to side
- Moving each leg forward, backward, and sideways

Later, the therapist or nurse may teach the resident a specific gait pattern. The bars are not used for a long time because residents may become dependent on them. They may be afraid of falling when they begin to ambulate without the bars. Before beginning an exercise, explain and demonstrate what you want the resident to do. Assist the resident by holding the transfer belt for support. Give simple, direct verbal cues.

Levels of Assistance

Restorative nursing has a special language. You must learn this language. These definitions apply to the level of assistance that residents need during transfers and ambulation. You will find references

PROCEDURE

19 USING THE TRANSFER BELT

1. Perform your beginning procedure actions.
2. Assist the resident to dress and put on nonslip footwear.
3. Apply the transfer belt snugly around the resident's waist. Lock the buckle. Check the fit with three fingers.
4. Stand in front of the resident. Keep your feet apart, knees bent, and back straight. Using an underhand grasp, place one hand under each side of the belt.
5. Move the resident to the edge of the bed so the feet are touching the floor. Tell the resident to separate the knees to provide a wide base of support.
6. Instruct the resident to lean forward on the count of three. Tell him or her to push up from the bed with the hands while you lift the belt. Place your knees and feet firmly against the resident's knees and feet for support.
7. Assist the resident to a standing position.
8. Complete the transfer. Guidelines for using the belt for ambulation are listed in Chapter 13.
9. Perform your procedure completion actions.

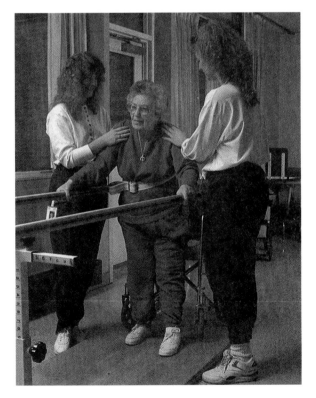

Figure 12–18 The parallel bars provide a stable support early in the resident's progressive mobility program. (Courtesy of Medline Industries, Inc. (800) MEDLINE)

to these terms on the care plan. Use the terms in your documentation.

▪ *Independent:* The resident can transfer or walk independently for a **functional distance.**

This is the distance required for a specific location or activity. The resident can **transition,** or move between surfaces independently. He or she can balance while standing. The resident can turn his or her body without falling. This term also applies to residents who use assistive ambulation devices.

▪ *Supervision* is also called **standby assistance.** This means watching the resident perform the activity. Provide verbal cues, if necessary. Give physical assistance only if necessary. Residents require supervision if one or more of the following considerations exists:

▪ Does not always use good judgment
▪ Unexpected loss of balance
▪ Cannot turn without falling
▪ Cannot transition between surfaces

▪ Residents require minimal to moderate assistance if one or more of the following considerations exists:

▪ The resident is weak or unsteady during transfers or ambulation. He or she requires a gait belt and physical assistance from one person.
▪ The resident's standing balance is good. Endurance may be poor. Transitions or turning are unsafe.

Residents requiring minimal to moderate assistance may benefit from an assistive ambulation device. They may require physical support in some situations. The care plan will list directions for safe ambulation.

▦ Moderate to maximum assistance means that one or more of the following conditions exists for the resident:

▦ Weak and/or unsteady

▦ Poor endurance

▦ Inability to transfer independently

▦ Inability to ambulate a distance of 100 feet

▦ Requires the assistance of one to two staff members and an assistive device for safe transfers and ambulation

▦ Requires continuous monitoring during transfers because of poor balance and frequent falls

▦ Inability to transition

▦ Inability to turn

The Minimum Data Set provides different definitions. Some facilities use these to describe the amount of assistance necessary. These terms are listed in Table 12–3.

Guarding Techniques

Guarding is positioning and using your body to keep the resident safe. Guarding supports the resident. It reduces the risk of falls if the resident is weak, loses his or her balance, slips, or begins to fall. Remember that the resident may be stiff when he or she first stands. Think of how you feel after riding in a car for a few hours. The resident will move more freely after a few minutes. Move your body as the resident moves. Avoid interfering with his or her movement. Always use guarding when moving residents.

A variety of guarding techniques are used during transfers:

▦ The **pivot technique** is used for moving residents who can bear weight on at least one leg. Use the pivot technique for transfers from bed to chair, wheelchair to toilet, and back. It involves positioning your knees and feet to keep the resident from sliding **(Figure 12–19).** Use your knee to brace the resident's strong leg. Place your foot against the side of the resident's foot. Your knee should touch the resident's knee. Position your other leg slightly behind the first leg. If you are sure that the resident can use the strong leg for support during transfers, use this technique for guarding the weak leg. This extra support enables the resident to use the weak leg during the transfer.

▦ The **sliding technique** is used for transfers when the resident cannot bear weight. Use this

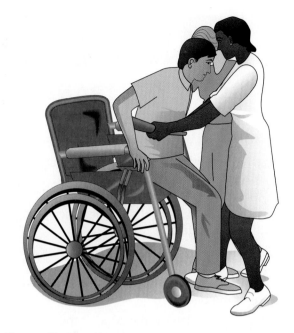

Figure 12–19 The restorative nursing assistant uses the feet and legs to guard the resident.

technique for moving residents on a sheet, such as from bed to stretcher. Use your body weight to hold the two surfaces (head and stretcher) together during the transfer. This keeps them from separating. One of more caregivers stand on each side of the resident. The sheet is rolled close to the resident's body. On the count of three, lift the sheet, pulling the resident over to the stretcher.

▦ The **lifting technique** is used when three or more staff members must physically lift a resident who is lying down. Cradle the resident against your body. Wrap your arms around the resident's back. Hold the resident close to your body.

Completing the Procedure

A transfer is not complete until the resident is safe and comfortable. He or she must be in good body alignment and properly supported. Avoid exposing the resident's body. Place the call signal and needed personal items within reach.

Transferring from Bed to Wheelchair and Back

The resident must master these skills when learning transfers. Your supervisor and the care plan will provide directions for each step. Before beginning, bring the wheelchair to the bedside. Position it on the resident's strong side at a 35° angle. Remove the leg rests or fold them back. Lock the brakes.

PROCEDURE

20 TEACHING THE RESIDENT TO TRANSFER FROM BED TO CHAIR

1. Perform your beginning procedure actions.

2. Provide verbal cues for the resident to dangle at bedside. Assist only if necessary. Bring the clothing, robe, or shoes to the bedside. Help the resident dress, if necessary.

3. Place the transfer belt around the resident's waist. Lock the buckle and check the fit.

4. Give the resident verbal cues to lean forward, place the unaffected hand on the bed, and push up to a standing position. Hold the belt with an underhand grasp, providing only the degree of support necessary.

5. Provide verbal cues and instruct the resident to take small steps toward the wheelchair.

Instruct him or her to turn on the strong foot until he or she feels the seat on the back of the legs. (In a dependent transfer, you would position the chair so that you could pivot the resident. The steps would be unnecessary. In an independent transfer, the resident will walk a few steps to reach the chair. Placing it too close to the bed may be unsafe.)

6. Instruct the resident to hold the arms of the chair, bend forward, and slowly lower the body into the chair.

7. Perform your procedure completion actions. Sincerely compliment the resident on this success.

To return the resident to bed, reverse this procedure. Move the wheelchair so the strong side is toward the bed. Apply the transfer belt. Give the resident verbal cues to slide his or her body forward in the chair. Next, cue the resident to pull the feet back slightly, lean forward, and push up using the hands. Remind the resident to keep the head forward over the feet. You may use the expression, "nose over toes." Hold the transfer belt with an underhand grasp. Provide only the amount of assistance necessary.

Assisting the Resident to the Front of the Chair

The resident must be able to move to the front edge of the chair before standing, and for most transfers. Sitting at the front of the chair moves the center of gravity over the base of support in the feet. This makes standing easier and safer. Several methods can be used for moving to the front of the chair. The care plan will list the method to use.

Side-to-Side Weight Shift (Procedure 21)

The side-to-side weight-shifting method is commonly used for moving residents with hemiplegia.

Pelvic Slide (Procedure 22)

The pelvic slide is used for residents with good arm strength and trunk control. This move works well for residents with paraplegia. Move the pelvis and trunk as separate units.

Wheelchair Push-Ups (Procedure 23)

Wheelchair push-ups relieve pressure on the hips, buttocks, and coccyx. They are helpful to residents who sit in a chair for long periods of time. Wheelchair push-ups increase upper body strength. This helps prepare the resident for transfer procedures. The care plan will list directions. The restorative nurse determines how often the resident should practice and the number of repetitions each time. Before the resident does the procedure independently, make sure he or she can do so safely.

Sitting Push-Up (Procedure 24)

The sitting push-up also requires good arm strength and trunk control. This method also works well for moving residents with paraplegia. Place your hands on the shoulders to balance the resident, if necessary. This keeps him or her from leaning too far forward.

PROCEDURE

21 MOVING TO FRONT EDGE OF CHAIR USING SIDE-TO-SIDE WEIGHT SHIFT

1. Perform your beginning procedure actions.
2. Lock the brakes.
3. Remove the chair legs or fold them back.
4. Position yourself in front of the resident.
5. Place one arm around the resident's shoulder. Place the other arm around the outside and under the thigh on the opposite side.
6. Assist the resident to shift his or her weight toward you. After shifting the resident's weight to the side, assist in moving the thigh forward with your hand.
7. Move to the opposite side of the body and repeat the procedure.
8. Repeat as many times as necessary until the resident reaches the edge of the seat.
9. Proceed to the transfer or ambulation.

PROCEDURE

22 MOVING TO FRONT EDGE OF CHAIR USING PELVIC SLIDE

1. Perform your beginning procedure actions.
2. Lock the brakes.
3. Remove the chair legs or fold them back.
4. Position yourself in front of the resident.
5. Place your hands around the resident's hips, then under the buttocks.
6. Instruct the resident to push on the armrests, lifting the hips off the seat.
7. Slide the buttocks to the front of the chair.
8. Place your hands behind the resident's shoulders. Assist the resident to move the shoulders forward until they are centered over the pelvis. The resident may be able to do this independently.
9. Proceed to the transfer or ambulation procedure.

PROCEDURE

23 TEACHING WHEELCHAIR PUSH-UPS

1. Perform your beginning procedure actions.
2. Position the small front wheels facing forward. Lock the brakes.
3. Remove the leg rests or fold them back. Place the resident's feet on the floor.
4. Position yourself in front of the resident.
5. Instruct the resident to place both hands on the armrests, push the body up, lock the elbows, and lift the hips off the seat **(Figure 12–20).**
6. If the resident can use one or both legs, instruct him or her to push with the feet while pushing up with the hands.
7. Instruct the resident to unlock the elbows, slowly flex the knees, and lower himself or herself gradually to the seat.
8. Repeat as instructed by the restorative nurse or therapist.
9. If the resident can perform the procedure independently, remind him or her to practice.
10. Perform your procedure completion actions.

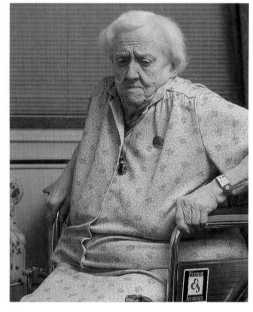

Figure 12–20   To perform wheelchair push-ups, the small front wheels of the chair face forward. The footrests are elevated and the resident's feet are on the floor. The brakes are locked. The resident relieves pressure on the buttocks by pushing on the armrests with the arms and lifting the weight of the body off the seat.

PROCEDURE

24 MOVING TO FRONT EDGE OF CHAIR USING SITTING PUSH-UP

1. Perform your beginning procedure actions.
2. Lock the wheelchair brakes.
3. Remove the chair legs or fold them back.
4. Position yourself in front of the resident.
5. Instruct the resident to place both hands on the armrests of the wheelchair, push up, lock the elbows, and move the hips forward.
6. If the resident has difficulty moving the hips or legs, place your hands around the hips. Pull them forward when the resident lifts.
7. Repeat the procedure until the resident reaches the edge of the chair.
8. Proceed to the transfer or ambulation procedure.

Toilet Transfers

A survey of long-term care facility workers revealed that toilet transfers are the most difficult. This is because the bathrooms in most facilities are small. Many meet the OSHA definition of "confined spaces." The wheelchair takes up a great deal of space. The toilet is close to the wall. There is little room for the assistant to move during the transfer. An elevated toilet seat and handrails **(Figure 12–21)** must be used when teaching this transfer.

Reverse this procedure to return to the chair. If possible, position the wheelchair on the resident's strong side. To rise from the toilet, the resident holds the rail. Provide verbal cues to slide forward slightly. After moving forward, cue the resident to pull the feet back and lean forward. He or she pushes up with the hands on the rails, or pulls up

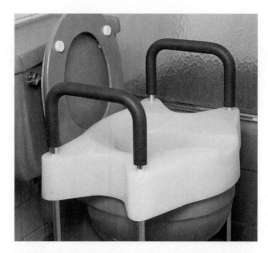

Figure 12–21   When working on toilet transfers, an elevated seat with hand rails is used for safety. (Courtesy of Briggs Corporation, Des Moines, IA. (800) 247-2343)

PROCEDURE

25   TEACHING THE RESIDENT TO TRANSFER FROM WHEELCHAIR TO TOILET

1. Perform your beginning procedure actions.

2. Position the wheelchair at a right angle to the toilet, if possible. Position the chair so that the toilet is on the resident's strong side, if possible.

3. Lock the chair brakes.

4. Remove the chair legs or fold them back.

5. Apply the transfer belt.

6. Assist the resident to unfasten clothing.

7. Cue the resident to place the hands on the armrests and slide forward in the chair.

8. Instruct the resident to pull the feet back under the body, placing them firmly on the floor.

9. Tell the resident to lean forward and push up, turning to the strong side **(Figure 12–22)** until feeling the toilet seat on the legs. Hold the transfer belt, but assist only to the degree necessary.

10. Instruct the resident to hold the grab rail, using the other hand to undress. Assist if the resident has hemiparesis.

11. Tell the resident to hold the rail and slowly lower his or her body to the toilet seat.

12. Remove the transfer belt.

13. Provide privacy. Instruct the resident to call for assistance when done.

14. Perform your procedure completion actions.

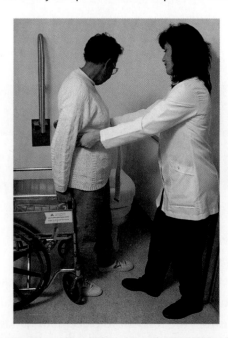

Figure 12–22   Assist the resident to stand, then pivot by holding the support rail.

using the rail on the wall. Remind the resident to face forward, keeping the head over the feet. After the resident is seated in the chair, assist him or her to the sink. Provide supplies for handwashing.

Tub Transfers

Most facility residents shower several times a week. However, some residents prefer a tub bath. If the resident will be going home, the restorative nurse will develop a program to teach transfers into and out of the bathtub. The type of procedure used is determined by the height and position of the tub. The procedure varies if the tub is in the middle of the room or against the wall. Because there are many variables, no specific steps are listed here. The care plan and your supervisor will provide directions to meet the resident's needs.

The bathtub should be disinfected before this procedure. Place a rubber mat in the bottom of the tub. Instruct the resident to leave the shoes on until he or she is ready to place the feet into the tub. Using an adaptive tub chair or stool **(Figure 12–23)** makes this procedure easier and safer for the resident. A sliding board may also be used for this transfer. Cover it with a pillowcase. Never use a sliding board against the resident's skin. If a chair or stool is available, place it next to the tub. The resident can transfer from the wheelchair to the chair. From there, he or she transfers into the tub **(Figure 12–24).** If no chair is available, the resident may transfer directly to the tub. Seat the resident on the side of the tub. Assist him or her to pivot and ease into the water.

Car Transfers

After residents have mastered transfers in the facility, they may learn car transfers. Teach the resident to transfer independently, if possible. A sliding board may be used. A transfer belt can be used, if necessary. The resident may have to transfer independently later in the trip, so learning how to move unassisted is best. Transfer the resident to the front seat. The door is wider and there is more space for the resident to move. A two-door car has wider doors than a four-door car. This transfer is easier if a wheelchair with removable armrests is used.

To get out of the car, reverse the procedure. The car seat is lower than a wheelchair seat. A transfer belt can be used to assist the resident to a standing position, if necessary. Have the resident hold the back of the seat or door frame for support.

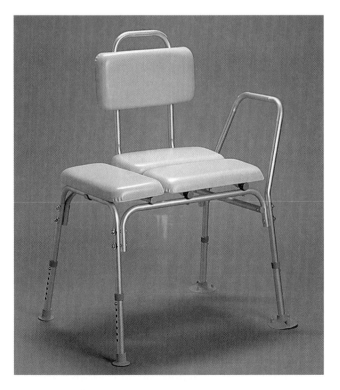

Figure 12–23 This long bench permits the resident to slide into the tub. (Courtesy of Briggs Corporation, Des Moines, IA. (800) 247-2343)

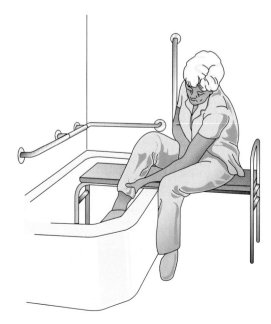

Figure 12–24 The resident sits on the bench and moves the feet into the tub.

PROCEDURE

26 TRANSFERRING THE RESIDENT INTO A CAR

1. Perform beginning procedure actions appropriate to the environment.

2. Open the car door. Position the wheelchair at a 45° angle to the door. Lock the chair brakes. Apply the transfer belt **(Figure 12–25A)**.

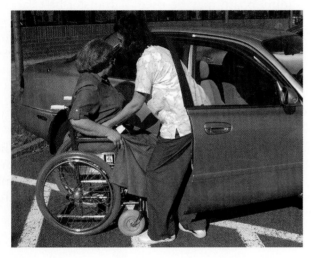

Figure 12–25A   Assist the resident to a standing position.

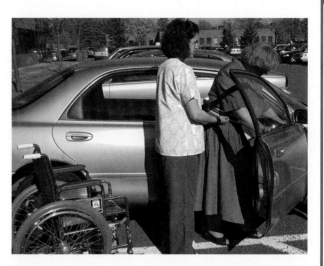

Figure 12–25B   Holding the back of the seat and open window frame for support, the resident pivots and sits down.

3. If moving to the weaker side, instruct the resident to hold onto the door frame. Opening the window makes this easier. Hold the door stable during the transfer. If the resident is moving to the stronger side, have him or her hold the back of the seat.

4. Assist the resident to stand. The resident pivots until he or she feels the door frame on the back of the legs. Tell the resident to sit gradually **(Figure 12–25B)**.

5. After the resident is seated, have him or her move one leg at a time into the car. Use the hands to pick them up, if necessary **(Figure 12–25C)**.

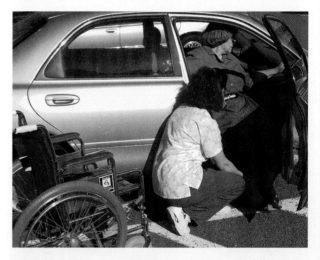

Figure 12–25C   The resident lifts one leg at a time into the car.

6. Perform your procedure completion actions appropriate to the environment.

▇ SPECIAL WHEELCHAIR PROCEDURES

When the resident is outside the facility, special wheelchair procedures may be necessary. You may use these procedures when assisting with trial home and community visits. For safety, practice these procedures with an assistant. Do not attempt them alone unless you are trained and know how to do them safely. Use good body mechanics. You must use a wheelchair designed for outdoor use. Inspect the handgrips carefully. They must be in good repair and fit tightly, and should not slip when you pull the chair backward.

Tilting the Wheelchair

Tilting the wheelchair backward is necessary in some places outside the facility. This procedure is used for curbs, ramps, and single steps. The procedure involves tipping the wheelchair until it reaches the balance point. You will be able to move the chair easily on the rear wheels in this position.

Ramps and Inclines

To transport a wheelchair up a ramp, instruct the resident to lean forward slightly. Push the resident up, from behind the chair. Two methods are used for moving wheelchairs down ramps. The first involves turning the chair backward and backing down the ramp. Position yourself behind the chair and walk backward. Guide the chair by using the handgrips. Walk slowly and use your body to guard the chair. For safety, avoid using this procedure on steep ramps.

The second method for going down a ramp involves tipping the chair to the balance position.

For this procedure, the resident does not lean forward. After the chair is balanced, guide it down the ramp, facing forward.

Curbs and Single Steps (Procedure 29)

This procedure is used for going up single steps and curbs. Use good body mechanics. Keep your back straight and knees bent. Use the strong muscles in your legs and arms to do the job.

Going Up and Down Stairs (Procedure 30)

Going up and down stairs should be avoided, whenever possible. Use this procedure only if an elevator or ramp is not available. Do not use this procedure on an escalator. At least two people must perform this procedure. Three assistants are recommended, if available. The assistants must have the strength and endurance to lift and move the chair up or down the stairs safely.

PROCEDURE

27 TILTING THE WHEELCHAIR BACKWARD

1. Explain the procedure to the resident. Make sure that his or her arms, legs, hands, and feet are within the chair frame, for safety.

2. Place one foot on the kickspur and press down. Pull back on the handgrips.

3. Slowly tilt the chair back until little effort is required to stabilize it. In this position, the back of the chair is at about a 30° angle.

4. To return the chair to an upright position, press on the kickspur with your foot. Lower the handrests slowly. Guide the chair down slowly, by applying pressure on the kickspur and lowering the handgrips.

PROCEDURE

28 USING A WHEELCHAIR ON RAMPS AND INCLINES

1. Explain the procedure to the resident. Make sure that his or her arms, legs, hands, and feet are within the chair frame.

2. Slowly tilt the chair into the balance position.

3. Hold the handrests to maintain the balance position. Guide the chair down the ramp slowly, facing forward.

PROCEDURE

29 MOVING A WHEELCHAIR UP CURBS

1. Explain the procedure to the resident. Make sure that his or her arms, legs, hands, and feet are within the chair frame.

2. Position the chair with the front wheels close to the curb. Slowly tilt the chair into the balance position.

3. Move forward slowly until the front wheels are over the curb. Move the rear wheels forward until they touch the curb.

4. Hold the back of the chair securely. Slowly lower the front wheels down to the sidewalk.

5. Stand close to the wheelchair. Lift the chair up by the handgrips. Roll it up and over the curb.

6. Step up onto the curb.

Reverse the procedure to go down the curb. You will move the chair down the curb backward.

7. Turn the chair and back the large, rear wheels to the edge of the curb. Step down onto the street as the wheels near the edge.

8. Stand in the street. Slowly pull on the handgrips, rolling the large wheels down, onto the street.

9. Tilt the chair to the balance point. Lift the front wheels off the sidewalk.

10. Step back until the front wheels have cleared the curb. Slowly lower the chair to the street.

11. Pull the chair backward until you have enough space to turn the chair around.

PROCEDURE

30 MOVING A WHEELCHAIR UP OR DOWN STAIRS

1. Explain the procedure to the resident. Make sure that his or her arms, legs, hands, and feet are within the chair frame.

2. To go up stairs, back the chair up until the rear wheels touch the bottom step. One assistant stands on the second step, the other at the bottom of the stairs. The strongest assistant leads. He or she stands at the resident's head.

3. The assistant near the legs grasps the lower sides of the chair frame. The assistant near the head tilts the wheelchair back to the balance point.

4. Work as a team. The assistant at the head gives the commands. On the count of three, lift and guide the chair up the step. The assistants each move up one step simultaneously. Keep the chair at the balance point.

5. Continue in this manner until you reach the top step. The assistant at the head backs the

chair up, allowing the assistant at the feet to step up to the landing.

6. The assistant at the head guides the chair around, returning it to an upright position.

To go down stairs, reverse the procedure. In this sequence, the stronger assistant should be at the resident's legs. He or she will give the commands.

7. The assistant at the feet stands three steps from the landing.

8. The assistant at the head tips the chair to the balance point, rolling it to the edge of the steps. The assistant at the legs grasps the sides of the wheelchair frame securely.

9. On the count of three, the large wheels are slowly lowered down one step. Both assistants move down one step.

10. Repeat until you reach the bottom of the stairs. The assistant at the head returns the chair to an upright position.

SLIDING BOARD TRANSFERS

A sliding board (**Figure 12–26**) transfer is used for residents with good upper body strength and sitting balance. The procedure is performed by doing a series of push-ups. The resident locks the elbows and pushes with the hands. After lifting the buttocks, he or she lowers onto the sliding board. He or she lifts and slides until the transfer is complete. The resident may have to do wheelchair and bed push-ups before using a sliding board. To transfer, the resident must be able to lift the buttocks off the bed. Sliding board transfers are commonly used for transferring residents with paraplegia.

The wheelchair must have removable armrests when a sliding board is used. The resident must have clothing on the lower half of the body. Blue jeans do not slide well on the board. Cotton or synthetic slacks are best. If the resident has difficulty sliding on the board, draping a pillowcase across the board may be helpful. Do not encase the board in the pillowcase as you would a pillow. The board can also be waxed to maintain a slippery surface. The resident may need assistance when learning

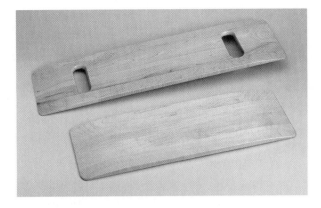

Figure 12–26 The sliding board can be used for independent or dependent transfers. (Courtesy of Briggs Corporation, Des Moines, IA. (800) 247-2343)

this procedure. Always use a transfer belt when the resident is learning the procedure.

Two assistants can move dependent residents by using a sliding board. One assistant stands in front and the other behind the resident. At the count of three, both assistants hold the belt and slide the resident across the board.

PROCEDURE

31 SLIDING BOARD TRANSFER FROM BED TO WHEELCHAIR

1. Perform your beginning procedure actions.

2. Remove the arm of the wheelchair closest to the bed. Remove the chair legs or fold them back.

3. Position the wheelchair parallel to the bed, or at a slight (about 35°) angle. Lock the brakes.

4. Apply a transfer belt. Check the fit with two or three fingers.

5. Instruct or assist the resident to move close to the edge of the bed.

6. Tell the resident to lean away from the wheelchair. Place the sliding board well under the buttocks. The beveled side of the board faces up. Avoid pinching the resident's skin between the board and the bed.

7. Place the opposite end of the board well onto the seat of the wheelchair.

8. Instruct the resident to push up with the hands, lock the elbows, and move across the board. Repeat until the resident is seated in the chair with one buttock on the board.

   The resident may push on the opposite armrest of the wheelchair with one hand. This will help achieve greater height in the push-ups. The resident may also push on the board. Caution the resident to avoid placing the fingers under the edges of the board.

9. Be prepared to assist by lifting the resident's buttocks during the sitting push-up. If the resident is having trouble balancing, place your hands on the shoulders for support.

10. Support the resident's legs with your hands, if necessary.

11. Instruct the resident to lean away from the bed. Remove the board.

12. Remove the transfer belt.

13. Perform your procedure completion actions.

PROCEDURE

32 SLIDING BOARD TRANSFER FROM WHEELCHAIR TO BED

1. Perform your beginning procedure actions.

2. Remove the arm of the wheelchair closest to the bed. Remove the chair legs or fold them back.

3. Position the wheelchair parallel to the bed, or at a slight (35°) angle. Lock the brakes.

4. Apply a transfer belt. Check the fit with two or three fingers.

5. Instruct or assist the resident to move close to the edge of the wheelchair. Block his or her knees with your knees.

6. Instruct the resident to lean toward the side opposite the bed. Place the sliding board well under the buttocks. The beveled side faces up. Avoid pinching the resident's skin between the board and the chair.

7. Place the opposite end of the board well onto the bed.

8. Guard the resident by standing in front of him or her.

9. Instruct the resident to push up with the hands, lock the elbows, lift the buttocks, and move across the board to the bed. Repeat until the resident is seated on the bed with one buttock on the board.

The resident may push on the opposite armrest of the wheelchair with one hand. This will help achieve greater height in the push-up. The resident may also push on the board. Caution the resident to avoid placing the fingers under the edges of the board.

10. Hold the transfer belt. Be prepared to assist by lifting the resident's buttocks during the sitting push-up. If the resident is having trouble balancing, place your hands on the shoulders for support.

11. Support the resident's legs with your hands, if necessary.

12. Instruct the resident to lean away from the wheelchair. Remove the board.

13. Remove the transfer belt.

14. Perform your procedure completion actions.

PROCEDURE

33 PUSH-UP TRANSFER FROM WHEELCHAIR TO BED

1. Perform your beginning procedure actions.

2. Remove the arm of the wheelchair closest to the bed. Remove the chair legs or fold them back.

3. Position the wheelchair parallel to the bed, or at a slight (35°) angle. Lock the brakes.

4. Apply a transfer belt. Check the fit with two or three fingers.

5. Instruct or assist the resident to move close to the edge of the wheelchair.

6. Instruct the resident to lean forward.

7. Guard the resident by standing in front of him or her.

8. Instruct the resident to place one hand on the bed, the other hand on the seat of the chair and push up with the hands, lock the elbows, and move from the chair to the bed.

The resident may push on the armrest of the wheelchair with one hand for greater height.

9. Be prepared to assist by holding the transfer belt.

10. Support the legs with your hands, if necessary, during the procedure.

11. Remove the transfer belt.

12. Perform your procedure completion actions.

Push-up Transfers

A push-up transfer may be used for moving some residents. This type of transfer is used for residents with good upper body strength, endurance, and sitting balance. Residents who use this procedure have usually mastered sliding board transfers. They can lift the buttocks clear of the sitting surface. The procedure is similar to the sliding board transfer, but the board is not used.

◼︎◼︎◼︎ POSITIONING THE RESIDENT IN A CHAIR OR WHEELCHAIR

You learned basic positioning and use of props and postural supports in your nursing assistant class. That information is not repeated here. Proper positioning is as important for residents sitting in chairs as it is for residents in bed. Some residents are in restorative programs to learn how to transfer to the wheelchair. The residents may never progress to ambulation.

Before leaving a resident seated in a chair, make sure that he or she is in good alignment. Good sitting posture begins with positioning the pelvis correctly. Position the resident upright in the center of the chair seat, with the hips to the back. If the resident leans to the side, use props to bring him or her to an upright position. Make sure the weight is evenly distributed on the buttocks. You should be able to place a flat hand between the armrests and the resident's hips. Position the resident's arms on the armrests. Check to make sure the shoulders are not pushed up. Check behind the knees. There should be three or four finger widths between the knees and the seat. Adjust the feet and legs so they are in line with the pelvis. Support the feet on the footrests.

The resident's hips and knees are positioned at a 90° angle when sitting in a chair. Support the feet so the legs do not dangle. Use foam or padding on the chair seat if the resident will be sitting for long periods. Assist the resident to stand or shift his or her weight periodically.

PROCEDURE

34 POSITIONING THE RESIDENT IN A CHAIR OR WHEELCHAIR

1. Perform your beginning procedure actions.
2. Seat the resident upright so the head is erect and centered over the spine. If the resident leans to the side, provide support with pillows, foam, or other props.
3. Position the resident's arms for comfort.
   a. Position the arms on the armrests if this does not push the shoulders up. If the shoulders are elevated, add a seat cushion. This will elevate the resident, preventing shoulder strain.
   b. If the resident's shoulders are hanging, support the arms on pillows, foam, or other props.
   c. Position the resident's hands in his or her lap.
4. The back of the wheelchair should be at the lower level of the resident's shoulder blades.
   a. If the chair back is too low, apply an extension or find another chair.
   b. If the chair back is too high, elevate the resident on a cushion.

5. The hips and back are positioned at a 90° angle. If the resident's hips slide forward, check the depth of the chair to make sure it fits. If the depth is correct, consult your supervisor for postural supports, a wedge cushion, or restraint alternatives. Gripper may be placed on the seat to keep the resident from sliding.
6. The edge of the seat should be two to three inches from the back of the resident's knees. Position the legs at a 90° angle. If the knees touch the seat, place a cushion behind the back to move the resident forward.
7. Position the feet and ankles at 90° angles. Support the feet on the floor or the footrests. If the resident's legs dangle:
   a. Elevate the feet on a stool.
   b. Use a commercial device made for this purpose.
   c. Check with your supervisor to see if the leg rest can be shortened to fit.
8. Perform your procedure completion actions.

Pressure Relief

Years ago, pressure ulcers were called decubitus ulcers. The term **decubitus** means lying down. Pressure ulcers can develop from sitting in chairs, so the name was changed. Residents who sit in chairs for long periods can develop skin breakdown. Anticipate this risk. Pad seats before transferring residents.

You will work with residents who are confined to chairs. Teach and remind them about pressure-relieving activities. When you begin teaching, stay with the resident and give verbal cues. Over time, residents will be able to perform the activity independently. The restorative nurse will recommend a frequency for the exercises. The ideal time frame is every 15 minutes. The type of activity is determined by safety factors and the resident's physical ability.

Wheelchair push-ups are the best method of relieving pressure when the resident is seated. Follow Procedure 23 for wheelchair push-ups. The resident places the palms on the armrests of the wheelchair. The feet are flat on the floor. Caution the resident against performing push-ups with the feet on the footrests. Instruct the resident to push down with the hands, extend the elbows, and lift the buttocks from the chair. This should be done at least five times, or the frequency specified by the care plan.

Some residents do not have the arm strength or trunk control to perform push-ups. You will teach these residents to lean to the sides and front of the chair to relieve pressure. For more dependent residents, have the resident grab your hands. Tell him or her to pull on your hands and shift the weight on the buttocks.

PROCEDURE

35 LEANING TO THE SIDE FOR PRESSURE RELIEF

1. Perform your beginning procedure actions.
2. Lock the wheelchair brakes. For extra security, back the wheelchair against a wall.
3. Instruct the resident to lean forward slightly, then lean back.
4. Have the resident lean from side to side. Teach him or her to lift as much weight off the buttocks as possible.
5. Perform your procedure completion actions.

KEY POINTS IN CHAPTER

Mobility programs teach residents to transfer and either propel a wheelchair or ambulate.

The wheelchair is an important piece of restorative equipment in the long-term care facility.

Fitting the wheelchair to the resident is very important.

The small, front caster wheels of the chair provide the ability to move in all directions. The large part of the small front wheel faces back when the chair is moving. It should face forward when the chair is parked.

Lock the brakes when the wheelchair is parked.

Always use a transfer belt for moving residents.

A transfer is not complete until the resident is safe and comfortable.

A sliding board transfer is used for residents with good upper body strength and sitting balance.

Position the resident in good alignment when seated in a wheelchair.

Residents can develop pressure ulcers when seated in chairs, so pressure-relieving activities are important.

CLINICAL APPLICATIONS

1. Mrs. Logan was recently admitted to your facility from the hospital. The resident lived in her daughter's home before the hospitalization. She walked about the house and cared for herself while her daughter was at work. Mrs. Logan has severe pain in her joints from osteoarthritis. She was on bed rest on admission. She cannot turn from side to side without assistance. The physician has ordered a progressive mobility program to restore her ability to ambulate. Mrs. Logan cannot move in bed or get up unassisted. What activities must she complete before beginning an ambulation program?

2. Mr. Ellis complains of dizziness when he moves quickly or transfers from the bed to the chair. What preliminary activity should be done before moving this resident?

3. Dr. Dyer is 6 feet 4 inches tall and weighs 165 pounds. You will assist the nurse in measuring him for a wheelchair. Describe how you will take these measurements.

4. Mrs. Muñoz has poor hand control. She frequently drops things on the floor. Although the resident has been cautioned not to pick things up, she reaches between her legs to retrieve items. Once, she overturned the chair. She has almost fallen several times. What advice can you give this resident?

5. Mr. Nguyen is a 71-year-old resident who had a CVA. He propels the wheelchair with his strong hand and foot. The resident is 5 feet 5 inches tall. He has trouble reaching the floor with his leg. What type of wheelchair could be used to make mobility easier?

OBJECTIVES

After reading this chapter, you should be able to:

Spell and define key terms.

State the purpose and benefits of ambulation.

Describe how to identify candidates for a restorative ambulation program.

State the objectives of goal-oriented ambulation.

List 12 guidelines for safe ambulation.

Define the five basic types of weight-bearing orders.

List three types of assistive devices and describe situations when each is used.

Describe the five basic gait patterns used with assistive devices.

Define guarding.

Explain five basic guarding techniques used when ambulating residents.

AMBULATION

Ambulation promotes good health. All body systems benefit from the exercise. Independent ambulation provides the resident with emotional satisfaction. It increases the resident's opportunities for socialization. The goal of some ambulation programs is to maintain the resident's current functional level. However, many residents progress to independent ambulation. Some progress to ambulation with minimal assistance because of the goal-oriented approach.

Identifying Residents for a Restorative Ambulation Program

The first step in the restorative ambulation program is to identify potential candidates for the program. Residents who are cognitively impaired can participate if they are cooperative and can follow simple directions. Do not limit screening to alert residents only. Many of these residents can learn new skills. However, learning may take longer than it does for others.

After residents have been identified, members of the interdisciplinary team will assess them. They will develop a program based on the assessment to meet the resident's needs. Residents may be candidates for a restorative ambulation program if:

- They can walk independently for short distances; for example, residents who ambulate in their rooms or those who walk to or from the bathroom.

- They require minimal to moderate assistance walking in their rooms or to or from the bathroom.

- They previously used wheelchairs only for going long distances or taking trips outside the facility. These residents have declined. They now spend most of their time using the wheelchair instead of walking.

- They are restrained because they are unsteady on their feet.

- They are anxious, agitated, or restless.

- They do not have contractures, but have not been walking because of medical problems, weakness, or an unsteady gait.

- Their ability to ambulate has declined.

- They are afraid of falling. They use wheelchairs rather than walking.

- They are depressed or sad and need encouragement to walk outside their rooms.

- They are receiving skilled physical therapy, after referral from the physical therapist.

They have been discharged from physical therapy, but will benefit from a maintenance program.

They can walk, but use a wheelchair most of the time

They are cognitively impaired, with limited safety awareness. They walk with limited assistance.

Their overall ability to ambulate has declined. If the decline has occurred since a recent admission or within the past three months, these residents may qualify for skilled physical therapy. They should be screened by a therapist.

They have recently recovered from an illness and are still weak.

Resident Assessment

After identifying potential candidates, the therapist or restorative nurse will assess each resident. He or she will evaluate the resident's strength, balance, and endurance. The licensed team member will determine the resident's ability to:

Move independently in bed

Perform active range-of-motion exercises

Bear weight

Transfer independently or with minimal assistance

Walk independently, with an assistive device or the assistance of staff

Follow directions

Goal-Oriented Ambulation

After the assessment, the interdisciplinary team develops a program for each resident. ⒮Team members consider goals that will be useful or functional.⒮ For example, going to the dining room is a functional skill. Teaching transfers to and from the toilet is another functional skill. The overall objectives of restorative ambulation are to:

Increase or maintain the resident's ability to ambulate

Ensure that the resident can ambulate safely

Prevent the loss of independence

Prevent **disuse atrophy,** or muscular wasting from lack of use

Provide a safe, consistent ambulation program for residents who otherwise would be unable or unwilling to ambulate regularly

Increase residents' endurance for ambulation outside of their rooms

Increase residents' confidence and sense of well-being

Team members will consider risk and safety tors. They will develop special approaches for res. dents with:

Poor balance

Poor posture

Pain

Weakness

Limited mobility

Cognitive impairment

Limited movement in joints

Edema

Shortness of breath

Fear of falling

Residents with these conditions may require more than one assistant for safe ambulation. The physical therapist or restorative nurse will determine if this is necessary. The therapist or nurse will also decide whether the resident would benefit from an assistive device.

⒮When developing ambulation goals, the team determines the distance that the resident can ambulate safely.⒮ Preventing increased pain, edema, shortness of breath, or weakness is important. If you observe these conditions during ambulation, stop the activity. Notify your supervisor or a nurse.

Ambulation Goals.

Examples of restorative ambulation goals are listed in **Table 13–1.** The goals must be measurable. The care plan will describe:

The number of feet the resident will ambulate

The duration, or length of time, of the activity

The destination to which you will ambulate the resident

The type of assistance the resident requires

Special techniques or adaptive devices

Frequency of ambulation

The purpose of the ambulation, such as walking to the dining room, activities, or the bathroom

Preparing the Resident for Restorative Ambulation

You have learned to do stretching exercises before physical activity. This helps you to warm up and protects your body from injury. The same principle also applies to residents. Assisting the resident with simple warm-up exercises before ambulation is a good idea. The therapist or restorative nurse will develop exercises for the resident. Remain in the room. Provide verbal cues while the resident exercises. Exercise with him or her, if desired. You will

Table 13–1 Examples of Restorative Ambulation Goals

Restorative Ambulation Goals

- Resident will ambulate 45 feet with moderate assistance of one using arm-in-arm technique, at least twice daily.
- Resident will ambulate 100 feet (from room to nurse's station for medication and back) with minimal assistance of one, gait belt, and quad cane, at least twice daily.
- Resident will ambulate 300 feet (from room to dining room and back) with minimal assistance and a standard walker, at least twice daily for meals.
- Resident will stand for 5 minutes with one person standby assist at sink for AM and PM oral hygiene daily.

benefit from the stretching as well! Allow him or her to be as independent as possible. Procedure 13 (Chapter 11) can be used for warming up before ambulation. The resident can sit in the chair and perform stretching and active range-of-motion exercises.

GAIT

The way a person walks is called the **gait.** Residents with certain musculoskeletal and neurologic problems have a gait that is peculiar to the illness. For example, residents with Parkinson's disease walk with a shuffling gait. This is because of muscle rigidity. Residents with neurological problems walk with an **ataxic gait.** The residents appear uncoordinated. Their movement is somewhat irregular. They may walk with jerking movements. They keep their legs farther apart to make them more stable. Residents with an ataxic gait need a very wide base of support to prevent falls. Residents having pain may walk slowly. The resident's body language and facial expression may appear strained. The resident may move the painful area differently or abnormally.

Normal Gait

The normal gait pattern consists of two steps. The resident begins with the feet flat on the floor. He or she raises a leg, dorsiflexes the foot, and begins walking. The heel strikes the floor first **(Figure 13–1A).** The resident rolls forward on the sole of the foot and moves ahead. The arms swing back and forth, in the same direction as the opposite leg **(Figure 13–1B).**

Gait Training

Before beginning an ambulation program, the physical therapist may provide **gait training.** This program teaches the resident to walk. Gait training also involves:

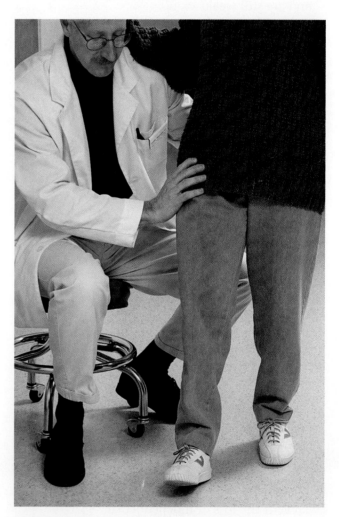

Figure 13–1A The heel strikes the floor first.

- Getting in and out of a chair
- Walking on uneven or irregular surfaces
- Going up and down stairs **(Figure 13–2)** and curbs
- Using assistive ambulation devices

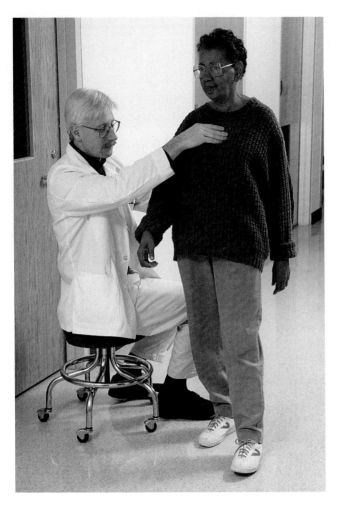

Figure 13–1B The arms swing in the same direction as the opposite leg.

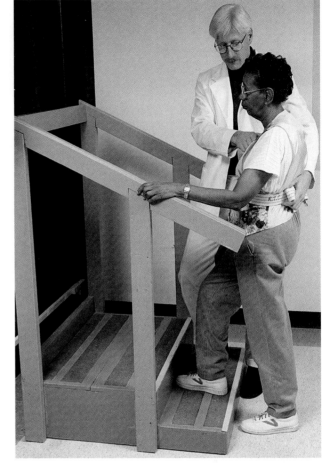

Figure 13–2 When discharge to home is anticipated, the licensed therapist will teach the resident to go up and down stairs and curbs.

Ambulation Guidelines

Ambulate residents on a tile floor whenever possible. Uneven surfaces such as carpeting, gravel, or grass make walking more difficult. They may also cause fatigue and loss of balance.

Use good judgment when ambulating residents. Safety is always a primary concern. Check for hazards on the floor, such as spills, or objects that could cause the residents to fall. Guidelines for ambulating residents are given on the next page.

Work with the resident privately if he or she is having difficulty, is frustrated, or is upset. As the resident progresses, consider his or her need for transportation to other areas of the facility. Instead of ambulating in the hallway, walk the resident to and from activities, meals, the bathroom, or the nurses' station for medications. If the program involves walking back and forth in the hallway, residents may continue to depend on their wheelchairs. This is because they view the activity as exercise. They do not see the functional purpose of the

ambulation. Privately ask other staff members to encourage residents when they see them walking. Marking the floor or wall in the hallway with the distance in feet is helpful. Measuring progress in feet encourages the resident. It also ensures a goal-oriented program.

Fatigue

In the early stages of the ambulation program, the resident may tire easily. The reasons for fatigue are:

- The resident has been physically inactive for a period of time.
- The resident has not performed the activity in a long time.
- The resident must use a higher degree of concentration to learn a new activity. The mental energy required, combined with increased physical activity, is tiring.
- The resident may suffer physiological effects related to the illness or injury, causing fatigue.

General Guidelines for Assisting Residents in Ambulation Programs

- Check the resident's shoes to make sure they have nonskid soles. Never ambulate a resident who has bare feet or is wearing only socks on the feet.
- Dress the resident in street clothes. If this is not possible, make sure the resident's body is covered. Avoid long pants, long robes, and slippers that could cause the resident to trip.
- Assist the resident to dangle, then stand at the bedside to balance before ambulating. If the resident feels weak, dizzy, or faint, return him or her to bed. Notify your supervisor.
- Always use a gait belt, even if the resident is steady on his or her feet.
- If the therapist orders an assistive device, have the resident practice using it. The therapist or restorative nurse will determine the gait pattern to use. Ambulate the resident with the device for the distance and time ordered.
- If the care plan or your assignment are not specific, ask for clarification.
- Practice good body mechanics.
- Teach the resident to use good body mechanics and practice safety.
- Monitor the resident for signs of pain, fatigue, or faintness. If noted, stop the activity. Notify your supervisor.
- Stay close, slightly behind and to the resident's side. Hold the center back of the gait belt with an underhand grasp **(Figure 13–3)**.
- Position your body so it moves with the resident's body. You should not interfere with the resident's movement.
- Have another assistant follow behind you with a wheelchair, if the resident's endurance is in doubt.
- Encourage the resident to stand upright when walking. The head, shoulders, hips, knees, and feet should be erect.
- Encourage the resident to take large, even steps. Teach him or her to maintain a wide

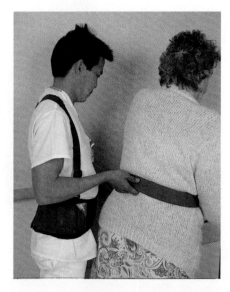

Figure 13–3 Stand slightly behind and close to the side of the resident. Grasp the belt in the center using an underhand grasp.

base of support. The distance between the feet should be equal to the resident's shoulder width.
- Allow adequate time for ambulation. Avoid making the resident feel rushed.
- Allow the resident time to rest, if necessary.
- Provide only the amount of assistance necessary.
- If the resident is not motivated, place a wheelchair ahead of him or her. Tell the resident the goal is to walk to the chair.
- Notify your supervisor if you believe the resident is unsafe.
- Stop ambulation immediately if the resident shows signs of illness, extreme fatigue, shortness of breath, dizziness, sweating, or anxiety. Notify your supervisor.
- Never leave the resident unattended during or after ambulation. When you are through, leave the resident safely sitting in a chair.

PROCEDURE

36 AMBULATING A RESIDENT WHO BEGINS TO FALL

1. Perform your beginning procedure actions.

2. Apply the gait belt. Check the fit with two or three fingers.

3. Assist the resident to stand, if needed.

4. Hold the center back of the belt with an underhand grasp.

5. Allow the resident to hold your free arm, if needed for balance and support.

6. Walk beside and slightly behind the resident. One leg is behind the resident's back. The other is at the resident's side. Keep the back leg directly behind the resident's knee.

7. If the resident begins to fall, push against the resident's knees with your knees. Control the fall with the gait belt.

8. Pull the resident close to your body with the gait belt. Ease the resident to the floor by sliding him or her down your legs **(Figure 13–4).** Use good body mechanics to avoid injury to your back.

   If the resident falls, try to decrease the impact of the fall. If you are near a wall, direct the resident toward it. You and the resident can slide gently down the wall to the floor. Protect the resident's head.

9. Call for help.

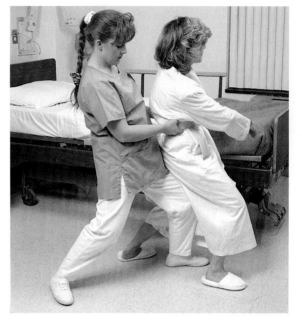

Figure 13–4 If the resident begins to fall, pull her toward your body and slide her down your leg. Bend from your knees to protect your back. Do not try to hold the resident up.

10. Stay with the resident until help arrives. Follow the licensed nurse's directions.

11. Perform your procedure completion actions.

▨ ASSISTIVE DEVICES USED FOR AMBULATION

Canes, crutches, and walkers provide support during ambulation. They redistribute the balance of the resident's weight. This shifts the center of gravity over a wider area. The device prevents loss of balance. Assistive devices often enable residents to be independent with ambulation.

Before ordering an assistive device, the therapist or restorative nurse assesses the resident. He or she will evaluate the resident's:

▨ Strength

▨ Coordination

▨ Range of motion

▨ Balance

▨ Stability

▨ Coordination

▨ General condition

The licensed professional will determine which type of device will best meet the resident's needs. The major indications for using an assistive device are:

▨ Structural deformity, injury, or disease that decreases the resident's ability to bear weight on the legs

▨ Muscular weakness or paralysis of the trunk or lower extremities

▨ Difficulty balancing

Some preliminary activities may be necessary before the resident can use the device. The therapist may use a **dynamometer (Figure 13–5)** to

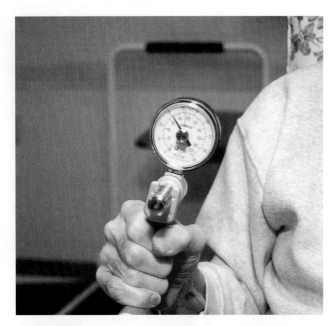

Figure 13–5 The dynamometer is used to test grip strength.

measure hand and grip strength. You may be asked to assist with the evaluation and preliminary activities. To use an assistive device, the resident must be able to:

- Grip the ambulation device with one or both hands
- Hold the hand and elbow in the correct position
- Support and elevate the body with the shoulder muscles
- Dangle unassisted with the feet on the floor or a footstool
- Push to a standing position using the arms and legs
- Stand at the bedside with minimal assistance
- Balance sufficiently to use the device

The resident must have sufficient strength in the hips and knees to walk. Strengthening exercises for the upper and lower extremities may be ordered.

SELECTING ASSISTIVE AMBULATION DEVICES

A variety of assistive ambulation devices are available. The device is selected based on the resident's coordination, degree of support, and stability. **Table 13–2** describes the features and resident requirements for ambulation devices.

Assistive devices come in a variety of sizes. Most are adjustable to fit the resident. Sometimes the res-

ident changes devices as his or her needs change. Residents with deteriorating conditions may go from devices providing less support to devices providing more. Residents with some conditions will improve. They will also change devices. Some residents will eventually be able to walk without the device. **Table 13–3** lists assistive devices from which the selection is made.

Walkers

Walkers are commonly used for and by elderly residents. Indications for using a walker are:

- Debilitating conditions
- Generalized weakness in one or both legs
- Need to reduce weight bearing on one leg
- Poor coordination
- Injury to one leg
- Inability to use crutches
- Difficulty balancing without support

The walker provides a sturdy base of support. The resident propels the walker by using elbow extension and shoulder depression. Residents who are recovering from hip fractures often begin ambulation using a walker. Several different types of walkers are available **(Figure 13–6)**. The therapist or restorative nurse will select the type that meets the resident's needs. The walker is adjusted so the handgrip is at panty-line height. If the shoulders are raised during ambulation, the walker is too high. Platforms may be attached to the walker to support the arms.

Walker height is adjusted by turning the device upside down. Each leg has a push-button lock. Depress the lock and push or pull the telescoping leg to adjust the height. All four legs must be the same height before the resident uses the device.

Types of Walkers. The most common types of walkers are pictured in Figure 13–6. The aluminum walker with rubber tips on all four legs is used most often. Walkers are also available with two and four wheels. These are used for residents who cannot lift a walker or have weak hands. The walkers have brakes on the wheels. The brakes lock automatically when weight is placed downward on the walker. A stair-climbing walker and several types of reverse walkers are also available. These are rarely used in the long-term care facility and are not discussed here. If a resident in your facility uses one of these devices, you will be given special instructions.

Safety Precautions for Ambulating Residents with a Walker. The therapist or restorative nurse will recommend a gait for the resident to use. The standard walker is picked up and placed a comfort-

Table 13–3   Selecting Assistive Ambulation Devices

The devices are listed here in order, from those providing the *most* stability and support to those providing the *least* stability and support.

parallel bars
walkers
axillary crutches
Lofstrand crutches (also called forearm or Canadian crutches)
two canes
one cane

The devices are listed in order, from those requiring the *least* resident coordination to those providing the *most* coordination.

parallel bars
walkers
one cane
two canes
axillary crutches
Lofstrand crutches

Some residents will use one crutch instead of two. Residents who have poor strength in the hand, wrist, and forearm, or those with poor grip strength, can have a platform attached to the walker or crutches.

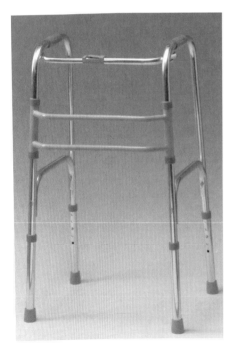 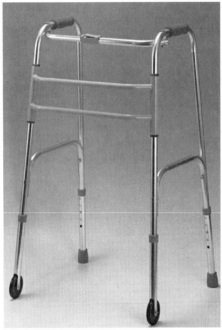 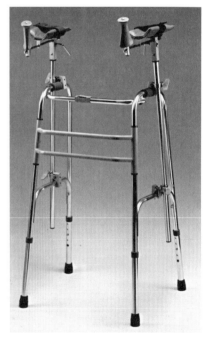

Figure 13–6   Many walkers are available. Platforms can be attached, if necessary, to support the arms. (Courtesy of Lumex Medical Products)

Table 13–2 Types of Assistive Devices

Assistive Device	Features	Resident Requirements
Walkers		
Standard	■ Adjustable ■ Rubber tips	■ Requires upper body strength ■ Provides maximum stability and support ■ Excellent for older persons
Rolling	■ Legs have wheels ■ Otherwise same as regular walker	■ Good for residents who only need walker for balance but not support
Crutches		
Axillary	■ Wooden or steel ■ Worn under axillae	■ Requires good upper body strength and balance ■ Not recommended for older persons ■ Best for younger persons with lower extremity or hip fractures that will heal in a short time ■ Provides greatest range of ambulation ■ Less stable than axillary crutches
Forearm (Lofstrand or Canadian)	■ Shorter than axillary crutches ■ Has metal cuff worn around upper arm	■ Best for long-term crutch use ■ Reduces stress on axillary vessels and nerves ■ Requires upper body strength and more stability and coordination ■ Provides most maneuverability of all crutches
Platform	■ Platform affixed to a crutch ■ Resident bears weight on forearm	■ Best for residents with severe arthritis or poor use of hands ■ Does not require as much upper body strength ■ Requires good balance
Canes		
Standard	■ Single leg ■ Curved handle ■ Rubber tip	■ Good for residents with only one good arm, lateral instability, or balance conditions
Quad (four-point)	■ Single cane resting on a platform with four legs ■ Rubber tips on legs	■ Better for residents with more severe conditions ■ Does not require as much coordination, but still requires balance and upper body strength in one arm
Walkcane or Hemiwalker	■ Has four legs that come all the way up to a handlebar ■ Rubber tips on all legs	■ Provides most stability of all canes ■ Best for hemiplegic residents who require extra support on one side

able distance ahead of the resident. Comfortable distance is important. If the resident must lean forward to reach the handles, the walker is too far away. All four legs of the walker should strike the floor at the same time. Some residents have a tendency to touch the back legs on the floor first. They rock the walker forward onto the front legs. This is a dangerous practice that causes falls. When all four legs are securely on the floor, the resident steps forward. If the resident has visual or cognitive deficits, assist with steering. Place one hand on the resident and one hand on the walker, guiding the resident.

Some residents pick up the walkers and carry them. This increases the risk of injury. The resident may not need the device, or may do better with a different type of device. Consult your supervisor.

Crutches

Crutches are used by extending the elbows and depressing the shoulders. Two types of crutches are

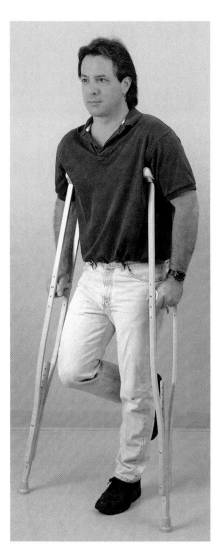

Figure 13–7 Axillary crutches are not commonly used by the elderly.

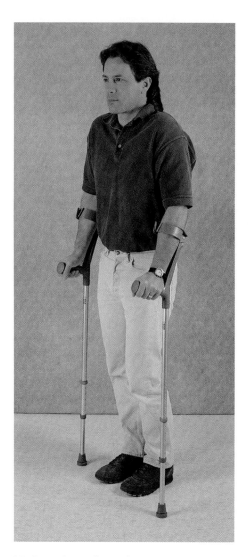

Figure 13–8 Lofstrand crutches are selected for individuals who will be using crutches over the long term.

available. **Axillary crutches (Figure 13–7)** are made of wood or aluminum. The crutches provide a moderate degree of stability. They are used by residents with weakness in one or both legs, those with leg injuries, and those needing extra trunk support. The correct height is two to three fingers-width below the underarm. Wooden crutches are adjusted by releasing the wing nut and removing the bolt. Metal crutches are adjusted by releasing the push-button lock and repositioning the telescoping legs. The elderly do not use crutches often. Most do not have sufficient arm strength to lift the body. Balance and coordination may also be a problem.

Lofstrand crutches (Figure 13–8) are also called forearm crutches or Canadian crutches. Residents using these crutches usually need them permanently, or for a long period of time. The crutches have a cuff that fits around the forearm. The resident can release the hand grip without dropping the crutch. They are used by residents with weak-

ness in both legs who have good trunk stability. Residents using Lofstrand crutches must have good coordination. They are slightly more difficult to use than axillary crutches. Lofstrand crutches have two adjustment mechanisms. The upper mechanism adjusts the hand grip height. The lower mechanism adjusts the crutch length. Both are adjusted by releasing the push-button lock and moving the telescoping mechanism. The hand grips are adjusted so they are at the panty-line level. The cuff should fit comfortably around the forearm. Platforms can be attached to support the forearms, if necessary **(Figure 13–9).** The platforms improve stability.

Canes

Canes are ordered for residents with balance problems, pain, or weakness in the legs. One or two canes may be used. Canes do not provide support. Many types of canes are available **(Figure 13–10).** The standard cane is shaped like the letter J. The

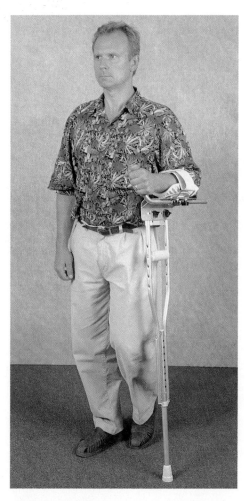

Figure 13–9 Arm platforms can be attached to Lofstrand crutches, if necessary.

quad cane has four feet. Of the canes available, it is the most stable. The resident can release the hand grip and it will not fall to the floor. The base of the quad cane comes in two sizes, small and large. The large base provides the greatest stability. The size may make maneuvering in tight spaces difficult. Canes are available with many different types of hand grips. Some have an offset shaft, which changes the center of gravity. This shifts the weight over the tip of the J cane or the center of the base of the quad cane.

The hand grip of the cane should be at the pantyline level. Wooden canes can only be adjusted by cutting them. Metal canes are adjusted by releasing the push-button lock and moving the telescoping shaft.

Teaching the Resident to Ambulate with a Cane. A number of gait patterns are used, depending on the resident's problem. The most common involves placing the cane in the hand opposite the weak leg. The cane and the weak leg move forward at the same time. This provides extra support on the weak side.

Safety Precautions. Be aware of safety factors at all times. Teach residents safe ambulation practices. Check the rubber tips before the resident ambulates. If the rubber is worn, replace the tip before the resident uses the device. If you feel a resident is not using an assistive device correctly, notify your supervisor.

Some residents may attempt to use the assistive ambulation device for transfers. They hold the device while getting into or out of the chair. This is an unsafe practice that may cause falls. Teach the

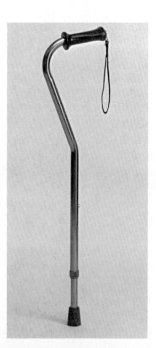
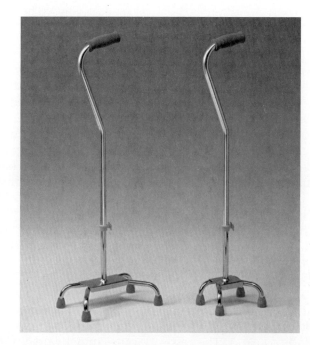
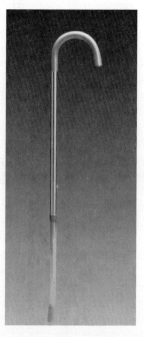

Figure 13–10 Many different canes are available. The therapist or restorative nurse will select one that best meets the resident's needs. (Courtesy of Lumex Medical Products)

resident to use the arms of the chair for support when sitting and standing.

GAIT PATTERNS

The therapist or restorative nurse determines the gait pattern to be used by the resident. He or she considers the physician's orders and the resident's ability to bear weight. The care plan will describe the type of weight bearing permitted. **Table 13–4** lists common phrases describing the degree of weight bearing.

Two-Point Gait

Residents using two assistive devices commonly use a two-point gait. The gait is used for residents with pain, muscle weakness, and difficulty balancing **(Figure 13–11)**. One assistive device and the opposite extremity are moved forward simultaneously. After the device is securely on the floor, the resident shifts his or her weight onto the support. The other assistive device and opposite extremity are moved forward. This sequence is repeated until the resident reaches the destination.

Three-Point Gait

The three-point gait **(Figure 13–12)** is used for residents with a weak, painful, or injured extrem-

ity. It may also be used when the physician orders decreased weight bearing. A walker or two crutches or canes can be used. The walker or both crutches or canes are moved forward at the same time. The resident moves the affected extremity forward. The resident shifts his or her weight to the upper extremities, then moves the strong leg forward. The resident shifts the weight to the weak leg, repeating the pattern until he or she reaches the destination. When the resident first learns this gait, he or she may move the unaffected leg forward between the assistive devices. Encourage the resident to step slightly ahead, simulating normal ambulation. As residents become more proficient, the assistive device(s) and affected extremity can be moved forward at the same time.

Four-Point Gait

The four-point gait **(Figure 13–13)** is also called the deliberate two-point gait. It is used with two canes or crutches. Residents using this type of gait have problems similar to those who use the two-point gait. However, the problems are more severe. The four-point gait is sometimes used when residents first begin using assistive devices. As the resident becomes proficient, he or she may graduate to the two-point gait.

Table 13–4 Weight Bearing

Type of Weight Bearing Ordered	Description
Full weight bearing (FWB)	The resident can bear full weight on the affected extremity. Assistive devices are used for balance, not to decrease weight on the affected extremity.
Weight bearing as tolerated (WBAT)	The amount of weight bearing is determined by the resident and can range from partial to full, depending on pain and the resident's tolerance.
Partial weight bearing (PWB)	A limited amount of weight bearing is permitted. If this amount is designated in pounds, the resident may practice using a spring scale to determine the feeling of this amount of weight on the affected extremity. If you are assisting with use of the spring scale, elevate the opposite foot to the same height as the scale to prevent falls.
Toe-touch weight bearing (TTWB)	The resident cannot bear weight on the affected extremity, but may touch the toes to the floor for balance.
Nonweight bearing (NWB)	The affected extremity cannot bear weight. Your facility policy may state that this extremity should not touch the floor.

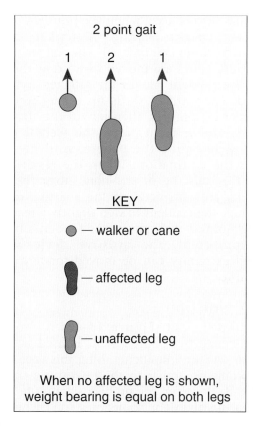

Figure 13–11 The two-point gait.

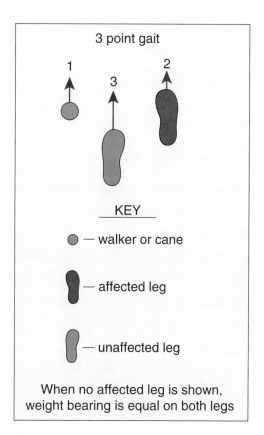

Figure 13–12 The three-point gait.

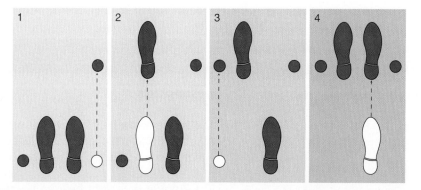

Figure 13–13 The four-point gait. The resident is bearing weight on both legs.

To use the four-point gait, one assistive device is moved forward and placed on the floor. The opposite leg follows. The other assistive device moves forward, and is placed on the floor. The other leg follows. The resident shifts weight to the three remaining supports each time an assistive device or leg is lifted from the floor. The cycle is repeated until the destination is reached.

Swing-to Gait

The swing-to gait **(Figure 13–14)** is used for residents with muscular weakness, paralysis, or paresis. Residents with decreased weight bearing on one leg may also use the gait. A walker or two crutches are

used. The resident moves the assistive device(s) forward, placing it on the floor. He or she shifts the weight to the arms. Both legs move forward together, until they are even with the assistive device. Then they are placed on the floor. The resident shifts weight bearing back to the legs. He or she moves the device forward, repeating the sequence.

Swing-through Gait

Two crutches are used for the swing-through gait **(Figure 13–15).** Some therapists teach this gait with a walker. This gait is rarely used for the elderly. The indications for using the swing-through gait

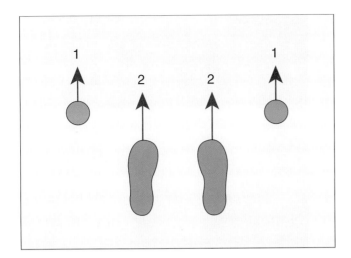

Figure 13–14 The swing-to gait. The resident is bearing weight on both legs.

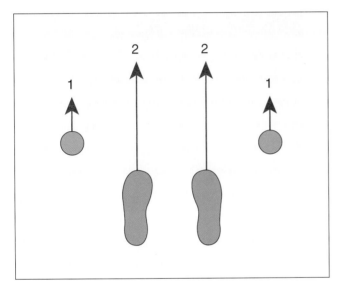

Figure 13–15 The swing-through gait. The resident is bearing weight on both legs.

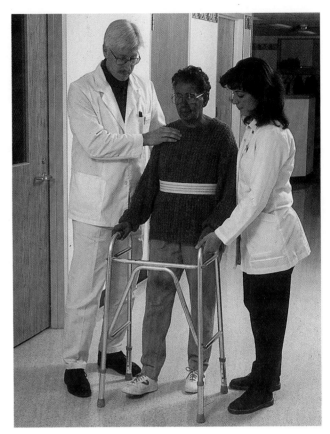

Figure 13–16 The therapist is guarding the resident by supporting her shoulder. The restorative nursing assistant is holding the gait belt with the right hand and the walker with the left hand.

are the same as for the swing-to gait. This technique is used for residents who have greater ability and confidence using assistive devices. The resident moves the assistive device(s) forward and places it on the floor. The weight is shifted to the arms. Both legs move forward simultaneously. When they are slightly ahead of the device, they are placed on the floor. The resident shifts weight bearing back to the legs. He or she moves the device forward, repeating the sequence.

Guarding

Use guarding techniques when assisting residents with ambulation. Using a gait belt is a form of guarding. Placing your hand on the resident's shoulder keeps him or her from falling forward

(Figure 13–16). Your supervisor may teach you to place one arm around the resident's waist. You will hold his or her arm with the other hand. The same technique is used if two assistants are ambulating the resident. Other forms of guarding are:

- Holding the resident's hand for balance or support
- Teaching the resident to use the hand rail with one hand while you stand on the opposite side holding the gait belt

When the resident is learning to ambulate, stand closest to the strong side. Standing on the strong side supports the weaker extremity. Residents tend to lean away from the injured or painful extremity when they begin to ambulate. If the resident starts to lean or fall, shift the resident's weight to the strong leg and your own body. As the resident's ability improves, you can guard from the opposite side. This encourages good posture and weight bearing on the affected leg.

Practice guarding residents by using your feet and body movements. Move your outside foot simultaneously with the assistive device on that side. Your inside foot is behind the resident. Move this foot when the resident moves the foot on the side you are guarding.

■ SPECIAL SITUATIONS

The following procedures will not be performed in the long-term care facility. However, you may work with residents learning these procedures in preparation for discharge.

Curbs

The therapist teaches residents to step on and off curbs. Before going up or down curbs, you must know the resident's:

■ Diagnosis

■ Weight-bearing status

■ Affected side

■ Ability to follow instructions

You must also learn special safety precautions to take. Always use a gait belt when assisting residents on curbs.

To go up a curb:

■ Stand in the street, behind the resident.

■ Hold the gait belt with an underhand grasp.

■ If the resident uses an assistive device, instruct him or her to place the device one-half to two-thirds of the way forward next to the curb.

■ Instruct the resident to step up with the stronger leg.

■ After the resident has stepped up, he or she shifts the body weight to the stronger extremity. Tell the resident to lean forward slightly and straighten the stronger leg.

■ Instruct the resident to move the weaker leg, push with the hands on the assistive device, and pull the leg and device up the curb.

To go down a curb:

■ Stand on the curb, behind the resident.

■ Hold the gait belt with an underhand grasp.

■ Advise the resident to move close to the curb, so the toes are near the edge.

■ If an assistive device is used, the resident bends the stronger leg and moves the assistive device and weaker leg down to the street. The device and the weak leg may be moved together. The device can be moved first, followed by the leg, if the resident prefers.

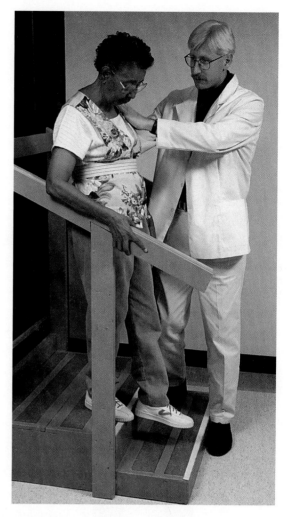

Figure 13–17 The licensed therapist will teach the resident to go up and down stairs. The same procedure is used for curbs.

■ Tell the resident to lean slightly on the assistive device and lower the stronger leg.

■ Instruct the resident to avoid leaning heavily on the device. This may cause loss of balance.

Stairs

Walking on stairs is difficult for many elderly residents. The physical therapist teaches residents this skill (**Figure 13–17**) if discharge to a home with stairs is anticipated. Remind the resident not to bend forward. Instruct him or her not to pull on the handrail to go upstairs. This position changes the center of gravity and increases the risk of falls.

Canes are carried in the strong hand or hooked in the resident's shirt pocket while the resident is using stairs. Residents who use crutches may hold the handrail with one hand and use a crutch in the other.

Going up and down stairs with a standard walker is impossible for most residents. This is also a dangerous practice. A specially designed stair walker should be used. This walker has an additional set of handgrips on the sides that are used on stairs. The walker is turned backward for going up stairs, and faces forward for going down.

Going up stairs:

- Remind the resident to use the handrail.
- Always use a gait belt.
- Have the resident place his or her hand on the handrail on the stronger side.
- Cue the resident to lead with the stronger leg, placing the foot on the first step.
- Have the resident lean slightly forward, push down on the handrail, and straighten the stronger leg.

- Have the resident raise his or her body, lifting the weaker leg to the step.
- Repeat for the remaining stairs.

Going down stairs:

- Remind the resident to use the handrail.
- Always use the gait belt.
- Have the resident place his or her hand on the handrail on the stronger side.
- Remind the resident to lead with the weaker leg. Cue him or her to bend the strong leg slowly, placing the weaker leg on the first step.
- After the weaker leg is firmly on the step, and the knee is straightened, tell the resident to step down to the same step with the strong leg.
- Repeat for the remaining stairs.
- Remind the resident to stand erect. Bending forward on stairs increases the risk of falls.

KEY POINTS IN CHAPTER

- *All body systems benefit from exercise and ambulation.*
- *The ability to ambulate provides residents with emotional satisfaction and opportunities for socialization.*
- *Ambulation programs are designed to maintain or improve function.*
- *The interdisciplinary team assesses the resident. They will design an ambulation program to meet his or her needs.*
- *Ambulation goals must be purposeful and functional for the resident.*
- *Residents should prepare for ambulation by doing warm-up exercises.*
- *Gait is the way a person walks. Residents with certain musculoskeletal and neurologic problems have gaits peculiar to the illness.*
- *Residents should be ambulated on a tile floor whenever possible.*
- *Residents should be ambulated for a functional purpose. Residents view walking in the hallway as an exercise. Because they do not see a purpose for walking, they may depend on the wheelchair for transportation.*
- *Use a gait belt and good body mechanics when ambulating residents.*
- *Canes, crutches, and walkers are assistive devices that redistribute the resident's weight, shifting the center of gravity over a wider area and providing greater support.*
- *Assistive devices must be adjusted so they are the correct size for the resident.*
- *Five different gait patterns are used when teaching residents to ambulate with assistive devices.*
- *Guarding techniques keep the resident safe during ambulation.*

CLINICAL APPLICATIONS

1. You are ambulating Mrs. Stanski in the hallway using a walker and a gait belt. She complains of dizziness and nausea. What will you do?

2. Mr. Stone is saddened over the death of his wife of 50 years. She was his roommate in your facility. Mrs. Stone became ill and died suddenly. Mr. Stone has been staying in his room most of the day. When he leaves the room, he uses a wheelchair. Before his wife's death, Mr. Stone was up and about in the facility. He used a walker and was active in the resident volunteer program. He visited with other residents often. Now he is staying to himself. How can you assist Mr. Stone? Should he be screened for a restorative ambulation program?

3. Miss Grubbs fell and fractured her ankle. Before the injury, she ambulated independently. Her balance was unsteady at times. Miss Grubbs has mild arthritic deformities in her hands. The physician applied a cast to her ankle. He ordered no weight bearing for six weeks. How will you assist this resident? What type of ambulation device do you think will work best for her?

4. You ambulate Mr. Sarrano to the dining room for meals with a walker twice a day. He sits in a wooden chair with arms at the dining table. Mr. Sarrano tends to fall into the chair. He sits forcefully. He has almost tipped backward several times. What do you recommend?

5. Mrs. Huynh recently returned to your facility. She was hospitalized for five days for a severe urinary tract infection. Before she was hospitalized, she ambulated about the facility independently using a cane. Now she is weak and unsteady. She remains in bed much of the time. She can turn herself in bed, but cannot get up without help. She is using a wheelchair for transportation to the dining room. What must be considered before beginning an ambulation program? From the information given here, do you think she will be able to walk around the facility again?

Restorative Approaches to Meeting Residents' Nutrition, Hydration, ADL, and Personal Care Needs

Restorative Approaches to Meeting Residents' Nutrition and Hydration Needs

After reading this chapter, you should be able to:

- *Spell and define key terms.*
- *Explain why nutrition is important for the elderly.*
- *List the signs and symptoms of malnutrition and dehydration.*
- *Describe the effect the environment has on residents' appetite.*
- *State how to manage a restorative dining program.*
- *Explain how to establish and maintain a restorative feeding program.*

NUTRITION IN THE ELDERLY

Nutrition is important to the longevity and quality of life in the elderly. Residents look forward to meals and snacks. Surveyors will tell you that if the food looks, smells, and tastes good, residents have fewer complaints about the facility overall. Some residents will tell you that food is one of the few things they look forward to. The need for food is at the bottom of the Maslow pyramid. However, eating meets needs on several levels. Look at eating as one of the most important activities of the day.

Malnutrition

Malnutrition is a serious problem in the elderly. Signs of malnutrition are listed in **Table 14–1**. Some residents are admitted with malnutrition. However, studies have shown that many residents develop malnutrition in long-term care facilities. A list of weights and calories needed for gain or loss is given in Appendix C of this book. Barriers to adequate nutrition are both physical and psychological. Residents on restricted diets and those who prefer ethnic and cultural foods may not eat enough. Young and middle-aged residents may prefer foods such as stir-fry, sandwiches on pita bread, and tacos. These items are not normally served in long-term care facilities.

Other issues that affect residents' use of nutrients are:

- Infection
- Activity
- Pressure ulcers
- Chronic diseases
- Cognitive impairment
- Inability to eat independently
- Sensory loss
- Poor oral hygiene
- Side effects of medications

Weight loss is a problem in the long-term care industry. Take this problem very seriously. A resident who is losing weight is not receiving adequate nutrients. This increases the risk of serious illness, infection, skin breakdown, and other conditions.

Many residents require assistance with meals. This is usually because of physical impairments and cognitive loss. Some residents require total feeding. Some need prompting and coaxing. Staff members spend a great deal of time serving meals and feeding residents. Ensuring that all residents receive adequate nutrition is a challenge.

Table 14–1 Signs of Possible Malnutrition

Body Part Affected	Signs of Possible Malnutrition
Face	pale color; dark, sunken appearance of eyes; edema
Eyes	dry, dull appearance; may have redness surrounding cornea; inflamed eyelids
Lips	dry, swollen, cracked, red
Hair	dull, dry; hair falls out excessively; thin; hair color uneven
Tongue	swollen, smooth; may have sores or abnormal color
Gums	sores; may bleed
Teeth	dental cavities; discolorations; teeth missing
Skin	dry, flaky, chapped, loose; subcutaneous fat lost, edema in feet and ankles
Nails	brittle, ridged; may be inverted into a spoon shape
Muscles	weakness; edema at joints; may have problems with coordination and balance
Bones	may fracture easily
Nerves	irritability and disorientation; mental confusion; tingling in hands and feet
Heart	rapid, irregular rate

FACTORS INFLUENCING RESIDENTS' APPETITE

Food service is a great responsibility. It is shared by many team members. Staff must pay careful attention to:

- Food preparation
- Attractive presentation
- Meal service
- Atmosphere
- Feeding independence

Some facilities serve family-style meals. Food is placed in serving bowls on the table. The residents help themselves to the food. Residents enjoy this type of meal service. They often eat better when family-style dining is used. Some facilities offer a selective menu. In this type of dining, residents choose their food in advance. Some facilities offer five or six small meals a day instead of three larger meals. Serving meals in this manner is more expensive for the facility. However, it pays off for residents and the facility. Residents report improved satisfaction and quality of life. The facility benefits from a good reputation in the community. This increases the census, which produces more revenue.

Food has emotional importance for many individuals. It is important to social activities, family gatherings, ethnicity, culture, and religion. This is an important consideration. The pleasure of eating greatly contributes to the resident's quality of life. The ability to choose food and eat independently affects the resident's appetite. Team members consider the emotional impact of food when planning approaches and dietary interventions. Planning meals to meet the resident's medical and emotional needs is a challenging task. Preparing many meals at once is also a challenge. Residents in the facility must be served food at the same time. The food must be at the proper temperature. There are many different diets. Residents have many personal food preferences. This is difficult for the dietary staff.

Environment

(SA)Appetite is affected by the environment. The OBRA '87 laws require facilities to maintain a homelike environment. This is particularly important in the dining room. A pleasant atmosphere improves the residents' appetites **(Figure 14–1).** Tablecloths, centerpieces, attractive dishes, and table decorations promote good intake at meals. Unpleasant odors and offensive behavior affect the appetite. They may cause residents to stop eating. Knowing how the environment affects residents is important. Managing incontinence, difficult behavior, and other problems immediately promotes a pleasant atmosphere.

Seating Arrangements.   Eating is a social activity. Residents eat at dining tables in small groups. Seating arrangements should be selected so residents can socialize and talk with others. For example, avoid seating an alert resident at a table with three confused residents. The alert resident will have no one to talk to. Residents should face each other. Avoid isolating them by seating them facing a wall or a window. Round or square tables work best. Long tables tend to isolate residents socially.(SA)

Cognitively impaired residents who are easily distracted may not eat well. They are busy monitoring the activity in the room instead of eating. Seat these residents in a quiet area. Reduce activity as much as possible. Avoid positioning their chairs facing the center of the room. If this is not possible, consider feeding them in another area. A corner of the dining room may be screened off for them. When working with cognitively impaired residents, bowls may work better than plates. Cups with large handles work well. Small, frequent meals may work better than larger ones.

Positioning.   (SA)Proper positioning is important at meal time.(SA) Food is not swallowed or digested if the resident is not upright. Poor posture increases the risk of choking. Many facilities have restorative ambulation programs at mealtime. The residents' wheelchairs are parked at the dining room door. The residents are ambulated to their tables. They are seated in regular dining chairs with arms. The residents benefit from the ambulation. Sitting in chairs improves their posture for meals. (SA)When residents sit in wheelchairs, monitor the distance of the chair from the table. Residents should not extend their arms more than 10 to 12 inches to reach the food. The elbows should be lower than the wrists.(SA) If the wheelchair is too low, the resident will have to reach up to eat. This causes strain on the shoulder and arm muscles. Reaching up to eat increases fatigue. Residents may become too tired to finish the meal.

Attention to seating arrangements at mealtime improves the residents' appetites and quality of life. Residents receive physical benefits from ambulation programs in the dining room. For residents in wheelchairs, a tray with Velcro® fasteners **(Figure 14–2)** may make eating easier. Position the wheelchair next to the table. (SA)This keeps the resident from becoming isolated.(SA) He or she

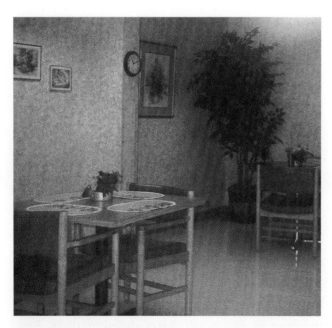

Figure 14–1 The restorative nursing assistants in this facility redecorated the dining room, creating a comfortable, homelike environment. (Courtesy of East Galbraith Health Care Community, Cincinnati, OH)

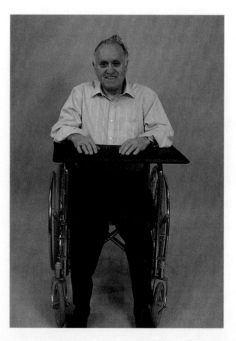

Figure 14–2 The lap tray is useful for residents who must remain in the wheelchair for meals. (Courtesy of Skil-Care Corporation, Yonkers, NY (800) 431-2972)

will benefit from socialization with others. If space does not permit the wheelchair to fit in at the table, try grouping three or four residents with trays in a circle. This will provide the socialization they would have at a table.

Vision Loss. Some residents have difficulty eating because of vision problems. They do not eat their meals because they cannot see them. Residents with vision problems may not know that they have not eaten all the food. Some are fed by staff because their visual problem is unrecognized and uncorrected. Some residents have a condition called hemianopsia. This is a complication of a CVA. These individuals have blindness in the visual field in one or both eyes. (SA)If you notice that a resident has eaten the food on only one side of the plate or tray, turn it around. The resident may finish the meal. He or she may not be able to see the food on both sides of the tray.(SA)

Some residents have uncorrected visual problems. Some need the prescription in their glasses changed. These individuals may have poor appetites. Upon closer monitoring, you will notice that they try to pick up the food several times before finally scooping it up. They may not be able to move the utensil to the mouth without spilling. This is related to the inability to see. After trying unsuccessfully to pick up the food, the resident becomes frustrated and stops eating. If you believe a visual problem is interfering with the resident's ability to eat, inform your supervisor. Attention to the residents' ability to see is very important. Vision affects many areas of residents' lives.

Food Substitutes. (SA)Long-term care facilities are required to have a substitute available if the resident refuses the meat or vegetable. If residents do not like food served, or are not eating, offer the substitute. Liquid nutritional beverages or commercial supplements are not substitutes. These are medically prescribed and require a physician's order. Do not offer liquid nutritional supplements as meal replacements. They are usually high in carbohydrates, but may not contain adequate protein. They contain sugar, which can be harmful to residents with diabetes and those on special diets.(SA)

Adaptive Devices for Eating. Some residents have poor appetites because they have difficulty feeding themselves. Others eat their food, but struggle with utensils. This is usually because of physical problems. Some residents regularly spill their beverages. Residents with these problems should be evaluated for adaptive eating devices. Improving their appetites and making it easier to eat or drink may be resolved with proper utensils and assistive devices. Notify your supervisor if you feel a resident should be screened for adaptive eating devices.

The most common adaptive devices are used for feeding. Many devices are available to meet residents' needs. Look through a catalog of these items so you know what is available. The most common devices are plate guards **(Figure 14–3A)**, plates with modified edges **(Figures 14–3B and C)**, cups **(Figure 14–3D)**, and adaptive silverware **(Figure 14–3E, F, and G)**. Other items, such as the straw holder, may be used. An alternative to a straw holder is taping the straw to the side of the cup. Some residents scoop the food away from the body, causing the plate to slide. A piece of gripper or a damp washcloth under the plate will hold it in place. Review Chapter 9 for additional information about adaptive devices.

ALTERNATIVE NUTRITION

Some residents receive nutrition by alternative methods. These include intravenous feedings **(Figure 14–4A, p. 225)**, total parenteral nutrition, and tube feeding **(Figure 14–4B, p. 225)**. Alternative nutrition is used when the resident has medical problems that prevent him or her from eating normally. (SA) The goal is always to return these residents to oral feeding.(SA) For some, this will not be possible. However, residents are assessed and a plan is developed to restore their eating ability whenever feasible.

Tube Feedings

Some residents who can consume food orally also receive tube feedings, because of weight loss. A plan will be developed to remove the tube at a later time. Some of these residents are served a tray at each meal. They receive tube feedings during the night. This is because the tube feeding solution fills the stomach. If it is given during the day, it suppresses the appetite and the resident does not eat. You may be assigned to work with the resident so that he or she does not lose the ability for self-feeding.

Some residents receive tube feedings because of severe swallowing disorders. Their condition causes **aspiration** of food and fluids. Aspiration is a serious condition in which food enters the lungs. Residents who aspirate may be permanently fed by tube. The speech therapist will assess their ability to swallow and make recommendations.

Sometimes a **modified barium swallow** is ordered. This study shows the resident's potential for aspiration on an x-ray. After the procedure, push fluids, if the resident can take fluids orally. Monitor the resident's bowel movements carefully. Barium will become solid in the colon, causing obstruction and other serious complications. Monitoring fluid intake and bowel movements is important. The nurse may administer laxatives to assist in removing the barium. Inform your supervisor if the resident is not taking fluids, or if he or she does not have a bowel movement daily.

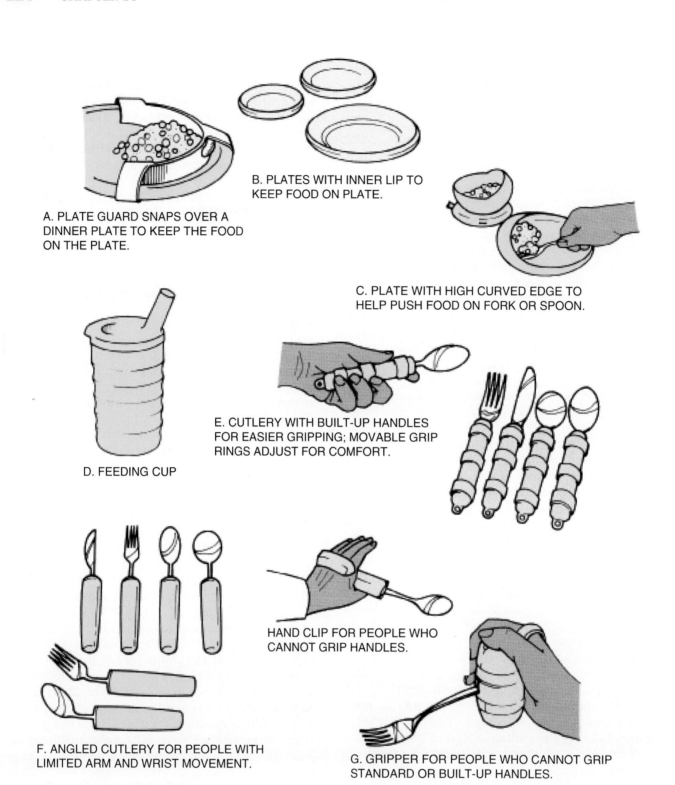

A. PLATE GUARD SNAPS OVER A DINNER PLATE TO KEEP THE FOOD ON THE PLATE.

B. PLATES WITH INNER LIP TO KEEP FOOD ON PLATE.

C. PLATE WITH HIGH CURVED EDGE TO HELP PUSH FOOD ON FORK OR SPOON.

D. FEEDING CUP

E. CUTLERY WITH BUILT-UP HANDLES FOR EASIER GRIPPING; MOVABLE GRIP RINGS ADJUST FOR COMFORT.

F. ANGLED CUTLERY FOR PEOPLE WITH LIMITED ARM AND WRIST MOVEMENT.

HAND CLIP FOR PEOPLE WHO CANNOT GRIP HANDLES.

G. GRIPPER FOR PEOPLE WHO CANNOT GRIP STANDARD OR BUILT-UP HANDLES.

Figure 14–3 Adaptive eating devices.

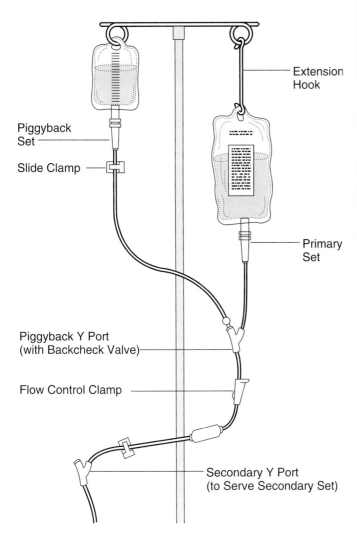

Figure 14–4A Residents who are fed by intravenous infusion may also receive a meal tray.

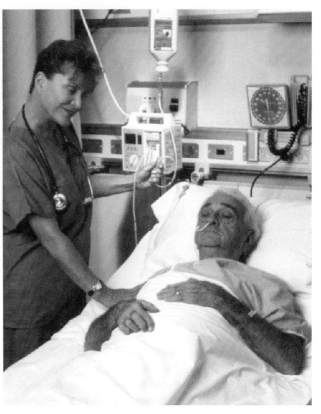

Figure 14–4B Whenever possible, the goal for residents who are tube-fed is to assist them to return to eating normally. (Photo used with permission of Ross Products Division, Abbott Laboratories, Columbus, Ohio)

▓▓ PLANNING NUTRITIONAL INTERVENTIONS

The MDS 2.0 assesses the resident's nutrition intake. The dietitian will review laboratory reports and assess the resident further. The resident and his or her family are invited to participate in the care conference. During the care plan, the team will plan nutritional approaches to maintain or increase the resident's weight. When planning nutritional programs, the team considers the resident's:

▓ Medical needs

▓ Cultural and religious practices

▓ Wishes

▓ Personal goals

▓ Food preferences

▓ Quality of life

▓ Medical prognosis

▓ Physician's orders

▓ Benefits of treatment

The team looks at the resident holistically. After the care plan is developed, staff uses the nursing process to implement and evaluate the effectiveness of the plan.

The dietitian plans the menu to meet the resident's medical needs. The occupational therapist works with residents who have feeding problems. The therapist may develop feeding plans for some residents. He or she also recommends adaptive devices to help residents eat independently. The speech therapist works with residents who have swallowing disorders. He or she also evaluates the resident's position. The therapist may recommend a change in posture or procedures to improve swallowing. The physical therapist works with the resident's posture. He or she recommends positions for residents with special needs. The restorative nurse develops restorative dining and feeding programs. You will assist residents with meal service. You will work with the feeding program, assist residents to use adaptive equipment, and teach residents to eat independently.

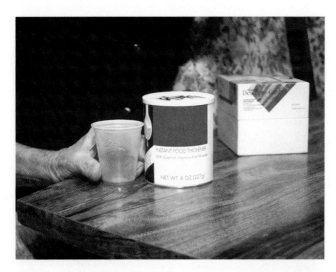

Figure 14–5 The speech therapist will order the type of thickener and consistency to mix.

Some residents have **dysphagia.** Residents with this condition have difficulty swallowing food and liquids. The speech therapist evaluates these residents. He or she may recommend using food thickeners **(Figure 14–5).** These are nonprescription products that are ordered from the food vendor. Thickeners do not change the taste of foods or beverages. Thickening food and liquids makes swallowing easier and prevents choking.

The speech therapist will recommend the type and amount of thickener to use. The therapist will order the texture of the liquids. You will mix the thickener to achieve the texture ordered. For example, the therapist may recommend that liquids be mixed to the consistency of peach juice or nectar. Add the thickener immediately before feeding. When adding thickeners:

- Use the correct product
- Use the correct amount
- Follow manufacturers' directions
- Stir the thickener well
- Follow the speech therapist's instructions for positioning and feeding

Feeding Techniques for Residents with Dysphagia

The speech therapist recommends techniques and positions for improving swallowing and preventing choking. Residents with dysphagia may require one-to-one assistance, prompting, or supervision at meals. Before beginning, make sure the resident is fully awake and alert. During the meal, reduce distractions. Focus the resident on eating. Position residents with dysphagia upright for meals. Use props, if necessary. The head should face forward, with the body flexed forward slightly. Prompt the resident to eat slowly, taking small bites. Remind him or her to chew the food well. The speech therapist may tell you to remind the resident to tuck the chin in when swallowing. This changes the position of the airway, reducing the risk of choking.

THE RESTORATIVE DINING PROGRAM

The restorative nurse develops the dining program. He or she will use the therapists as consultants, if necessary. The nurse will evaluate the dining room and meal service for:

- Atmosphere
- Assistance given to residents
- Seating arrangements
- Table height
- Food acceptance
- Resident need for adaptive devices

Grouping Residents with Similar Needs

The nurse will evaluate seating in the dining room. He or she will group residents with similar needs together. Alert, independent residents will sit together. Residents with feeding problems are also grouped together. Residents needing limited physical or verbal assistance form one group. Residents who require spoon-feeding form another group. The objective is to group the residents according to the level of assistance they need. This enables the nurse to concentrate staff according to the residents' needs. Residents get more individual attention when this is done.

(SA)Residents must be monitored at mealtime because of the risk of choking.(SA) One staff member can supervise a group of alert residents. He or she will serve coffee, offer substitutes, and monitor for choking. Two or more staff members may be used for a group needing limited physical or verbal assistance. Staff circulates between the tables, prompting the residents to eat. Offering residents a drink may prompt them to begin eating again. Allow residents to eat independently as much as possible. If a cognitively impaired resident stops eating, provide verbal cues. If this is ineffective, try hand-over-hand technique. If this is ineffective, spoon-feed the resident. Encourage him or her to begin eating independently again.

Two or more staff members work with the group that must be fed. One-to-one feeding is ideal. However, this may not be realistic, because of staffing. Nevertheless, one staff member should feed no more than two or three residents at once. Special

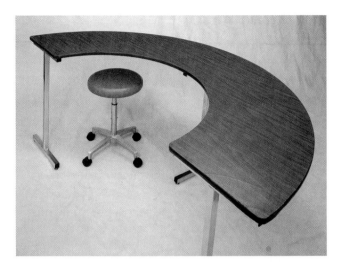

Figure 14–6 The feeding table is horseshoe-shaped. One nursing assistant can feed two or three residents at one time using this table. (Courtesy of Medline Industries, Inc. (800) MEDLINE)

feeding tables **(Figure 14–6)** are used. Encourage residents to eat finger foods and drink beverages.

▨ RESTORATIVE FEEDING RETRAINING

Restorative feeding retraining is a special restorative dining program. Facilities have many different names for this program. The overall objective is to restore resident independence. The benefits of the program include:

▨ Improved socialization

▨ Increased coordination

▨ Prevention of nutritional declines

▨ Prevention of weight loss

▨ Improved appetite

▨ Improved self confidence

Identifying Potential Candidates for the Restorative Feeding Program

Candidates for a restorative feeding group are residents who have:

▨ The physical ability to move one or both hands to the mouth

▨ Problems eating because of limited range of motion, poor eye-hand coordination, or sensory deficits

▨ Weakness that interferes with the ability to eat

▨ Visual limitations that interfere with the ability to eat

▨ Been spoon-fed for a long time, but staff is unsure of the reason why

General Guidelines for Assisting Residents to Eat Independently

▨ Provide a pleasant atmosphere.

▨ Provide adaptive dishes, cups, and utensils if needed **(see Figure 14–7).**

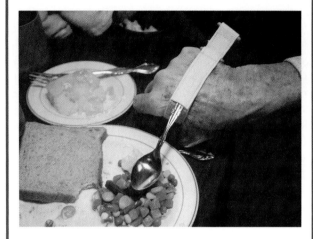

Figure 14–7 Many residents use adaptive utensils.

▨ Position residents comfortably in an upright position, using props if necessary.

▨ Monitor the height and distance of the table in relation to the resident.

▨ Describe the food when serving it; comment that it looks or smells good.

▨ Move the food within the resident's reach.

▨ Offer seasonings and condiments.

▨ Provide only one dish at a time, if the resident is overwhelmed with the amount of food or is easily distracted.

▨ Provide simple verbal cues to eat, one step at a time.

▨ If the resident does not respond to verbal cues, use hand-over-hand technique.

▨ Repeat the instructions as often as necessary.

▨ Praise the resident's efforts.

▨ Encourage the resident to keep trying.

Residents with cognitive impairments can participate in a feeding retraining program. Cognitively impaired residents who can follow simple directions should be further evaluated. Some residents who are spoon-fed do well in a restorative feeding program.

Residents who are not candidates for a restorative feeding program are those who:

- Are at high risk for choking
- Are unwilling or unable to follow directions
- Are combative when care is given
- Display socially inappropriate behavior, such as spitting or throwing food, during meals
- Cannot sit upright

After residents' needs and abilities have been identified, the restorative nurse assesses them further. He or she will determine if the residents are appropriate for the program. A feeding assessment is time-consuming. It involves observing one or more meals. After the assessment, team members will meet to establish individual goals for each resident. Like other restorative programs, residents will start with small goals and build on their successes. Some residents will progress to independence. Others may always require supervision with meals. Complete feeding independence may not be a realistic goal for some residents. However, improving their ability follows the intent of OBRA. It provides residents with greater independence, confidence, and self-esteem.

▓▓ ESTABLISHING THE RESTORATIVE FEEDING PROGRAM

Establishing a feeding program takes planning and coordination. Many team members are involved. You are an important contributor to this team. You must understand how to establish and maintain a successful program. Other team members include the:

- Restorative nurse
- Director of nursing or assistant
- Dietary manager
- Licensed dietitian

The administrator and maintenance supervisor may participate if environmental modifications are necessary. Other team members may be appointed by the director of nursing or restorative nurse. For example, the charge nurse and CNAs may be invited to participate.

Staff must be committed to the restorative feeding program and believe that it will work. Nursing staff involvement is important. Staff members bring a working knowledge of the residents and unit operations. Involving staff in planning and developing the program creates ownership, commitment, and the desire to make the program succeed.

Considerations for a Successful Restorative Feeding Program

Establishing and maintaining a restorative feeding program requires attention to detail. A successful program is created by following the nursing process. The feeding committee will assess:

- Residents
- The environment
- Nursing and dietary department operations relating to feeding
- Staffing
- Scheduling
- The need for staff training

After the assessment, a plan is developed. The plan is implemented, evaluated, changed, and improved upon.

Staffing and Scheduling Considerations. Restorative feeding programs may fail if they are not scheduled and coordinated between restorative staff, nursing staff, and the dietary department. Residents receive the most benefit if they participate in the program three meals a day, seven days a week. This means that additional staff must be trained and available to assist with the program. The director of nursing or other nurse manager selects staff members. He or she also oversees the schedule. A trained staff member must be on duty to cover 21 meals a week. The restorative nurse will teach team members their responsibilities. Another scheduling concern involves the staff working on the nursing unit. They must see that residents in the program are dressed, toileted, prepared for meals, and transported to the dining area on time.

Group Size. A successful restorative feeding group is limited in size. One staff member assists three or four residents. Effectively managing a larger group is difficult or impossible. Large groups may defeat the purpose of the program. Residents in the program will have varying levels of difficulty eating. One or two residents may be totally dependent. The others should have only mild or moderate problems eating. Balance the number of residents and their abilities with the number of staff available. Assigning a whole group of totally dependent residents sets the scene for failure. The feeding program is intense, and staff cannot adequately assist the entire group. A session for 3 or 4 residents will take one staff member 50 to 60 minutes.

Location. The feeding program works best if residents eat in a private area. The room should be free from distractions. A large dining area does not work as well as a smaller room. The room should not be used for any other purpose during meals. The table should be large enough to accommodate three or four residents. Avoid using a long table, if possible. Long tables make assisting residents difficult. They also create social isolation. Seat residents in regular dining chairs whenever possible. Residents in wheelchairs using lap trays may join, but should be placed close to the group. Make the atmosphere pleasant and comfortable. Use a tablecloth or placemats. Provide seasonal table decorations, if possible.

Scheduling Meals. Working with a restorative feeding group takes a long time. Many facilities serve this group 30 to 60 minutes ahead of the main dining room group. This should not create a hardship on well-organized dietary and nursing staff. Serving the feeding group early allows time for the assistant to work with the group. When finished, he or she can assist with meal service or work with a maintenance group in the dining room. Some facilities need many staff members in the dining room at mealtime. Serving the feeding group early may be critical to program success.

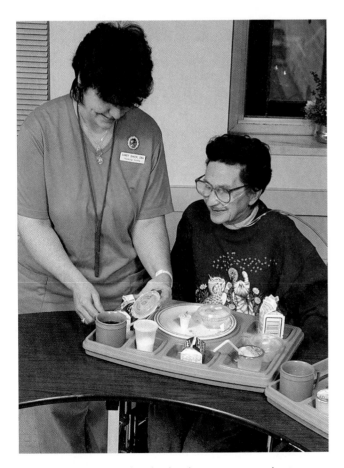

Figure 14–8   Describe the food as you set up the tray.

Plan to serve the group meals at a time that works best for your facility.

Restorative Meal Service

Resident needs can change from day to day. Keeping a record of individual approaches for each resident on an index card is helpful. The cards can be delivered on meal trays. They can be kept in a file box in the dining area as well. Update the cards whenever there is a change. You will quickly learn the approaches to use with residents. Relief staff may not be as familiar with residents' changing needs. The cards provide continuity of care. The card can include information such as:

- The resident's feeding goal(s)
- Special positioning needs
- Adaptive devices
- Special preferences, such as two packets of creamer in coffee
- Order, positioning, or placement of food items, if any
- Techniques that do or do not work with the resident
- Cues to use and when to use them
- Other special techniques to use

When serving food, remove the dishes from the tray. Place them in front of each resident. Offer seasoning and condiments. Present the food pleasantly **(Figure 14–8).** Describe the meal as you serve it. Comment that the food looks or smells good. Provide the necessary adaptive utensils. Prepare the dishes for residents with visual impairments by using the clock method **(Figure 14–9).** Placing food in separate bowls makes it easier for visually impaired residents to find and eat their food.

After serving residents, give verbal cues to encourage them to eat. Encourage them to be as

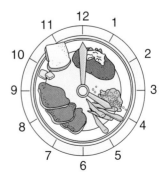

Figure 14–9   Describe the food to the resident compared with the positions on a clock face.

independent as possible. Recognize and praise progress, even if small. Some residents will require a cue for each step of the meal. This takes patience and time. Give simple, direct cues, one at a time. For example, you will say:

▦ "Pick up the spoon."

▦ "Put the spoon in the mashed potatoes."

▦ "Scoop the potatoes onto the spoon."

▦ "Put the spoon in your mouth."

▦ "Chew."

▦ "Swallow."

▦ "Good!" or "Great!"

If verbal cues are ineffective, use hand-over-hand technique **(Figure 14–10).** Tell the resident what you are doing. Use simple, direct terms. Encourage the resident to try again after using hand-over-hand technique once or twice.

Circulate around the table, providing verbal cues and hands-on assistance as needed. If a resident's food gets cold, reheat it. Offer to refill beverages.

Communication.   The restorative nurse will monitor the group regularly. Communicate with the nurse frequently. Report your observations, suggestions, comments, and concerns. The nurse will reassess residents. He or she revises residents' goals and modifies the program as needed.

Maintenance.   When residents reach their maximum potential, the nurse develops a maintenance program. Residents will remain in the feeding group for approximately four more weeks. During this time, they will follow the maintenance plan. Some facilities have a separate feeding area for residents on maintenance programs. Giving residents extra time in the feeding program strengthens their skills. After four successful weeks of maintenance, they are moved to the regular dining area. Staff is given instructions for maintaining the residents' independence. As one resident leaves the group, another is added.

Documentation.   The documentation for a restorative feeding program is somewhat different from other documentation.

You will document the amount (percentage) of food the resident eats independently. ⓢⒶYou will also document the total amount of food each resident consumes.ⓢⒶ For example, the resident fed herself 60% of the meal. Her total intake was 90%. This tells the reader that the resident did not eat 10% of the meal. Follow your facility guidelines for calculating the percentage each resident eats **(Figure 14–11).** Make a narrative note of any special circumstances daily. For example, document refusal to cooperate, physical illness, significant improvements or declines.

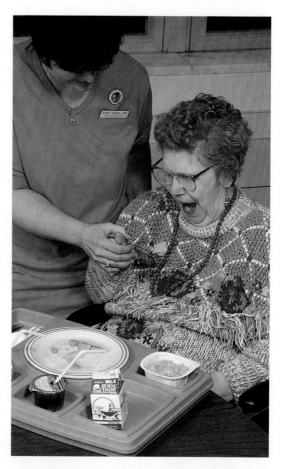

Figure 14–10   If the resident does not respond to verbal cues, try hand-over-hand technique.

Consider this example of a significant change. A resident is not doing well with restorative feeding. She has trouble getting the food to her mouth. She spills often. The resident gets new glasses. The next day she eats her meal unassisted, without spilling. This is a significant improvement. Document it in your daily notes and report it to the restorative nurse. Record food refusals, substitutes, calorie count, and intake and output according to your facility policy. Read the charting from the previous day. This will give you an overview of the resident's progress when other staff was on duty.

You may be required to complete a weekly summary of the resident's progress. Summarize the resident's:

▦ Level of participation

▦ Motivation

▦ Reality orientation

▦ Special techniques

▦ Progress

▦ Regression

The restorative nurse will also complete a weekly note and monthly summary.

DIETARY INTAKE GUIDE

MEALS/SUPPLEMENTS/LIQUIDS CONSUMED
Directions: Record amount of the total meal consumed using the following guidelines.

R ### REFUSED – 0%
Refused meal completely,
or consumed only one
or two bites of each item.

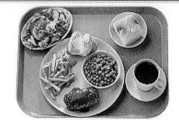 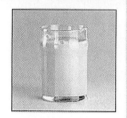

P ### POOR – 25%
Approximately 25% of entree,
or 50% of one item consumed.

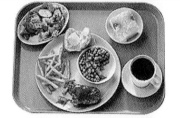 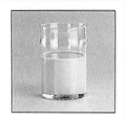

F ### FAIR – 50%
Approximately half of food is
consumed (ie, 50% of entree,
25% of vegetable and soup left).

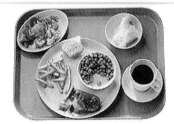 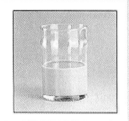

G ### GOOD – 75%
Majority of the meal is consumed,
but a significant amount of one
or more items is left (ie, 25%
of entree, or 75% of vegetable left).

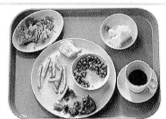 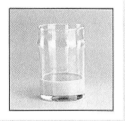

A ### ALL – 100%
Entire meal is consumed except
for a minimal amount of food
(ie, less than 25% of vegetable left).

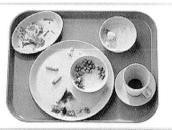 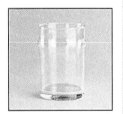

Common Errors Made Estimating Dietary Intake
- Overestimating the total consumption (ie, total entree is consumed, but no other food is touched. Record as Poor/25%—not Fair/50%).
- Overestimating the total consumption when food is pushed around the tray.
- Letting how much a resident normally consumes influence the actual consumption.

Figure 14–11 Follow your facility policy for recording total meal consumption. (Photo used with permission of Ross Products Division, Abbott Laboratories, Columbus, Ohio)

Patience—A Key to Success.   Restoring residents' ability to feed themselves takes a long time. Some residents will take as long as several months before reaching their maximum level of independence. Be patient. Restorative feeding programs work. They improve the quality of the residents' lives. Feeding programs make the staff's work easier at mealtime. Your commitment to making the program successful is a valuable investment of your time and energy. The feeding program makes a difference in the operation of the facility, quality of life, and residents' well-being.

▣ HYDRATION

⑤The elderly are at risk of **dehydration.** Dehydration is a serious condition.⑤ Residents become dehydrated when the liquid taken in is not adequate to maintain body functions. Untreated, it can lead to many complications, including death. The elderly do not feel thirst as acutely as younger persons. Many factors contribute to dehydration. These include normal aging changes in the kidneys and inadequate intake. Many residents restrict fluids because they fear incontinence. Other risk factors for dehydration are:

▦ Immobility

▦ Cognitive impairment

▦ Physical inability to pour liquids

▦ Physical inability to pick up the cup and drink

▦ Infection

▦ Fever

▦ Medical problems

Signs and symptoms of dehydration are:

▦ New onset of mental confusion

▦ Sudden worsening of confusion in a cognitively impaired resident

▦ Dry mucous membranes

▦ Weight loss

▦ Weakness and fainting

▦ Dark circles under eyes; eyes appear to be sunken in

▦ Decreased blood pressure

▦ Increased pulse and respiration

▦ Loss of elasticity in skin, tenting when skin is pinched gently, poor skin turgor

▦ Decreased urinary output

▦ Urine appears dark and concentrated

Most adults consume 2,000 cc to 3,000 cc of liquids each day. This is approximately 8 to 12 glasses, or 2 to 3 quarts. At a minimum, residents need 2,000 cc, or 8 glasses each day. The licensed dietitian calculates each resident's minimum fluid needs. The amount needed is based upon the resident's weight and activity. All residents should meet or exceed the intake amount recommended by the dietitian each day. Many facilities write this amount on the care plan. ⑤All staff should offer residents fluids when they are in the room.⑤

Fluid Restrictions

Sometimes residents with heart or kidney disease, or other medical problems are put on **fluid restrictions.** Residents on fluid restriction can take in a very limited amount of fluid each day. The total liquid allowed in a 24-hour period is calculated carefully. Usually, the total is divided by three shifts. The care plan lists how much fluid the resident may consume each shift. The fluid includes fluids served on meal trays and liquids consumed on the nursing unit. The largest quantity is usually given by the day shift. The night shift usually gives the least, because the resident is asleep during the night.

Restorative Hydration Programs

Many facilities have restorative hydration programs. Some pass hospitality carts to provide fluids. These programs are usually very informal. Facilities may provide sugar-free beverages in the dining room or other area of the facility **(Figure 14–12).** This enables residents to help themselves throughout the day. Sugar-free beverages are used because the area is not always monitored by staff. Some res-

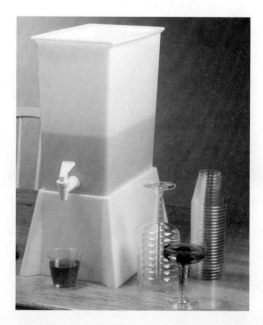

Figure 14–12   Many facilities make beverages available so residents can help themselves during the day. (Courtesy of Briggs Corporation, Des Moines, IA. (800) 247-2343)

idents have diabetes and other conditions in which sugar is harmful.

(SA)Some facilities make coffee available as well. If your facility makes coffee available, the area should be monitored. Surveyors have written deficiencies for this. Unsupervised residents can spill the hot coffee, causing serious burns.(SA)

Some facilities distribute juice or other liquids several times each day. Staff members stop to offer each resident a drink. They provide assistance drinking, if needed. All staff are responsible for providing fluids. Offer fluids during and after restorative care. Monitor for signs of inadequate fluid intake. Report problems to the nurse, if noted.

KEY POINTS IN CHAPTER

Nutrition is an important factor in longevity and quality of life in the elderly.

Most residents look forward to meals and snacks.

Food has emotional importance for many individuals. The relationship of food to social activities, family gatherings, ethnicity, culture, and religion is important.

Malnutrition is a serious problem in the elderly.

Barriers to adequate nutrition are both physical and psychological.

The mealtime environment can influence the appetite. A homelike environment is important.

Eating is a social activity. Seating is arranged so residents can socialize with others.

Proper positioning at mealtime is important. Good positioning improves swallowing and digestion and reduces the risk of choking.

Monitor residents' position in relation to the distance and height of the table.

The most common adaptive devices are used for eating.

The goal for residents receiving alternative forms of nutrition is to return to oral feeding whenever possible.

The registered dietitian plans the menu to meet the resident's medical needs.

The occupational therapist works with residents who have feeding problems. He or she recommends adaptive devices and feeding techniques.

The speech therapist works with residents who have swallowing disorders.

The speech therapist may recommend the use of food thickeners. He or she also recommends techniques and positions to promote easy swallowing and prevent choking.

The restorative feeding program is developed by the restorative nurse. The restorative nursing assistant and other designated staff members implement the program.

Developing restorative dining and feeding programs requires a team approach and commitment.

At a minimum, residents should consume 2,000 cc of liquid each day.

The registered dietitian calculates the amount of fluid the resident requires each day. The nursing staff is responsible for seeing that the resident consumes this amount.

Offer residents liquids and monitor for signs and symptoms of dehydration during care.

CLINICAL APPLICATIONS

1. Mrs. Lauer is a 77-year-old resident with COPD. She had a CVA which left her with right-sided hemiparesis. She was right-handed. Before admission, she was cared for in her daughter's home. The daughter states that she fed Mrs. Lauer because the dominant hand was paralyzed. She requests that her mother be spoon-fed to prevent weight loss. Weight has been a problem for this resident in the past. Mrs. Lauer propels the wheelchair in her room. She uses her left hand and left foot. Staff push the chair in the hallway because her endurance is poor. She becomes short of breath from pushing the chair. Is this resident a candidate for a restorative feeding program? Why or why not? If you think she should be evaluated, who will you report to? What will you report?

2. Mr. Bernstein has a urinary tract infection. He is alert. He normally propels his wheelchair about the facility, visiting with other residents. You assist with his restorative ambulation program. When you prepare to ambulate him, he seems confused and very weak. There is 100 cc of dark, concentrated urine in his catheter bag. What action will you take? What is one potential cause of this problem? What other observations should you make and report to your supervisor? What will you do first?

3. Mrs. Wayne is spoon-fed by staff. The tray is placed to the side. Mrs. Wayne throws food on the floor and at other residents. She can wash her own upper body each morning without difficulty. Should she be evaluated for a restorative feeding program? Why or why not?

4. Mr. Chiang is a resident in the restorative feeding program. When his meal is served, he grabs his bread and eats it quickly. He sits and waits for you to spoon-feed him the rest of his meal. He opens his mouth when he sees the spoon coming. He can drink a glass of milk without spilling. What approaches will you take with this resident? How will you develop his self-care skills?

5. Miss McGill is 4 feet 9 inches tall. She weighs 76 pounds. She usually eats 50% of her meals and refuses substitutes. The resident has lost 5 pounds in the past month. Miss McGill is frail and tires easily. She sits in her wheelchair for meals. She is mildly confused, but enjoys visiting with residents and staff. Miss McGill likes being complimented on her appearance. The resident sits at the dining table with two other residents who are quiet and speak little. A third resident at the table had a CVA and is unable to speak. You notice that Miss McGill must reach about 18 inches to get her food. The table height comes almost to the resident's shoulders because she is so short. After eating 50% of the meal, Miss McGill puts her fork down and falls asleep in her chair. How can you assist this resident?

CHAPTER 15

Restorative Self-Care

OBJECTIVES

After reading this chapter, you should be able to:

- Spell and define key terms.
- State the purpose and principles of restorative self-care ADL programs.
- State the goals and objectives of restorative ADL programs.
- Identify residents who are potential candidates for ADL programs.
- Define the levels and types of assistance used in ADL programs.
- List the guidelines for restorative ADL programs.
- Explain why continuity of care is important.
- Describe how to meet the needs of residents with CVA, hip surgery, arthritis, Parkinson's disease, and COPD.
- List the guidelines for restorative dressing programs.

RESTORATIVE ADL PROGRAMS

Most restorative care is given to assist residents with activities of daily living. Observe the resident carefully. A resident may tell you that he or she is interested in mastering a specific ADL. Inform your supervisor. The information you contribute is very important. Because you spend so much time with residents, you may make observations that others miss.

Restorative ADL programs maintain or improve the residents' ability to complete hygiene and grooming procedures. Independence in self-care improves self-esteem. It promotes self-confidence and dignity. Remember, the activities in this chapter are things we do each day. They are very personal. Most people prefer to do them alone. Nevertheless, many residents require assistance. Some depend entirely on others for ADLs. Dependence on staff can cause residents to become depressed, lose self-esteem, feel isolated, and lose hope.

Goals of Restorative Self-Care

The interdisciplinary team considers several types of goals when developing self-care programs. Some goals improve the resident's ability. Others delay loss of independence in residents with deteriorating conditions. Some programs maintain the resident's present level of self-care. Overall objectives of self-care programs are to:

- Restore maximum function
- Replace total care with a program of task segmentation and verbal cues
- Restore the resident's ability to function with fewer supports
- Reduce the time required for providing assistance
- Prevent or delay further loss of independence
- Support the resident who is certain to decline
- Reduce the risk of complications

Principles of Activities of Daily Living

Understanding the principles of ADL programs will help you to assist residents. The basic principles of all ADLs are the same, and are listed in **Table 15–1**.

Self-Care Adaptive Devices. Many adaptive devices are available to enable residents to be independent with ADLs **(Figure 15–1A, p. 237** and **15–1B, p. 238).** If adaptive devices are ordered, use them consistently. Teach residents to use them correctly.

Identifying Candidates for Restorative ADL Programs

A key to developing a successful program is staff participation. All staff members observe the residents for clues that they can improve self-care. Many residents are candidates for ADL programs. Staff should not complete procedures for the sake of

Table 15–1 Principles of Assisting with Activities of Daily Living

1. Recognize the resident's potential. Try to determine why the resident is not using skills he or she is able to do.

2. Each self-care skill is composed of many steps. If the resident cannot do one of the steps, he or she will not be able to complete the skill.

3. Learn which ADL skill is most important to the resident and begin the restorative program with this skill.

4. Schedule the restorative program at the normal time of day for the activity.

5. Allow enough time for the resident to complete the activity.

6. Provide clear, brief, simple verbal cues. Repeat if necessary.

7. If verbal cues are ineffective, use hand-over-hand technique.

8. Practice safety. Teach the resident safety and provide frequent reminders.

9. Allow residents to be as independent as possible. If the resident has difficulty, allow him or her to struggle briefly before intervening. Avoid letting the resident struggle to the point of frustration. Break the task into smaller steps, if necessary.

10. Use adaptive equipment if necessary. The care plan will direct you.

11. Patience, persistence, and consistent care are essential.

12. Restorative teaching should be provided by all staff, any time the activity is completed. The care plan provides specific instructions. All staff must know how to prompt the residents in ADL skills.

13. Advise other staff members to use the care plan for guidance and consistent approaches.

14. Update the care plan as the resident progresses, if the resident's condition changes, or if the approaches change. Keeping the care plan current is important.

saving time. If the resident can complete a task, he or she should be permitted to do it. This is part of the OBRA '87 philosophy. For example, staff bathes a cognitively impaired resident. However, when given the washcloth and verbal cues, the resident washes her face and upper chest. Encourage the resident to do this routinely. Staff will complete only those tasks that the resident cannot do. Report your observations about residents' self-care ability to your supervisor.

Any resident with a deficit in self-care skills should be screened for restorative self-care programs. Residents with the conditions listed in **Table 15–2** should be evaluated by a licensed nurse or therapist.

Residents who have had a recent exacerbation of a chronic illness may be able to return to their former level of function. An *exacerbation* is an aggrava-

tion of symptoms or an increase in the severity of a chronic condition. If returning to the former level is not realistic, the program is used to maintain the resident's current level. Licensed personnel will determine what is realistic for the resident, based on an assessment. Examples of conditions that have exacerbations that cause a decline in self-care ability are:

- all types of arthritis
- multiple sclerosis
- chronic obstructive pulmonary disease (COPD)
- cystic fibrosis

Residents who have recently been admitted from home or the hospital, and who plan to return home after a short stay, are also good candidates for ADL programs. Because they have been at home, they

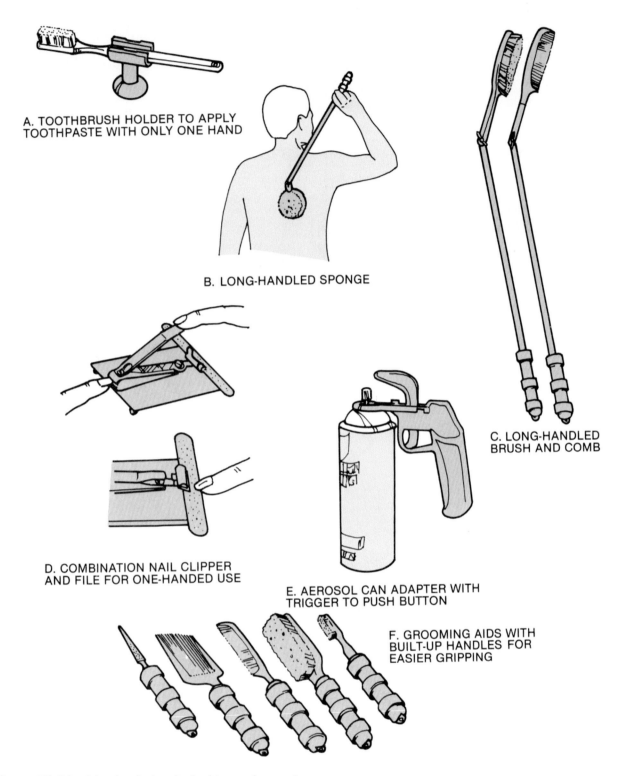

A. TOOTHBRUSH HOLDER TO APPLY TOOTHPASTE WITH ONLY ONE HAND

B. LONG-HANDLED SPONGE

C. LONG-HANDLED BRUSH AND COMB

D. COMBINATION NAIL CLIPPER AND FILE FOR ONE-HANDED USE

E. AEROSOL CAN ADAPTER WITH TRIGGER TO PUSH BUTTON

F. GROOMING AIDS WITH BUILT-UP HANDLES FOR EASIER GRIPPING

Figure 15–1A Adaptive devices for bathing and grooming.

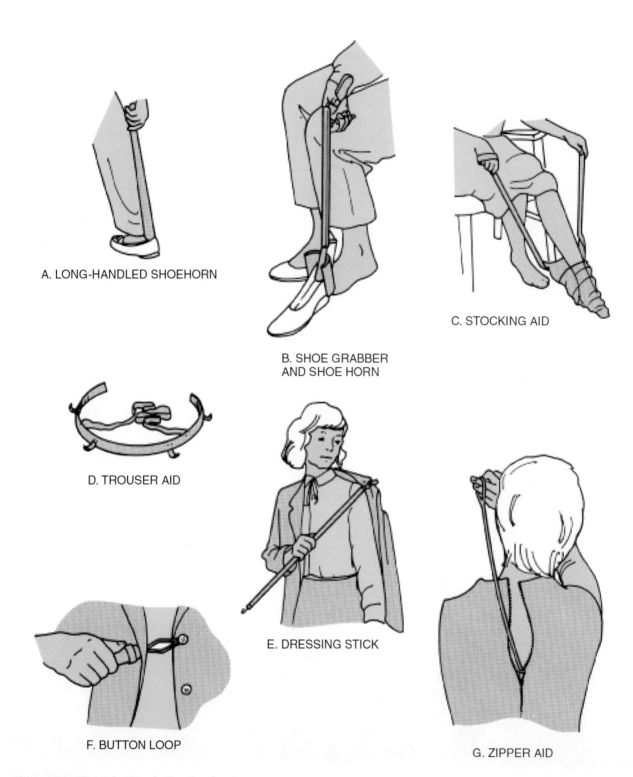

A. LONG-HANDLED SHOEHORN

B. SHOE GRABBER
AND SHOE HORN

C. STOCKING AID

D. TROUSER AID

E. DRESSING STICK

F. BUTTON LOOP

G. ZIPPER AID

Figure 15–1B Adaptive devices for dressing.

Table 15–2 Potential Candidates for Restorative Self-Care Programs

Candidates for self-care programs include residents who:

- Have the potential to increase their level of self-care
- Have the ability to learn, even if cognitively impaired
- Can follow directions
- Have recently had restraint reduction, improving their mobility
- Have recently had surgery
- Are motivated to relearn self-care skills
- Are recovering from injuries related to accidents
- Have recent paralysis or a neurologic condition
- Have had recent amputation(s)
- Have had a CVA
- Are recovering from pneumonia
- Are recovering from heart attack
- Are recovering from hip or other fractures
- Are recovering from a stroke
- Have recently fallen
- Have generalized weakness because of an acute illness
- Have cognitive impairments but are able to follow simple directions, have good motor functioning, and show potential for increasing self-care skills

have probably been caring for themselves. A restorative program will maintain their ability, or improve their ability if they are weak following an acute illness. Table 15–2 lists potential candidates for a grooming or hygiene program.

THE RESTORATIVE ADL PROCESS

After residents are identified, the restorative nurse assesses their abilities. Part of the assessment involves determining the resident's desire to participate. The nurse will identify tasks that the resident wants to work on. The nurse will talk to staff about the resident. Next, a task analysis is completed. This identifies the resident's ability to complete each step of the task. The nurse has the resident try adaptive devices during the assessment. He or she determines if using the device makes the task easier for the resident. **Table 15–3** is a sample task analysis. As you can see from this example, there are many steps in most ADLs.

In addition to the task analysis, several other tools may be used to assess self-care ability. A written evaluation is completed. **Instrumental activities of daily living** (IADLs) are higher-level tasks required for living in the community. These include paying bills, planning a menu, making a shopping list, and driving a car. If the resident has discharge plans, the nurse will assess his or her IADLs.

During the assessments, the restorative nurse evaluates the resident's ability to follow directions. The nurse determines if the resident has the physical and mental ability to participate in the program.

DEVELOPING THE CARE PLAN

Following the assessment, the interdisciplinary team meets to develop goals. Goals may involve completing all or part of the procedure independently. The principle here is that doing something is better than doing nothing. The team determines if special equipment or adaptive devices are necessary. If so, team members arrange to make or obtain them. Environmental modifications are considered and completed if possible. Simple changes, such as moving furniture, may be all that is necessary. For example, a resident fears falling. Personal items and furnishings are in the path between her bed and the bathroom. Staff will move these items so the resident has a clear route to the bathroom. Structural changes to the building may not be possible. Structural changes must be cost-effective and beneficial to all residents. If not, they will not be made.

The team develops approaches for staff to use when assisting residents. When developing approaches, they review the task analysis. The program begins by working on the steps that the resident cannot complete. The information is recorded on the care plan. Residents in restorative programs

Table 15–3 Showering Task Analysis

Key: **+ = Resident can complete task**
           0 = Resident cannot complete task
      N/A = Not applicable

Date	Key	Initial	Step
			1. Identifies equipment for bathing.
			2. Gathers equipment.
			3. Turns on cold water first, hot water last.
			4. Regulates water temperature.
			5. Undresses (dressing and undressing is a separate task analysis). Puts on shower cap (washing hair is a separate task analysis).
			6. Enters shower (transfer is a separate task analysis).
			7. Pulls shower curtain or establishes privacy.
			8. Adjusts shower head, if necessary.
			9. Wets washcloth.
			10. Washes face (resident may prefer not to use soap).
			11. Rinses and wrings out washcloth.
			12. Applies soap to washcloth.
			13. Washes neck and ears.
			14. Rinses and wrings out washcloth.
			15. Rinses soap from neck and ears.
			16. Rinses and wrings out washcloth.
			17. Wets washcloth.
			18. Applies soap to washcloth.
			19. Washes one shoulder, axilla, arm, and hand.
			20. Rinses and wrings out washcloth.
			21. Rinses shoulder, axilla, arm, and hand.
			22. Wets washcloth.
			23. Applies soap to washcloth.
			24. Washes other shoulder, axilla, arm, and hand.
			25. Rinses and wrings out washcloth.

(continues)

Table 15–3 Showering Task Analysis, *continued*

Key: **+ = Resident can complete task**
                  0 = Resident cannot complete task
                  N/A = Not applicable

Date	Key	Initial	Step
			26. Rinses shoulder, axilla, arm, and hand.
			27. Wets washcloth.
			28. Applies soap to washcloth.
			29. Washes chest and abdomen.
			30. Rinses and wrings out washcloth.
			31. Rinses chest and abdomen.
			32. Wets washcloth.
			33. Applies soap to washcloth. (A long-handled bath sponge may be substituted for the washcloth for the legs and back.)
			34. Washes one leg and foot.
			35. Rinses and wrings out washcloth.
			36. Rinses leg and foot.
			37. Wets washcloth.
			38. Applies soap to washcloth.
			39. Washes other leg and foot.
			40. Rinses and wrings out washcloth.
			41. Rinses leg and foot.
			42. Wets washcloth.
			43. Applies soap to washcloth.
			44. Washes back.
			45. Rinses and wrings out washcloth.
			46. Rinses back.
			47. Wets washcloth.
			48. Applies soap to washcloth.
			49. Washes groin and perineum.
			50. Rinses and wrings out washcloth.

(continues)

Table 15–3   Showering Task Analysis, *continued*

Key: + = **Resident can complete task**
         0 = **Resident cannot complete task**
       N/A = **Not applicable**

Date	Key	Initial	Step
			51. Rinses perineum.
			52. Wets washcloth.
			53. Applies soap to washcloth.
			54. Washes buttocks and rectal area.
			55. Rinses and wrings out washcloth.
			56. Rinses buttocks and rectum.
			57. Turns off hot water.
			58. Turns off cold water.
			59. Dries body, following bathing sequence.
			60. Steps out of shower.
			61. Dresses.
			62. Removes personal items from shower.
			63. Places towels in hamper.

will have one long-term goal. This goal describes the end result, or what the program will accomplish. Short-term goals are used to break the long-term goal into small steps. The resident builds on each small step until he or she reaches the long-term goal.

Restorative goals and approaches may change quickly. The care plan is reviewed every three months. Residents may take less time to meet some goals. As the resident achieves a goal, the restorative nurse develops a new goal. He or she lists approaches for the next step. Thus, the care plan may change several times before the next care conference. Some facilities use a separate attachment to the care plan because of the frequent changes. Check the care plan frequently to stay up to date.

Understanding the Care Plan

When assisting residents with self-care, provide the least amount of assistance necessary. This may be difficult for you, but it is best for the resident. Limiting your assistance takes practice and experience.

The care plan will describe the level (amount) and type of assistance the resident needs. You may also use verbal cues and hand-over-hand technique. Facilities use different terms for describing the degree of help necessary. Definitions for the levels of assistance are listed in **Table 15–4.** The most common terms and descriptions for the type of assistance you will provide are listed in **Table 15–5.** Some facilities use the MDS definitions. These are listed in **Table 15–6.** You will use these terms in documentation. They are defined according to documentation guidelines.

▇▇▇▇ WORKING WITH THE RESIDENT

The restorative assistant is the primary caregiver for ADL retraining programs. You will be teaching, reinforcing, and reminding residents to use the

Table 15–4   Type of Assistance Provided with ADLs

Type of Assistance	Description
Setup	Preparing equipment and supplies for an activity. The resident is given items needed for the task, or the items are placed on a table or other location where the resident can reach them.
Positioning	The resident is assisted with proper positioning to complete the task. This may include assisting the resident to sit or stand at the edge of the bed or sink. In some cases, you will transfer the resident into a wheelchair. You will position the resident in the designated location and provide supports, such as pillows or props, to assist in maintaining the position for the duration of the activity.
Physical assist	The type of assistance necessary for most ADL tasks is confined to helping the resident begin a task and completing a procedure when the resident is unable to do so. Use discretion in providing assistance. Avoid doing things that the resident is able to perform independently.
	In most cases, the care plan will specify the type of assistance to provide. The plan is developed for one staff member. In some cases, two or more staff members may be required. If this is necessary, the plan will specify the number of assistants.
Verbal cues	Brief, clear, and concise directions or hints that prompt the resident to do something. These may also be called *prompts* or *hints*.
Hand-over-hand technique	Placing your hand over the resident's hand and guiding him or her to perform the desired action.
Coaching	Gently urging or encouraging the resident to perform the task.
Pacing	Allowing the resident to perform the task at his or her own rate of speed, without rushing. Allow for rest, if needed.
Giving or receiving feedback	Acknowledging that you understand what the resident is telling you; having the resident show or tell you that he or she understands your directions.
Encouragement and/or support	Giving emotional support. Provide positive reinforcement and praise. Making comments about the resident's progress or ability motivates the resident. A positive attitude is important. Give the resident confidence that he or she can do the task.

Table 15–5 Levels of Assistance

Level of Assistance	Description	Example
Independent	The resident completes the task with no help or staff oversight; or staff help/oversight was provided only one or two times in the last seven days.	The resident bathes independently. She was weak and dizzy one day last week. A nursing assistant gave her a bed bath on that day. The following day, she washed herself.
Standby or Observation Guarding	The resident is probably independent; however, for safety, a staff member should be close when the resident performs the task.	The resident prefers to stand at the sink to bathe. Her balance is poor. Staff stand next to her to provide support if she becomes unstable.
Supervision	Oversight, encouragement, or cueing was provided three or more times during the last seven days, or supervision plus physical assistance was provided only one or two times during the last seven days.	The resident is mentally confused. He has the physical ability to bathe himself, but forgets what he is doing. He is easily distracted. Staff remain in the room while he is bathing and give him verbal cues. They redirect his attention if he becomes distracted.
Light Contact or Guarding Assistance	The resident begins the activity, but an assistant must stand by, maintaining light contact with the resident's body for safety and assistance, if needed.	The resident prefers to take a partial bath while standing at the sink to bathe. Her balance is poor. Staff stand next to her to hold the gait belt for support while she washes herself.
Limited Assistance	The resident is highly involved in the activity; received physical help in guided maneuvering of limbs, and/or other non-weight-bearing assistance three or more times; or help was provided only one or two times during the past seven days.	The resident is in a bathing retraining program. The nursing assistant used hand-over-hand technique four times in the past week to assist her with the bath.
Moderate Assistance	The resident begins the activity, but needs physical help in completing it.	The resident's goal is to wash her upper body. After washing her face and arms, she becomes tired and cannot finish bathing. The nursing assistant completes the bath.
Extensive Assistance	Although the resident performed part of the activity, over the previous seven-day period, the resident required the following help three or more times: ■ Weight-bearing support ■ Full staff performance during part (but not all) of the week	The resident's goal is to wash her upper body. She can usually complete this task. The resident was very confused last week. She refused to bathe. The nursing assistant bathed the resident five days out of seven.
Maximum Assistance	The resident is dependent. One or two staff members must complete the major part of the activity.	Mrs. Long is obese. She is confused and has hemiparesis. She is given a bed bath daily by staff. She washes her face, but staff bathe the rest of her body. Two staff must turn her and wash her back and lower body.
Total Dependence	The resident required full staff performance of the activity over the entire seven-day period. This term may be used interchangeably with maximum assistance.	Mrs. Long is obese. She is confused and has hemiparesis. She is given a bed bath daily by staff. She washes her face, but staff bathe the rest of her body. Two staff must turn her and wash her back and lower body.

Table 15–6 MDS Definitions of Assistance with ADLs

Type of Assistance	Description
Independent	No help or staff oversight. Can also mean that staff help or oversight was provided only one or two times during the past seven days.
Setup	For dressing—retrieving clothes from the closet and laying out on the resident's bed; handing the resident a shirt. For eating—cutting meat and opening containers at meals; giving one food category at a time. For toileting—handing the resident a bedpan or placing articles necessary for changing ostomy appliance within reach. For personal hygiene—providing a wash basin and grooming articles. For bathing—placing bathing articles at tub side within the resident's reach; handing the resident a towel upon completion of the bath.
Supervision	Oversight, encouragement, or cueing provided three or more times during the past seven days. Can also mean that supervision (three or more times) plus physical assistance was provided only one or two times during the past seven days.
Limited assistance	The resident is highly involved in the activity. He or she received physical help in guided maneuvering of limbs or other nonweight-bearing assistance on three or more occasions. Can also mean limited assistance (three or more times) plus more help provided only one or two times during the last seven days.
Extensive assistance	Although the resident performed part of the activity over the last seven days, help of the following type(s) was provided three or more times: ■ Weight-bearing support provided three or more times. ■ Full staff performance of activity three or more times during part, but not all, of the last seven days.
Total dependence	Full staff performance of the activity during the entire seven-day period. Complete nonparticipation by the resident in all aspects of the activity.

skills. You may also be asked to show other nursing assistants how to assist the residents.

When planning your day, schedule care at the time that the task would normally be done. Relearning ADLs takes time. Allow enough time for the activity. Avoid rushing the resident. Gradually, the resident's skills will improve.

Report changes in the resident's progress to the restorative nurse. Progress may be inconsistent from day to day. Everyone has an off day occasionally. Do not become discouraged if the resident has a temporary setback. If the resident meets a goal, wait a few days to see if he or she maintains it. If so, report to the restorative nurse. The nurse will revise the care plan, advancing to the next step. By working on one small goal at a time, the resident will eventually master the task.

Role of the Certified Nursing Assistant

To be effective, restorative care must be given 24 hours a day, 7 days a week. This is an OBRA '87 requirement. The nursing assistants caring for the residents when you are off duty must follow the program as well. For example, the residents brush their teeth at bedtime. You will work on toothbrushing with the resident during the day.

General Guidelines for Assisting Residents with Restorative ADL Procedures

- Keep stress and distractions to a minimum.
- Become familiar with the procedure and the directions for completing it.
- Establish a routine to decrease stress.
- Adapt to normal changes in the resident's cognitive function.
- Follow the care plan.
- Allow enough time for the activity.
- Provide enough space for the activity.
- Modify the environment, if necessary.
- Make sure the resident is safe and positioned in good body alignment.
- Provide a chair so the resident can sit during the activity, if appropriate. Sitting makes tasks easier and conserves energy.
- Keep distractions to a minimum.
- Be consistent. Perform the procedure at the same time, in the same way, and in the same environment.
- Stress the resident's ability, not the disability. (Say, "You *can* do this with your left arm." instead of, "You *can't* do this with your right arm.")
- If family members are (or will be) involved in the resident's care, teach them how to help. Advise them of how much they should and should not do. Always explain why.
- Be patient and persistent with the resident.

- Keep your instructions simple. Tell, show, and ask. Give simple, one-step commands. Repeat, if necessary.
- If necessary, begin by giving physical assistance. Allow the resident to complete the step. For example, guide the resident's arm to the sleeve. Allow the resident to place his or her arm in it.
- Be flexible.
- Adapt the procedure to the resident. Avoid trying to adapt the resident to the procedure.
- Guide the resident in developing his or her own safe method of completing the task.
- Complete the task using the same sequence of steps each day. For example, assist the resident to dress by putting on clothing in the same order.
- Communicate with the resident during the task, if this is not distracting.
- Support, encourage, and praise the resident. If he or she completes a step successfully, provide immediate feedback and praise. Use praise and rewards that are most important and effective for the resident. For example, after the task is complete, take the resident for a walk outside, if this is important to him or her. A cup of coffee and cookies may be an effective reward for another resident. Individualize the reward to the resident.

The second-shift nursing assistants will follow the restorative care plan in the evening. This provides continuity of care. It gives the resident additional opportunities to practice the skill. The practice reinforces the resident's learning and ability.

Documentation

The restorative nurse will describe the program in the progress notes. ⓈⒶYou will document your daily care on a flow sheet. You will also complete a weekly summary. Document the level of assistance the resident requires in the weekly note. Address the resident's progress, or lack of progress, toward the care plan goals. Make your notes direct and concise.ⓈⒶ

They need not be lengthy. A sample note is shown in **Figure 15–2.** The restorative nurse will

> Resident is motivated and participating in his self-care program. In the past 7 days, he has progressed from requiring hand-over-hand technique to supervision with verbal cues. Goals and approaches are effective. Will continue present plan.
>
> *John Morrison, CNA, RNA*

Figure 15–2 This brief note describes the program, the resident's progress, the assistance needed, and plans for continuing.

meet with you weekly. He or she will also write a progress note. The nurse will write a monthly summary of the resident's progress, describing plans for continuing or modifying the program.

SPECIAL RESIDENT CONDITIONS AND NEEDS

Residents with certain conditions have special needs. The most common conditions affecting ADLs are discussed in this section. These principles can be adapted to all other residents.

Residents with CVA

Residents who have had a CVA have problems related to brain damage from the stroke. The resident may be able to move one or both sides of the body. Some residents are weak. Using the affected extremity may be painful. Some have very tight, spastic muscles. If the resident has hemiparesis, he or she will not be able to use one side of the body. Residents with CVA may have problems balancing. Make sure residents are stable, safe, and positioned correctly.

Special Conditions

Residents with CVA experience many problems affecting their ability for self-care. You must understand these conditions. You must know how to work with them to provide restorative care. The resident may be impulsive. Judgment may be poor, including judgment about personal safety. Knowing this, try to anticipate what will happen next. Plan care with safety in mind. Common problems of CVA affecting ADLs are:

- Loss of feeling and muscular weakness on the affected side
- Balancing difficulty and poor muscular control
- Pain, particularly in the shoulders
- Poor endurance; resident fatigues easily
- Fluid retention, especially the affected hand, wrist, foot, and ankle
- Visual field deficits
- Denial
- Memory loss
- Confusion

Residents with right hemiplegia respond best if the procedure is demonstrated before beginning. Residents with left hemiplegia are easily distracted. They respond best if the procedure is divided into many small steps. Keep explanations brief. Provide verbal cues. You may need to redirect the resident's attention during the procedure.

Unilateral Neglect. Unilateral neglect was defined in Chapter 7. Residents with this condition ignore one side of the body. Approach the resident from the affected side. Touch and stimulate that side of the body. Encourage the resident to look toward that side. Position the bed and chair so that there is activity on the affected side. Remind the

---

> ## General Guidelines for Assisting Residents with Hemiplegia with Restorative ADL Programs
>
> - Plan your care by considering the resident's condition and needs.
> - Position the resident in good body alignment.
> - Support the paralyzed extremities, using props or pillows if necessary.
> - Practice safety.
> - Approach residents and work from the affected side. This reverses the effects of unilateral neglect.
> - Encourage the resident to use the affected side to hold and support items.
> - Set up supplies and equipment on the strong side.

resident to pay attention to the affected side and use it, if possible.

Associate Reactions. **Associate reactions** are muscle spasms. They are caused by an increase in muscle tone. Insecurity, excitement, fear, and overactivity trigger spasms. If spasticity occurs, stop the activity. Allow the resident to rest and regain control, then begin again. Increase the assistance you are providing. Attention to proper positioning will decrease the risk of associate reactions.

Apraxia. **Apraxia** is the inability to plan a motor activity. Although residents lack planning skills, they have the motor ability to complete the task. When working with a resident with apraxia, you may need to help begin movement. Use hand-over-hand technique when necessary. After beginning, the resident may continue independently. Hands-on assistance may also be necessary.

Residents with Hip Surgery

Hip surgery is common in the elderly. Total hip joint replacement is the most common surgical procedure in this age group. (SA)When a resident has had hip surgery, he or she must follow certain precautions for up to six months. This prevents hip dislocation **(Figure 15–3).**(SA) The resident must avoid:

- Bending forward past 90 degrees
- Crossing the knees or ankles

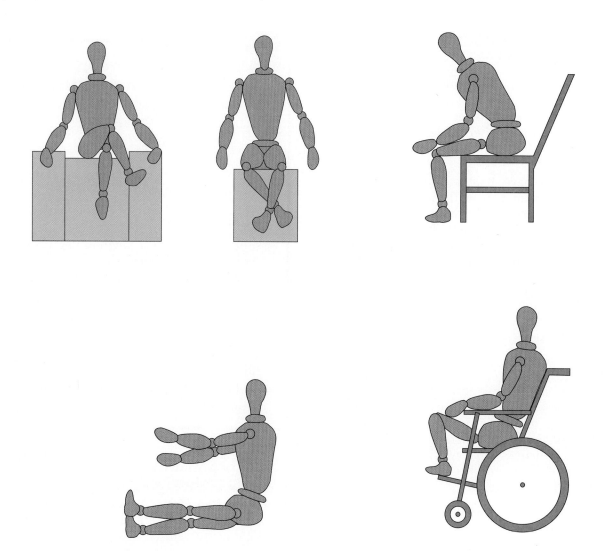

Figure 15–3 Hip precautions are an important part of care for residents who have had hip surgery.

■ Raising the knee higher than the level of the hip

■ Turning the foot of the operative leg inward

Hip precautions make dressing and bathing the legs difficult. Assistive devices are available to help residents complete tasks without bending. These devices are also useful for residents with back pain or limited ability to bend forward or raise the legs.

Residents with Arthritis

Residents with arthritis have weakness and limited range of motion. The restorative program is designed to conserve energy and avoid stress on the joints. Performing ADLs when sitting is usually easier. Adaptive devices are useful.

Residents with Parkinson's Disease

Residents with Parkinson's disease have tremors of the extremities. Their muscles are rigid. They lean forward when walking. They walk with a shuffling gait. The tremors and rigidity increase the risk of falls. Sitting in a chair to complete ADLs is safer and easier than standing. Residents with Parkinson's are very slow. Allow extra time and be patient. Avoid showing impatience with your body language.

Residents with COPD

Residents with COPD use most of their energy to breathe. They tire easily. Allow frequent rest periods. The supine position may cause respiratory distress. Consult your supervisor before using the supine position.

Problems with Bathing

Resistance to bathing is a common problem in residents with cognitive impairments. The resident may have forgotten the purpose of bathing. Residents may resist undressing in front of you. Wrapping a towel around the shoulders and pinning it may help. Leave the towel in place during the bath. Some residents may be afraid of water. The resident may not be able to feel the water temperature. Bathing is a complex task involving many steps. Taking a bath may be too overwhelming for the resident.

🆂🅰Be flexible and avoid forcing the resident.🆂🅰 If the resident becomes agitated and refuses to bathe, leave and try again later. Make sure the room is warm and private. Ask the resident to feel the water. Say something like, "This feels good." Explain what you are going to do. Tell the resident what you want him or her to do, one step at a time. Giving many directions at once is overwhelming. It may trigger a catastrophic reaction. Noise from the whirlpool, shower, heater, or other equipment may frighten the resident. Washing the hair may also be frightening. Use the resident's responses to guide your actions. Modify your behavior according to the resident's responses.

▰▰▰ ASSISTING RESIDENTS WITH DRESSING

Dressing is an important restorative program. Like personal hygiene, dressing is a very private, personal activity. Being able to dress independently is important to many residents.

Dressing Tips for Residents with Hemiparesis

Teach residents with hemiparesis to dress the affected extremity first. Teach them to undress the strongest extremity first.

Dressing Tips for Residents with Arthritis

Clothing with large buttons, pullovers, and elasticized pants are best. Hemiplegic dressing techniques may be used if one hand or arm is deformed or not functional. Avoid stress on finger joints by replacing zippers, hooks, and buttons with Velcro®.

General Guidelines for Selecting Clothing for Restorative Dressing Procedures

▰ Encourage the resident to select the clothing.

▰ Apply loose-fitting garments; clothing that is one size larger is easier to apply.

▰ Garments should fasten in front, whenever possible.

▰ Attach a ring to zippers.

▰ Elastic thread may be used to sew on sleeve buttons.

▰ Use Velcro® fasteners on clothing, whenever possible.

▰ Socks with loose tops are easier to put on than stretch tops.

▰ Large buttons are easier to fasten than small **(Figure 15–4).**

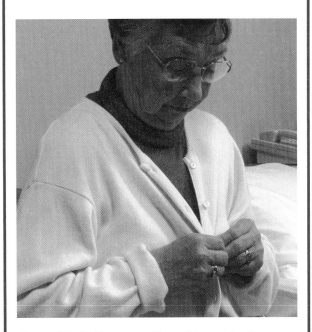

Figure 15–4 Encourage the resident to button the sweater by herself, even if this is more time-consuming.

▰ Use slip-on shoes; shoes with elastic laces or Velcro® are easier to put on.

▰ Sewing one side of the shoe tongue down prevents it from sliding down or curling under.

General Guidelines for Assisting Residents with Restorative Dressing Procedures

These guidelines are for residents with hemiparesis. They may be adapted to any resident.

▓ Putting on underwear and pants while lying down may be easier.

▓ Make sure shoes are on before transfers.

▓ Assist the resident to sit down for dressing.

▓ If balance is good, placing the feet on a stool makes it easier to dress the legs.

▓ Lay out clothing in easy reach, in order of use.

▓ Show the resident labels, pockets, or other landmarks for positioning the garment.

▓ Spread the shirt or dress on the resident's lap. Tell him or her to use the strong hand to put the weak arm into the sleeve, pulling it up.

▓ When the garment reaches the shoulder, pull the sleeve completely up and throw the shirt across the back **(Figure 15–5).**

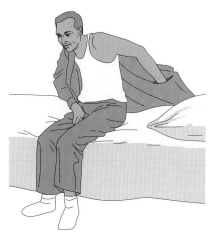

Figure 15–6   Using the strong arm, reach behind and slip the hand into the sleeve.

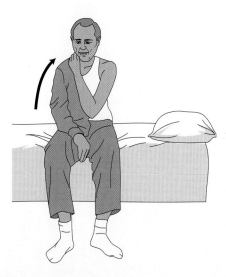

Figure 15–5   Throw the garment over the shoulder to the back.

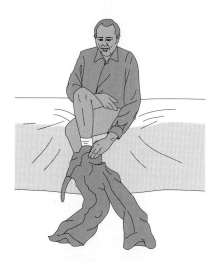

Figure 15–7   Place the weak leg into the pants first.

▓ Reach behind, using the strong hand. Place the strong arm into the armhole, positioning the sleeve **(Figure 15–6).**

▓ Teach the resident to button from the bottom up, so the buttonholes match.

▓ While sitting, place the strong hand across the weak leg, pulling the pants over the foot **(Figure 15–7).**

▓ Place the strong leg in the pants. Pull the pants up over the knees.

▓ Stand or lie down to pull up pants and fasten; if lying down, bend the strong leg at the knee, pushing with the foot to lift buttocks off the bed **(Figure 15–8).**

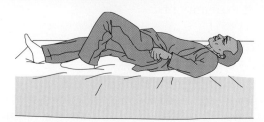

Figure 15–8   Push with the foot to lift the buttocks off the bed, pulling the pants up with the strong hand; roll to the side if necessary to pull the pants up on the affected side.

General Guidelines for Dressing Residents with Hip Precautions

▥ Dress the legs first by sitting in a chair. Use a dressing stick to pull pants over the feet and legs **(Figure 15–9).**

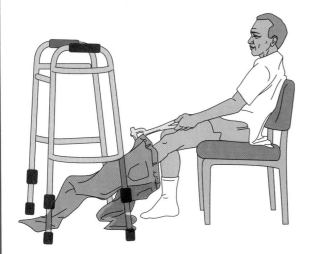

Figure 15–9 Using a dressing stick, slip the underwear or pants over the operative leg first.

▥ Put on undergarments first; catch the waist of underwear or pants with the dressing stick, lowering the stick to the floor.

▥ Slip the garment over the foot of the operative leg; repeat with other leg.

▥ Pull the slacks (or underwear) up to the knees.

▥ Place the walker in front of the resident. Tell him or her to stand **(Figure 15–10).**

▥ Have the resident hold the walker with one hand while pulling pants up with the other.

▥ When undressing, remove garments from the nonoperative or stronger leg first.

▥ Knee-high socks are recommended for both men and women.

▥ Slide the sock into the stocking aid, securing it correctly.

▥ Drop the sock to the floor in front of the operative foot, while holding the cords **(Figure 15–11).**

▥ Slip the foot into the sock, pulling it on. Release the garters.

▥ Repeat with the other foot, or put the sock on in the usual manner.

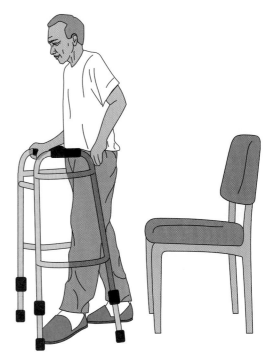

Figure 15–10 Stand to pull the pants up at the waist. Instruct the resident not to use the walker for pulling himself up.

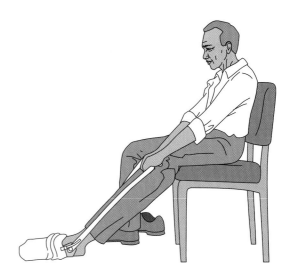

Figure 15–11 Using the stocking aid, slip the sock over the operative foot first.

▥ Use the dressing stick or long-handled shoe horn to put on shoes. Slip-on shoes work best.

Dressing Tips for Residents with Parkinson's Disease

Large buttons, Velcro® fasteners, and cuff buttons sewn with elastic are more manageable. Shoes with Velcro® fasteners are easier to manage. Residents may be unable to put on shoes because of stiffness.

Dressing Tips for Residents with Hip Precautions

Lower extremity dressing may be very difficult for residents with hip precautions. Use adaptive devices, if possible.

■ ASSISTING RESIDENTS WITH RESTORATIVE HYGIENE AND GROOMING PROGRAMS

ADL programs are highly personalized. This makes it impossible to provide general procedures for assisting residents. You will begin the program with the first step of the task analysis that the resident is unable to complete. Rather than following approaches in a textbook, you will follow the care plan and the directions of the restorative nurse.

Before beginning the task for the first time, explain what you want the resident to do. Demonstrate the task. During the task, cue the resident or use hand-over-hand technique. Friendly conversation may be helpful if it does not distract the resident. Discuss the weather, current events, or approaching holidays. This shows that you care about the resident and provides reality orientation. If the resident has tremors, weakness, or shakiness, bracing the elbow on the sink, table, or counter top will provide more control.

Restorative Bathing Tips

You may need to set up for bathing programs. Bring the resident to the sink whenever possible. If you are using a wash basin, carry it to the overbed table. Residents are encouraged to do their own setup whenever possible. However, carrying a full basin of water is not safe.

Restorative Grooming Tips

Complete grooming tasks in front of a mirror. The resident can sit in a chair in the bathroom. A small mirror can be used on the overbed table. A magnifying mirror is helpful for makeup or contact lens insertion. Instruct the resident to gather the necessary articles. Place them in a sack or walker bag to carry to the sink. Provide verbal cues, if necessary. Place a towel, washcloth, soap, and needed articles within reach. Begin makeup and shaving procedures by instructing the resident to wash and dry the face. Remember that residents prefer to do grooming activities a certain way. This may not be the way you would do it. Respect the resident's wishes.

Shaving Tips

When assisting with shaving, encourage residents to apply the shaving cream or preshave lotion independently. An adaptive dispenser handle is available. This can be used for residents who cannot press the valve on the can. Residents with arthritis in their hands or wrists may have difficulty grasping the razor. Using an electric razor or adaptive razor handle will solve the problem.

Oral Hygiene Tips

Set the resident up at the sink. Place the needed articles within reach **(Figure 15–12).** Residents who have difficulty grasping small objects may benefit from a built-up toothbrush handle. Residents with hemiparesis may benefit from suction cups. These hold items on the counter so the residents can brush their teeth or dentures independently.

Some residents cannot control water in the mouth. If the resident coughs, chokes, or cannot control the water, flex the neck slightly forward. Position the face over the sink. This will keep liquids away from the back of the throat. If the resident cannot rinse the mouth after toothbrushing, dip a sponge-tipped applicator (Toothette®) in water or mouthwash. Wipe the inside of the mouth.

Dressing and Grooming Problems

Some cognitively impaired residents resist dressing. Keep the morning routine consistent and familiar. Once you start, avoid interruptions. This can cause the resident to forget what he or she is supposed to

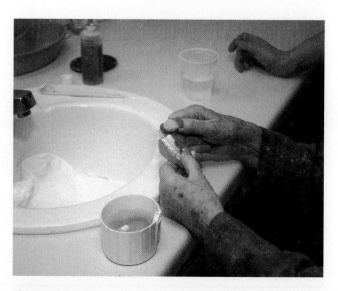

Figure 15–12 Set the resident up, then give her verbal cues.

General Guidelines for Assisting Residents with Behavior Problems with ADLs

Approaching the resident:

- Tell the resident who you are and what you will do. Do not ask if the resident remembers you.
- Focus on what the resident can do instead of what he or she cannot do.
- Laugh with the resident.
- Use hugs if the resident responds to this approach, and if appropriate for the resident.

Dressing programs:

- Do not ask what the resident wants to wear. Ask the resident to choose one of two items.
- Lay out clothes in the order of use.
- Hand the resident one article at a time.

Grooming programs:

- Avoid placing many articles in front of the resident at once.

Bathing programs:

- Residents may do better in a tub than a shower. Perceptual deficits may make the tub look very deep. Try using bubble bath.
- The resident may not be able to feel the water temperature. After running water, place the resident's hand in. Tell the resident that the water feels good.
- Follow the same bathing schedule the resident used at home.

---

be doing. Be understanding if the resident does not want to undress in front of you. Compliment the resident's appearance.

Lack of Progress

If the resident does not make the progress you expect, do not give up. The resident may be taking smaller steps, or may have other personal goals. Consult the restorative nurse. He or she may ask the occupational therapist to evaluate the resident. The therapist may suggest assistive devices or other techniques.

When the resident is not progressing, evaluate the goals and approaches. Try to learn why the resident is not progressing. Are the goals realistic? Can they be reduced or changed? Are the approaches practical? Revising the goals and approaches may restore the resident's progress. Consider making changes before abandoning the program. Discuss your thoughts and suggestions with the restorative nurse, who will make any changes to the program.

KEY POINTS IN CHAPTER

- *Dependence on staff for ADLs can cause depression and low self-esteem.*
- *Restorative ADL programs maintain or improve the ability to complete personal hygiene and grooming procedures. This improves resident dignity and self-esteem.*
- *ADL goals are designed for different purposes. They improve the resident's ability, delay loss of independence, and maintain the resident's level of self-care.*
- *Self-care programs are developed to restore the resident to maximum function.*
- *The restorative nursing assistant must understand the principles of ADLs.*
- *Many long-term care facility residents are candidates for restorative ADL programs.*
- *Staff should not perform procedures that residents can complete themselves.*
- *A task analysis identifies the resident's ability to complete each step of a procedure.*
- *The interdisciplinary team designs long-term goals that describe outcomes. Short-term goals enable residents to complete small parts of larger tasks. As residents meet the goals, the goals are advanced until an entire task is completed.*
- *The care plan describes the level and type of assistance the resident requires.*

(continues)

**KEY POINTS
IN CHAPTER
continued**

Restorative care is given 24 hours a day, 7 days a week. All staff members follow the care plan.

Residents who have had a CVA have many problems with ADLs.

Residents with unilateral neglect ignore one side of the body.

Associate reactions are muscle spasms caused by an increase in muscle tone.

Residents with apraxia lack planning skills, but have the motor ability to complete ADLs.

Total hip joint replacement is the most common surgical procedure in the elderly.

Residents with hip surgery must take special precautions for six months to avoid dislocating the hip.

The restorative program for residents with arthritis focuses on conserving energy and avoiding stress on the joints.

Residents with Parkinson's disease take longer to complete ADLs because of muscular rigidity. Residents may be taught to sit in a chair for ADLs. This prevents falls related to poor balance.

When assisting residents with COPD, allow frequent rest periods.

Before beginning an ADL, explain what you want the resident to do. Use demonstration, verbal cues, and hand-over-hand technique. Limit hands-on assistance as much as possible.

Friendly conversation during ADLs shows that you care and provides reality orientation.

If the resident does not make progress, do not abandon the program without additional assessment.

CLINICAL APPLICATIONS

1. Mr. Raines is a 68-year-old resident with hemiparesis. He is in a dressing program. Explain how you will teach this resident to put his affected extremities into his shirt and pants. Explain how you will teach him to remove his affected extremities from his shirt and pants.

2. Mrs. McAndrew has Parkinson's disease. She has tremors. The tremors are improved by taking regular medication. The resident takes pride in her appearance. She dresses well and has her hair styled in the beauty shop each week. She is in a restorative program for toothbrushing and applying makeup. When applying cosmetics, she becomes frustrated. The tremors interfere with her ability to put on lipstick and mascara. When she attempts these tasks, the makeup ends up elsewhere on her face. How can you decrease her frustration? What advice can you give her to control the tremors? Can you adapt the

environment to make these tasks easier for the resident?

3. Mr. Choi has severe arthritis. He has pain and limited movement in his fingers. The resident is in a dressing program. He has trouble buttoning his shirt. The buttons and buttonholes rarely match up. The resident is determined to do this by himself. How can you help him?

4. Mrs. Bayer is cognitively impaired, but follows simple directions. The resident feeds herself and propels her wheelchair short distances. The CNA dresses this resident each day. Is this resident a candidate for a restorative dressing program? Why or why not?

5. Mr. Zimmer had hip replacement surgery eight weeks ago. He will be going home when he can be independent. The resident is in a dressing program, but has trouble dressing his feet and legs. What advice can you give him?

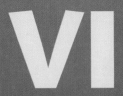
Restorative Care of Residents with Special Needs

Restorative Care of Residents with Respiratory Disorders

OBJECTIVES

After reading this chapter, you should be able to:

Spell and define key terms.

Describe the role and responsibilities of the restorative nursing assistant in assisting residents with respiratory disorders.

Explain why the resident with pneumonia needs to be well-hydrated.

Describe methods of conserving energy during daily activities.

Explain why conserving energy is necessary for residents with COPD.

State the purpose of coughing and deep breathing exercises.

State the purpose of pursed-lip and diaphragmatic breathing.

Explain the similarities and differences of pursed-lip and diaphragmatic breathing.

State the purpose of postural drainage.

Explain why using the incentive spirometer is a method of goal-directed therapy.

Describe how to assist the resident in using an incentive spirometer.

ROLE OF THE RESTORATIVE NURSING ASSISTANT IN CARE OF RESIDENTS WITH RESPIRATORY DISORDERS

ⓈⒶYou will have a limited role in the care of residents with respiratory conditions. The respiratory therapist and nurses will care for residents with acute and chronic conditions.ⓈⒶ Usually, you will care for the respiratory equipment. These procedures were described in Chapter 4. You may also assist residents with relaxation exercises. These were addressed in Chapter 3. Always apply the principles of standard precautions when working with residents who have respiratory conditions.

CARING FOR RESIDENTS WITH RESPIRATORY CONDITIONS

Being unable to breathe is a frightening experience. Breathing is on the lowest level of the Maslow pyramid, making it basic to survival. Residents with respiratory disorders need a great deal of emotional support **(Figure 16–1)**. They must have confidence in the skills of those who care for them.

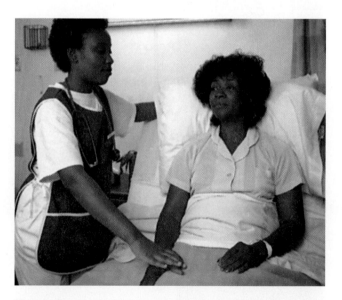

Figure 16–1 Residents with respiratory problems need a great deal of emotional support.

Pneumonia

Pneumonia is a serious infection of the lungs, caused by a pathogen. Residents with AIDS may develop a condition called *Pneumocystis carinii*

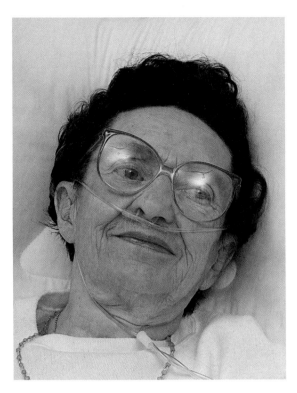

Figure 16–2 Residents with COPD use an oxygen cannula.

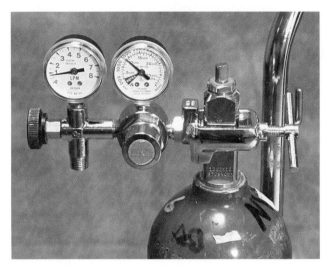

Figure 16–3 Check the flow rate each time you are in the room; notify a licensed nurse if it is set above 2 liters.

pneumonia (PCP). Pneumonia is a potentially life-threatening condition. It is treated with antibiotics and respiratory therapy.

In the acute stages of the illness, the resident may be hospitalized. Upon admission to the facility, nurses will administer antibiotics and other medications. Nebulizer treatments may also be given by nurses or respiratory therapists. The resident may be receiving oxygen therapy.

When caring for residents with pneumonia, adequate hydration is important. Liquids help to liquefy and eliminate secretions from the lungs. Recording intake and output is also important. This ensures that the resident takes in enough fluids. Residents with some heart or kidney conditions may be on fluid restrictions. Check the care plan for special fluid needs or limitations.

Chronic Obstructive Pulmonary Disease (COPD)

COPD refers to any chronic respiratory disorder hindering air flow out of the lungs. Examples of this condition are emphysema, chronic bronchitis, and asthma.

Medical Treatment. COPD is treated with medications and respiratory therapy. Oxygen therapy may also be used. Residents with COPD usually receive oxygen through a nasal cannula **(Figure 16–2)**. The flow rate is normally set at 2 liters per minute. Always check the flow rate **(Figure 16–3)**

when you are in the room. **SA**If the liter flow is greater than 2 liters, or the rate ordered for the resident, notify your supervisor.**SA** Oxygen is a prescription drug. Too much oxygen can be harmful to a resident with COPD.

ADLs. Residents with COPD must pace their activities. Allow frequent rest periods. Avoid completing all ADL care at once. Bring the clothing to the bedside. Allow the resident to dress in bed to save energy. Provide a chair at the sink so the resident can wash the face and hands or brush the teeth while sitting. This also conserves strength. Avoid activities that involve raising the arms above the head, such as using a hair dryer or curling iron. Avoid using aerosol sprays or talcum powder. Hair spray, deodorant, air freshener, and talcum powder are very irritating to the lungs. If air freshener is necessary, use a solid instead of a spray.

▨ BREATHING TREATMENTS AND TECHNIQUES

Several techniques make breathing easier for residents with conditions causing airway obstruction. Residents will be taught how to use these techniques. This takes practice, repetition, and concentration for the resident. These procedures may be practiced in combination with relaxation therapy. Provide verbal cues, demonstrations, and moral support. Apply the principles of standard precautions when handling secretions.

Coughing and Deep Breathing

Coughing and deep breathing exercises may be ordered. These activities reduce the risk of pneumonia. They decrease complications in bedfast residents and those who are recovering from surgery.

PROCEDURE

37 COUGHING AND DEEP BREATHING EXERCISES

1. Perform your beginning procedure actions.
2. Gather equipment:
   pillow (if needed)
   emesis basin
   tissues
   mouthwash
   cup
   straw
   disposable gloves
3. Assist the resident to the high Fowler's position.
4. Instruct the resident to hold a pillow across the abdomen or chest to splint the incision, if he or she had recent abdominal surgery **(Figure 16–4).**
5. Instruct the resident to breathe in slowly through the nose. Next, cough twice in a row to clear the airway.
6. Tell the resident to place a hand on the abdomen and inhale. Make sure the hand on the abdomen rises on inhalation.
7. Tell the resident to hold the breath for three seconds, then slowly exhale through pursed lips.
8. Repeat this exercise 5 to 10 times, or as ordered.
9. You may be instructed to include coughing with the deep breathing exercises. Tell the resident to take two slow breaths through the nose. Follow

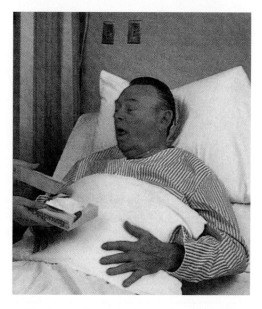

Figure 16–4 A pillow can be used to splint the abdomen.

with a deep breath through the nose. Tell the resident to keep the mouth open slightly. Have the resident hold the breath for three seconds, then cough twice during exhalation.

10. Offer tissues and an emesis basin if the resident coughs up secretions.
11. After the procedure, offer mouthwash to rinse the mouth.
12. Perform your procedure completion actions.

Pursed-Lip Breathing

Residents with COPD are taught to use **pursed-lip breathing** when they are short of breath. When done correctly, this exercise slows rapid respirations. It allows the resident to exhale more completely. Slow, complete exhalation helps keep the airways open. It reduces the feeling of shortness of breath.

Diaphragmatic Breathing

Diaphragmatic breathing slows the respiratory rate. It increases the ability to take a deep breath.

Postural Drainage

Postural drainage is a technique in which gravity is used to help drain and remove secretions from the

lungs. Current respiratory care standards recommend using this technique only for residents with cystic fibrosis or certain types of pneumonia. However, some physicians order the treatment for other respiratory conditions. The procedure is contraindicated if the resident has cancer in the area being treated, osteoporosis, unstable vital signs, or cyanosis. ⓢⒶYou will not be permitted to perform this procedure. You will assist with positioning, monitoring, and comfort measures. Know and follow your facility policy and state laws.ⓢⒶ

The nurse or respiratory therapist will listen to the lungs before and after the procedure. The licensed person determines if the resident can safely be repositioned. He or she will administer medications if necessary. You will be instructed on the

PROCEDURE

38 PURSED-LIP BREATHING

1. Perform your beginning procedure actions.

2. Assist the resident to the high Fowler's position, or **orthopneic position.** The orthopneic position is used for residents with respiratory conditions. It is the same as high Fowler's, with the arms extended across an overbed table. Or the resident can sit in a chair or on the side of the bed with the feet flat on the floor. Place an overbed table in front of the resident. Instruct him or her to lean forward, placing the arms on the table for support. This increases the chest space for lung expansion.

3. Tell the resident to keep the mouth closed and inhale slowly through the nose.

4. Instruct the resident to purse the lips as if he or she were whistling. Tell the resident to keep the abdominal muscles tight (contracted), and exhale. Exhalation should take at least twice as long as inhalation.

5. Repeat the exercise as directed.

6. Perform your procedure completion actions.

7. When the resident is proficient, remind him or her to use the exercise during ambulation and other forms of exertion.

PROCEDURE

39 DIAPHRAGMATIC BREATHING

1. Perform your beginning procedure actions.

2. Assist the resident to a comfortable position. The supine position may be the most comfortable. Using this position makes it easier to feel the abdomen moving.

3. Instruct the resident to place one hand across the abdomen. Place the other on the middle of the chest.

4. Tell the resident to inhale very slowly through the nose, while pressing the abdomen outward against the hand.

5. Count to three, then tell the resident to tighten (contract) the abdominal muscles. Use pursed-lip breathing to exhale slowly.

6. Repeat the exercise as ordered.

7. Perform your procedure completion actions.

position to use **(Figure 16–5).** Positioning the resident exactly as ordered is very important. Some positions involve placing the head and chest lower than the legs. Change the position immediately if the resident shows signs of respiratory distress. The resident remains in each position for 5 to 10 minutes. Using a tilt table in the therapy room **(Figure 16–6, p. 261)** is best. If your facility does not have a tilt table, the resident can be positioned in bed using foam, pillows, and props.

You may be directed to bring the suction machine to the room. Set it up before beginning the procedure. If the resident cannot cough, the licensed person will suction to remove secretions. Bring the suction unit to the room before you begin

positioning the resident. Apply the principles of standard precautions when assisting.

Some facilities also use **percussion** during postural drainage **(Figure 16–7, p. 261).** The resident's back is covered with a towel. The licensed person cups the hands and claps against the resident's chest wall. This loosens secretions. You will be given specific instructions for positioning the resident. ⑤The licensed person will perform the procedure.⑤

Monitor the resident closely after the procedure. The resident will cough up secretions. ⑤Do not leave the room until you are certain the resident is stable. Notify the licensed professional immediately if the resident shows signs of respiratory distress.⑤ Report complaints of pain or exhaustion after the

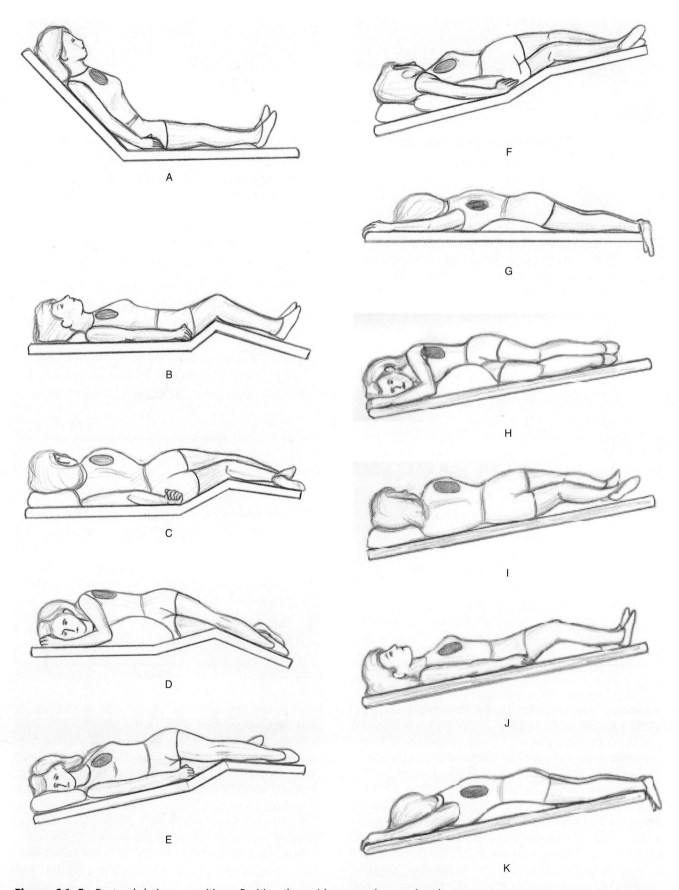

Figure 16–5 Postural drainage positions. Position the resident exactly as ordered.

PROCEDURE

40 ASSISTING WITH POSTURAL DRAINAGE

1. Perform your beginning procedure actions.
2. Gather equipment:
   emesis basin
   tissues
   mouthwash
   cup
   straw
   pillows
   props
   disposable gloves
   plastic bag

3. Position and support the resident as directed, using foam wedges or pillows.
4. Provide an emesis basin, tissue, and bag in which to discard secretions.
5. Remain in the room with the resident during and after the procedure. Monitor for signs and symptoms of respiratory distress. Monitor vital signs as directed. Provide comfort measures as necessary.
6. Offer the resident mouthwash to rinse the mouth.
7. Perform your procedure completion actions.

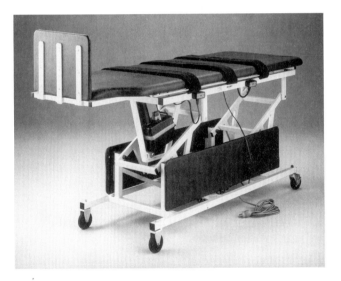

Figure 16–6 The tilt table is used for positioning residents for postural drainage, whenever possible. (Courtesy of Medline Industries, Inc. (800) MEDLINE)

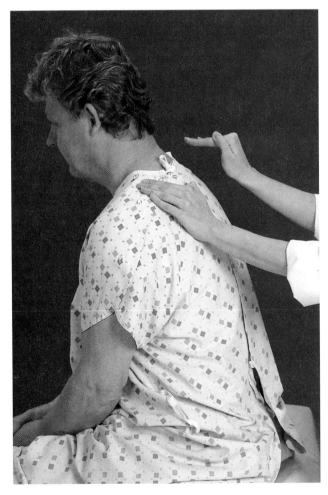

Figure 16–7 A licensed respiratory therapist or nurse will perform chest wall percussion. You will assist with positioning the resident and providing emotional support.

treatment. Notify the licensed practitioner immediately if the vital signs are unstable, the resident is cyanotic, or the resident shows signs of cardiopulmonary distress. Provide tissues, an emesis basin, and mouthwash. Make the resident as comfortable as possible.

Incentive Spirometry

Incentive spirometry is a form of goal-directed therapy. The purpose is deep breathing. The goals for incentive spirometry are individualized for the resident. The restorative nurse or respiratory therapist will develop the goals. The licensed person will specify the frequency of spirometer use. The goals will be achievable for the resident, but only after some effort. The incentive is for the resident to visualize how much air he or she is taking in with each inhalation **(Figure 16–8).** This is accomplished by inhaling from the spirometer. The resident watches the position of the ping pong balls inside. Apply the principles of standard precautions when assisting with this procedure.

The incentive spirometer is usually left at the bedside. The resident will be prompted to use it throughout the day. He or she is instructed to take four to five slow, deep breaths using the spirometer, or as ordered. If the resident becomes dizzy or complains of tingling in the fingers, he or she may be breathing too fast. Have the resident relax and breathe normally until the sensation passes. Monitor the resident's breathing before and after the treatment. Report your observations to your supervisor.

Other Types of Breathing Activities

Activities that emphasize forced expiration are very important in the elderly. Some restorative programs use activities in which residents blow up balloons or inflatable toys for exercise. Whistling games can be fun, and help residents' breathing. Some activi-

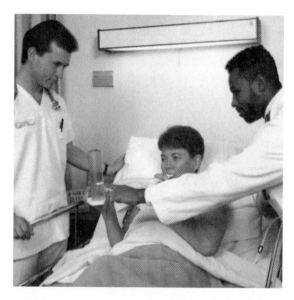

Figure 16–8 The resident inhales into the mouthpiece of the incentive spirometer, lifting the ping pong balls.

ties use straws for breathing exercises. This involves cutting a straw in half and asking the resident to sip juice. If the resident can do this, another half straw is added. After the resident drinks, another straw is added. This continues until the resident can no longer drink from the straws.

PROCEDURE

41 INCENTIVE SPIROMETRY

1. Perform your beginning procedure actions.
2. Gather equipment:
   incentive spirometer
   tissues
   emesis basin
   mouthwash
   cup
   straw
   disposable gloves
3. Assist the resident to sit in the high Fowler's position.
4. Instruct the resident to exhale slowly, emptying the lungs as much as possible.
5. Instruct the resident to place the mouthpiece between the teeth, closing the lips around the device.
6. Tell the resident to take a slow, deep breath, using the diaphragm. (See Procedure 39 on

diaphragmatic breathing.) Tell the resident to keep breathing in until the indicator on the device reaches the goal position.
7. Instruct the resident to hold the breath for three to five seconds.
8. Tell the resident to exhale normally.
9. Provide the emesis basin and tissues if the resident coughs up secretions.
10. Instruct the resident to rest briefly between breaths, then repeat the procedure.
11. Offer the resident mouthwash to rinse the mouth.
12. Perform your procedure completion actions.
13. Report the volume the resident reached and the resident's response to the treatment.
14. Report frequency of deep breathing, cough, and any complaints to your supervisor.

KEY POINTS IN CHAPTER

Licensed nurses and respiratory therapists provide most of the treatments for residents with respiratory disorders.

Pneumonia is a serious infection of the lungs. It is caused by a pathogen and is treated with antibiotic therapy.

Good hydration is important for residents with pneumonia.

When caring for residents with COPD, pace activities. Conserve their energy as much as possible.

When caring for residents with COPD, minimize activities that involve raising the arms over the head. Avoid exposing residents to aerosol sprays and powder.

Coughing and deep breathing exercises are ordered to reduce the risk of pneumonia. They also decrease lung problems in bedfast residents and those recovering from surgery.

Pursed-lip breathing slows rapid respirations. This enables the resident to exhale more completely.

Remind residents to use pursed-lip breathing during exercise and ambulation.

Diaphragmatic breathing slows the respiratory rate. It increases the ability to take a deep breath.

Postural drainage uses gravity to help loosen and remove secretions from the lungs.

Incentive spirometry is a form of goal-directed therapy. It improves the resident's ability to breathe deeply.

CLINICAL APPLICATIONS

1. Dr. Jaffe is a retired college professor. She was recently admitted to your facility after hospitalization for pneumonia. She is on a low-sodium diet. The care plan states that you must push fluids for this resident. Dr. Jaffe tells you she dislikes drinking water. What can you do to ensure adequate fluid intake?

2. Mr. Braddock is a 66-year-old resident with COPD. He gets tired during morning care. He cannot usually complete the activity. How can you help him conserve energy?

3. Miss Gabbert has COPD. She takes pride in her appearance. She will not leave her room until her hair is styled perfectly and she is wearing makeup. Her clothing must be adjusted perfectly. The resident uses a curling iron to style her hair each day. This activity is very tiring to the resident. Describe a plan of care to help the resident conserve strength and energy.

4. Mr. Gunn was recently readmitted to your facility after having his gallbladder removed. You are assigned to assist the resident with deep breathing exercises. The resident complains of pain in his incision. He refuses to do the exercises. What will you do?

5. Mrs. Fanelli was admitted yesterday after hospitalization for a blood clot in her leg. She has an incentive spirometer in her room. She tells you that she used the device in the hospital. There is no care plan for using this device. Should you consult someone to see if the order was overlooked? What action will you take?

6. The nurse checks with the physician who ordered the incentive spirometer for Mrs. Fanelli. The order states that the resident must use it four to six times a day. The resident tells you she has forgotten exactly how to use the device. How can you assist her?

CHAPTER 17

Bowel and Bladder Management

OBJECTIVES

After reading this chapter, you should be able to:

- Spell and define key terms.
- List three aging changes to the urinary system.
- List 10 causes of incontinence.
- List six types of incontinence and describe each type.
- Explain how behavior problems may be related to the need to use the bathroom.
- List at least three ways of modifying the environment to make it easier for residents to use the toilet.
- Compare and contrast incontinence management programs with restorative retraining programs.
- Describe the incontinence assessment process and state the restorative nursing assistant's role.
- State the purpose of Kegel exercises.
- Describe how to assist residents with Kegel exercises.

PROBLEMS RELATED TO THE URINARY SYSTEM

We eliminate waste from our bodies daily through urine and feces. Problems with elimination are common in the long-term care facility. Aging, medications, and many diseases affect elimination. Residents may have problems eliminating wastes, or may have lost control and become incontinent. Elimination is a very private matter for most people. It causes anxiety and embarrassment to many. Most residents prefer to care for this very personal body function independently. They do not like to ask for assistance. Changes in elimination affect the residents' self-esteem. You can help them by being sensitive, understanding, and professional. Always consider the residents' feelings when assisting with elimination. Do everything possible to avoid embarrassing the resident.

Aging Changes in Urinary Function

The aging process affects all systems of the body. As people age, the kidneys cannot filter the blood as effectively. Less urine is produced. Another aging change is decreased muscle tone. Because the bladder is a muscle, the capacity is reduced. It cannot hold as much as it did previously. The bladder stores a smaller quantity of urine. This causes increased frequency of urination. There is also a decreased time between the urge to void and the need to pass urine.

Incontinence is not a normal consequence of aging. It usually suggests a medical problem. Incontinence is common in cognitively impaired residents. Many lack the communication skills to express the need to use the bathroom. Most, however, do not forget this basic activity of daily living. If they are assisted to the bathroom, they will almost always urinate.

Prostate Enlargement. A common aging change in males is an enlarged **prostate gland (Figure 17–1).** The prostate surrounds the urethra just below the bladder. It secretes fluid in semen. As the prostate gland enlarges, it presses on the urethra. This causes **urinary retention,** or inability to empty the bladder completely. Some men have constant dribbling of urine. In extreme cases, they cannot urinate at all. Men normally stand to urinate. Assisting them to stand will help them empty the bladder more efficiently.

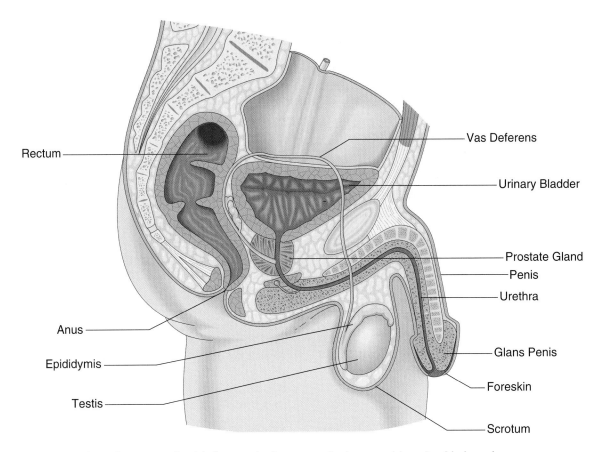

Rectum
Anus
Epididymis
Testis

Vas Deferens
Urinary Bladder
Prostate Gland
Penis
Urethra
Glans Penis
Foreskin
Scrotum

Figure 17–1 An enlarged prostate gland is frequently the cause of urinary problems in elderly males.

Chronic Diseases. Many diseases affect the urinary system. Blood does not circulate as well in residents with heart disease. Less urine is produced, resulting in edema. High blood pressure damages the kidneys. Strokes, trauma, multiple sclerosis, and other diseases affect sensation. This causes residents to be unaware of the urge to urinate. Some have an immediate need when they realize that the bladder is full. They may not know the bladder is full until it has reached its capacity. If the resident must wait, he or she will become incontinent.

▢ URINARY INCONTINENCE

Urinary incontinence can be temporary or permanent. Common causes of incontinence are:

▢ Medication reactions
▢ Disease
▢ Trauma
▢ Surgery
▢ Infection
▢ Stress and anxiety
▢ Tumors

▢ Mental confusion
▢ Difficulty getting to the bathroom
▢ Problems with clothing
▢ Loss of muscle control
▢ Vaginal problems in women
▢ Constipation or fecal impaction
▢ Inability to communicate the need to use the bathroom

Incontinence is a medical problem. Long-term care facilities use underpads, incontinent pads, chux, and briefs **(Figure 17–2)** to contain urine. Properly used, these garments prevent skin breakdown. ⑤They also avoid embarrassment to the residents. Select your words carefully. Do not call these medical aids *diapers*. Avoid using terms that are demeaning. Appropriate terms include *adult brief, garment protector,* and *clothing protector.* Your facility may have special names for these products. Catheters are avoided whenever possible. They increase the risk of infection, which can be serious in the elderly.⑤

Resident Assessment

Several conditions on the RAI will trigger urinary incontinence. When incontinence is triggered, the

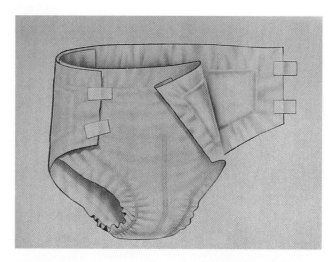

Figure 17–2 Wings® contoured adult brief. Avoid using demeaning terms for this type of garment. (Wings® is a registered trademark of Professional Medical Products, Inc.)

team will review the RAP. The urinary incontinence RAP guides them through an evaluation to determine:

- The cause of the incontinence, including reversible factors
- Whether the incontinence is acute or chronic
- The type of incontinence

The urinary incontinence RAP recommends several tests. It provides guidelines for referral to other health care providers for assessment. You have learned that the MDS is not an all-inclusive evaluation of the resident. Sometimes additional assessments are necessary. This is true with urinary incontinence. The RAP does not evaluate voiding patterns, habits, or the frequency, volume, and circumstances of incontinent episodes. This information is important. It helps determine the type, frequency, and severity of incontinence. Several additional assessments are necessary to provide proper treatment.

Types of Incontinence

A complete assessment of the resident will reveal the type of incontinence. Knowing the correct type is important. This helps staff plan the treatment program. **Table 17–1** lists some observations you can make to help identify the type of incontinence.

Stress Incontinence. Some female residents have a condition called **stress incontinence.** This is caused by weak muscles, having multiple children, and aging. In stress incontinence, the bladder leaks urine when the pelvic muscles are strained. This occurs when the resident moves, laughs, coughs, sneezes, or lifts. Some residents may pass urine when they stand up.

Urge Incontinence. **Urge incontinence** may be caused by infection. Some residents must use the bathroom immediately after taking a drink. Others have an immediate urge to void if they hear running water. Tumors, neurological problems, reproductive problems, and constipation can also cause urge incontinence. Residents have little warning of the need to urinate. They void many times each day. When the urge is felt, the need is immediate. If the urine begins to escape, the bladder empties involuntarily. The resident cannot control it.

Functional Incontinence. **Functional incontinence** occurs in residents who cannot get to the bathroom in time. **SA** This may be due to a mobility problem, such as stiff knees or inability to get out of the chair. This type of incontinence often occurs in residents who are restrained. It is common in residents who are disoriented and cannot find the bathroom. Functional incontinence is the easiest to treat. Take the resident to the bathroom regularly, before he or she has the urge to void. Answering call signals quickly often solves the problem. **SA**

Mixed Incontinence. **Mixed incontinence** is a combination of urge and stress incontinence.

Overflow Incontinence. **Overflow incontinence** occurs when the bladder is very full. Some residents with this condition may have a neurogenic bladder. They feel as if the bladder never empties completely. When the bladder becomes full, urine leaks out. This relieves the pressure. The resident may pass a small amount of urine without feeling the urge to void. Residents may need to void again shortly. In men, overflow incontinence is usually a sign of prostate problems.

Reflex Incontinence. **Reflex incontinence** is loss of urine that occurs without awareness. It is seen in residents with paralysis or neurologic problems.

Types of Continence

Researchers in Australia have divided bladder control into three categories. Some long-term care facilities in the United States use these terms.

- **Independent continence** is the ability to maintain continence without assistance.
- **Dependent continence** applies to residents who are physically or mentally impaired, but are kept dry by staff.
- **Social continence** applies to residents who cannot maintain continence independently, even with regular toileting by staff. The residents depend on absorbent products and other measures to contain urine.

Table 17-1 Observations of Incontinence

Type of Incontinence	Observations
Urge Incontinence	The resident may leak urine: ■ when he or she notices the need to use the bathroom ■ on the way to the bathroom ■ after drinking a small amount of liquid ■ when he or she hears water running The resident uses the bathroom many times throughout the day and night.
Stress Incontinence	The resident may leak urine: ■ when sneezing, coughing, or laughing ■ when he or she moves or exercises a certain way ■ when getting up from the bed or chair ■ when walking or lifting Stress incontinence is most common in women.
Overflow	The resident feels as if the bladder never empties completely. Passes a small amount of urine without feeling the urge to void. Urinates shortly after voiding the last time.

This type of incontinence may indicate prostate problems in men. Residents who are incontinent are often overflowing. They are not emptying the bladder completely. Taking the resident to the bathroom or offering the bedpan or urinal often results in additional urination.

Cognitively Impaired Residents

Residents who are cognitively impaired are challenging. Many will urinate if they are taken to the toilet. Some have behavior problems that may be caused by the discomfort of needing to use the toilet. The residents cannot express themselves verbally. Instead, they yell, scream, hit, or cry **(Figure 17–3)**. Some become restless. They pull at or remove their clothing. After they have urinated, the behavior stops. It takes an alert caregiver to recognize that the problem is related to elimination. Ⓢ Anticipate the need for toileting. Ⓢ Take residents to the bathroom every two hours. Some residents wander because of the need to eliminate. When they wander, they may be looking for the bathroom. If they see it, they will use it. They are incontinent when they cannot find the bathroom.

Ⓢ Managing incontinence requires good observation, planning, and effort. However, the results are gratifying. They benefit the residents and make your work easier. Warm, wet clothing or linen is an ideal breeding ground for bacteria. This increases the risk of skin and bladder infections. Preventing incontinence also prevents skin breakdown, discomfort, odor, and loss of self-esteem. Ⓢ

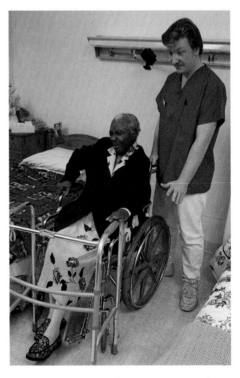

Figure 17–3 Behavior problems are frequently caused by the inability to communicate the need to eliminate.

BOWEL INCONTINENCE

Involuntary passage of stool is *bowel incontinence*. The causes are varied. The most common are:

- Trauma
- Neurological disease
- Inability to reach the toilet in time
- Cognitive impairment

Fecal material is very irritating to the skin. Exposed areas will break down quickly. Bowel incontinence lowers the resident's self-esteem. Your professionalism and compassion are important.

Bowel retraining is often combined with bladder management. Knowing the history and pattern of incontinence is useful. This helps staff to plan a bowel management program. Regular toileting to prevent bladder incontinence often results in the return of bowel continence.

Some residents have bowel incontinence only. In these residents, fluid intake, fiber in the diet, and exercise are increased. Bowel retraining is managed by giving suppositories at the same time each day. During the first week, the suppository is given daily. Later, the number of suppositories is gradually reduced. The resident is assisted to use the toilet at the same time each day. You may administer the suppositories, if permitted.

THE RESTORATIVE TOILETING PROGRAM

Studies have shown a relationship between improved mobility and reduction of incontinence. The studies suggest that a walking program increases mobility. Episodes of incontinence also decrease. Adaptive equipment such as walkers and wheelchairs should be available for residents with ambulation problems.

Environmental Considerations

Toilet seats must be at least 17 inches from the floor. Toilets should have arm or wall supports. Some residents may be unable to reach the bathroom because of distance. Other barriers, such as furniture placed in the way and poor lighting, may also be a problem. Chairs designed for ease in rising are helpful. In one study of chair-bound residents, 77 percent could stand up from chairs that were 17 inches at seat height, with arms 10 inches above the seat. Physical and chemical restraints also contribute to incontinence.

Restorative Care of Residents in Elimination Programs

You will work with residents who have many different elimination needs. Certain guidelines apply to assisting residents with elimination programs.

General Guidelines for Assisting with Elimination Programs

- Apply the principles of standard precautions. Anticipate your needs. Select the correct personal protective equipment.
- Ensure that the urinal, bedpan, or commode is within the resident's sight. These items should be in easy reach, if the resident uses them independently.
- Make sure the signal cord is within reach.
- Provide a safe, clear pathway to the bathroom.
- Keep the path to the bathroom well lit and obstacle-free.
- Follow the care plan exactly.
- Avoid scolding the resident for accidents. Praise him or her for using the toilet and for staying dry.
- If the resident cannot use the toilet, assist with the bedpan, urinal, or commode.
- If the resident uses a wheelchair, walker, or cane, keep it close to the bed.
- Keep the resident's skin clean and dry.
- Assist residents to adjust their clothing, if necessary.
- Assist residents to transfer on and off the toilet, if necessary.
- Provide privacy. Close the door and privacy curtain. Close the bathroom door even if you must remain in the room for safety.
- Avoid rushing residents when toileting.
- Assist residents to cleanse the perineum. Assist with handwashing, if necessary.
- Consult your supervisor if you think a resident would benefit from adaptive equipment, a raised toilet seat, or support rails for the toilet.

BOWEL AND BLADDER MANAGEMENT

Incontinence is a decline, as defined by OBRA. If a resident is admitted with bowel and bladder control, the facility must assist him or her to maintain control. If the resident becomes incontinent, the facility must be able to prove that the decline was unavoidable. Residents who are incontinent upon admission should be evaluated for a management program. If the resident is ill at the time of admission, wait until the condition improves.🆂🅰

Acute illness and declines in mental status may cause incontinence. Remember that it is not a normal part of aging. It must be prevented and treated aggressively. Managing incontinence is unpleasant. View it as a medical problem, beyond the resident's control. Conduct yourself professionally. Avoid affecting the resident's self esteem. 🆂🅰Assisting residents to be clean, dry, and odor-free is part of the facility routine.🆂🅰 Some, however, will benefit from active management programs. Bowel and bladder management initially may be a great deal of work for the staff. Over the long term, your efforts will pay off. Assisting residents to use the bathroom is much less work.

Incontinence Management Programs

Incontinence management programs are not active restorative programs. They are designed for residents who:

- Are very confused
- Have behavior problems related to toileting
- Cannot communicate the need to eliminate
- Can sit on the toilet or commode
- Will recognize the need and use the toilet after they are seated

A management program involves taking residents to the bathroom regularly. Most are toileted every two or three hours. A trial of incontinence management should be used on confused residents who can use a toilet. The resident is not actually "trained" to use the toilet. However, the results are the same. The resident and staff both benefit.

Scheduled Toileting. **Scheduled toileting** is used for residents who require physical assistance. The residents recognize the urge to use the toilet. However, they cannot get to the bathroom without help. Staff toilet the resident according to a schedule, usually every two to four hours. The schedule is adjusted for high intake periods, such as after meals. The resident is toileted 24 hours a day. He or she is prompted to void, even if the urge is not present. The goal is keeping the resident dry. Staff do not tell the resident to delay voiding or resist the urge to void. Studies have shown a notable decrease in incontinence in as little as two weeks.

Prompted Voiding. Some residents know or can learn to recognize that the bladder is full. They will respond when prompted to use the bathroom. These residents may benefit from a **prompted voiding** program. Residents in this program may be confused and cannot participate other types of programs. When you enter the room, ask the resident if he or she is wet or dry. Assist and encourage

the resident to use the toilet. This is called *prompting.* Praise the resident for remaining dry and for trying to use the toilet. Tell the resident when you will take him or her to the bathroom again. Most residents are successful if they are toileted every two to three hours. Prompted voiding may be done with habit training. The programs reinforce the resident's ability to recognize the urge to void and request assistance.

Habit Training. **Habit training** is used for residents with poor recall and short attention span. They urinate at fairly predictable times. The resident's voiding habits are studied until a pattern emerges. The restorative nurse develops a toileting schedule from this information. Praise the resident for being dry and using the toilet. Habit training will not be successful immediately. Residents may not regain complete control. However, over several months, it has been shown to reduce incontinence.

Residents with Catheters. Some residents are placed on bladder programs to remove an indwelling catheter. Facilities manage these programs differently. Some remove the catheter and begin an assessment. Studies have shown that this is the preferred method of retraining. Some facilities clamp and unclamp the catheter at regular intervals. This allows the resident to get used to the sensation of urine in the bladder. You may be asked to clamp and unclamp the catheter. This does not involve opening the closed system. Urine remains in the bladder when the catheter is clamped. It empties into the drainage bag when the clamp is opened. The catheter is reclamped immediately after emptying. The interval for catheter draining is increased slowly. Report to your supervisor if the resident complains of discomfort. Be prompt when unclamping the catheter to prevent bladder overfilling.

▓ RESTORATIVE BOWEL AND BLADDER RETRAINING

Bladder retraining involves using one or more techniques to assist residents to regain control. Many types of programs are used. The programs described previously were management programs. The programs in this section are active retraining programs. All require the resident to resist or delay the urge to void. He or she urinates on a schedule instead of the urinary urge. The schedule is based on an assessment of the times the resident has voided over the previous two weeks.

Some facilities adjust fluid intake. They delay voiding to allow the bladder to fill. Over time, the interval between voids is increased. Initially, the goal is to wait for about two hours to void. The goal is to void every three to four hours. Some facilities do not practice retraining during the night.

Residents may be taught relaxation or distraction techniques. Used correctly, these will help resist the urge to void. The resident uses the technique when the urge occurs. If he or she cannot delay voiding, the nurse readjusts the schedule. The new interval is reset from the time of the last void. Instead of resetting the schedule, some facilities continue with the regular schedule. They disregard the unscheduled urination. Bladder retraining may continue for several months. During this time, staff provides positive reinforcement. Never scold the resident for incontinence. Encourage him or her and reinforce that retraining takes time.

Developing an Individualized Program

Bowel and bladder retraining programs are designed for residents who have become incontinent because of:

▨ Acute illness
▨ Trauma
▨ Infection
▨ Medications

Residents with overflow incontinence are usually not good candidates for retraining, because of neurological problems. Residents do not have to be mentally alert for such programs. However, they must be able to follow directions.

For best results, bowel and bladder programs are developed as early in the illness as possible. The resident should be stable and not acutely ill. The nurse assesses the resident's physical condition, mental status, and ability to participate. An environmental assessment may be completed. This determines access and distance to the toilet. The resident's mobility is also assessed. This shows whether the resident can get to the bathroom independently. After all data are collected, a program is developed to meet the resident's needs.

Part of the assessment involves identifying factors that contribute to or cause the incontinence. A plan is developed to modify or eliminate these factors. A history of the resident's previous habits and routines is considered when the program is developed.

Restorative Assistant Responsibilities. A detailed analysis of the resident's incontinence over 7 to 14 days is completed. You will check the resident hourly. However, you will not prompt the resident to use the bathroom. If he or she requests assistance, comply. This part of the assessment involves checking to see whether the resident is wet, soiled, or dry. ⑤Ⓐ You will record the results on a form like the one shown in **Table 17–2**.⑤Ⓐ A pattern of fairly regular incontinent episodes will emerge. Accurate completion of this analysis is very

important. The resident's toileting schedule will be developed from the information on the form. Notify the nurse if the resident shows a pattern of urge, stress, or overflow incontinence, or if you believe other conditions are affecting elimination.

The Retraining Plan. After the assessment, the nurse analyzes the information. He or she develops a plan for the resident. The plan is based on the resident's:

▨ Previous habits
▨ Routines
▨ Recorded times of incontinent episodes **(Figure 17–4, p. 272** and **p. 273)**

The nurse will write a schedule with times to toilet the resident. Because the schedule is based on the resident's needs, the times may be irregular. Some people can wait for six hours before urinating. Others urinate every hour or two. Before retraining begins, the environment is modified to eliminate barriers.

The toileting schedule will be implemented by nursing staff. The nurse will reassess the schedule every few days. Staff takes the resident to the bathroom at the designated times. Each elimination is recorded. Success and failure are recorded. Praise the resident for success. Avoid scolding him or her for failures. The nurse continues to adjust the schedule until success is achieved. Flexibility, consistency, punctuality, a positive attitude, and being available at toileting times helps guarantee success. In addition, believe that the program will succeed. Maintain your motivation to help the resident. It may take several months for the resident to reach the highest level of independence. Be empathetic, patient, and supportive. Encourage the resident's success. ⑤ⒶYour efforts will help maintain the resident's dignity and self-esteem. Your facility will remain in compliance with the OBRA '87 requirements.⑤Ⓐ

Kegel Exercises

Some residents must exercise to strengthen the bladder muscles. These exercises are called **Kegel exercises.** Restorative nurses work with these residents. You will remind the resident to exercise. Kegel exercises are also called pelvic floor exercises or pelvic muscle exercises (PMEs).

Research has shown that Kegel exercises prevent incontinence. Over time, they strengthen pelvic floor muscles. Kegel exercises are helpful for women with stress incontinence. They may be used by men and women, combined with a management program for urge incontinence. Kegel exercises may also be effective for men who become incontinent after prostate surgery.

Table 17–2   Assessment for Bowel & Bladder Training

Patient: <u>Frank Martin</u>   **Room No. <u>629C</u>**

Date	Day 1 10/2/XX	Day 2 10/3/XX	Day 3 10/4/XX	Day 4 10/5/XX	Day 5 10/6/XX	Day 6 10/7/XX	Day 7 10/8/XX
7 AM	D	IU	IU	D			
8 AM	IU	D	D	D			
9 AM	D	IU	D	IU			
10 AM	D	D	D	D			
11 AM	D	D	IU	IU			
12 AM	IU	D	D	D			
1 PM	IU	IU	IU	IU			
2 PM	D	D	D	D			
3 PM	D	D	D	D			
4 PM	IBM	D	D	IU			
5 PM	IU	IBM	D	IBM			
6 PM	D	IU	IU	D			
7 PM	D	D	D	IU			
8 PM	IU	IU	IU	D			
9 PM	D	D	D	D			
10 PM	D	D	D	IU			
11 PM	D	IU	IU	D			
12 AM	D	D	D	D			
1 AM	IU	D	D	D			
2 AM	D	IU	IU	IU			
3 AM	IU	D	D	IU			
4 AM	D	D	D	D			
5 AM	D	D	IU	D			
6 AM	IU	IU	D	D			

CODE: D = DRY   TBM = TOILET BM
         IBM = INCONTINENT BM   TU = TOILET URINE
         IU = INCONTINENT URINE

EVALUATION FOR INCONTINENCE

RESIDENT _Martin, Frank_   ROOM NO. _629C_

DATE _10/1/xx_   PHYSICIAN _S. Neil, D.O._

CURRENT LEVEL OF INCONTINENCE:

_____ Is incontinent more than four times per day with no predictable voiding pattern.

__✔__ Would be soiled without staff efforts to keep dry. Staff has established a toileting schedule that prevents most episodes of incontinence.

_____ Is on an active Continence Management Program.

_____ Has an indwelling catheter.

_____ Is continent, no further evaluation needed at the present time.

OBSERVATIONS AND ACTIVITIES:

_____ Is incontinent more than four times per day with no predictable voiding pattern.

_____ Re-evaluate for other inventions once the following issues have been resolved:

    _____ medical evaluation for UTI

    _____ recovery from acute illness

    _____ healing pressure sore/decu

    _____ improved transfer skills

    _____ decreased combativeness

__✔__ If toileted on a regular basis, can usually remain dry.

_____ Continue catheter use [indicate why]

    _____ obstructive uropathy

    _____ chronic renal failure

    _____ CHF/fluid restriction

    _____ acute illness

    _____ pressure sores/decubs

    _____ dialysis

    _____ tube feeding

    _____ terminal illness

INTERVENTIONS:
Check frequently; change as needed; provided good skin/peri care; enter in care plan.

1. Ask if he needs to use the toliet when OOB.
2. Offer urinal when in bed.
3. Wears adult brief when up.
4. Provide peri-care after each incontinent episode.

Enter toliet schedule in care plan; schedule as follows:

6:30/am, 9:00/am, 10:30/am, 1:00/pm,
3:45/pm, 5:00/pm, 6:30/pm,
9:00/pm, 12:00/am, 3:00/am

Full assessment for Continence Management Program: RECOMMENDATIONS

B & B program established based on obvious pattern of incontinence during 14 day assessment. Schedule above reflects individual plan. Will implement x7da, then re-evaluate.

RESTORATIVE NURSE: _Laura Marschak, R.N._   DATE: _10/1/xx_

Figure 17–4 The restorative nurse gathers the previous elimination history and reviews the incontinence monitoring record. He or she will develop an individual toileting schedule for the resident based on this information. The plan will be reviewed and revised until the resident reaches his or her highest level of continence.

ASSESSMENT FOR BOWEL & BLADDER TRAINING

RESIDENT: _____ ROOM NO.: _____

	DAY 1	DAY 2	DAY 3	DAY 4	DAY 5	DAY 6	DAY 7
DATE							
7 AM							
8 AM							
9 AM							
10 AM							
11 AM							
12 N							
1 PM							
2 PM							
3 PM							
4 PM							
5 PM							
6 PM							
7 PM							
8 PM							
9 PM							
10 PM							
11 PM							
12 M							
1 AM							
2 AM							
3 AM							
4 AM							
5 AM							
6 AM							

CODE
D = DRY
IBM = INCONTINENT IBM
IU = INCONTINENT URINE
TMB = TOILET BM
TU = TOILET URINE

Figure 17–4 continued.

Kegel exercises strengthen the muscles surrounding the urethra and vagina. These muscles contribute to the closing of the urethra. They support the pelvic structures.

The first step is teaching the resident awareness of pelvic muscle function. The resident is taught to draw in, or lift up, the muscles surrounding the vagina and anus. This is the same as the action used for controlling urination and defecation. Residents are instructed to contract the muscles. They hold the contraction for at least 10 seconds, then release for 10 seconds. The exercises are done about 30 to 80 times a day for at least 8 weeks. They may need to be continued indefinitely. More time may be required with the elderly before seeing results. Over time, the exercises condition the muscles to contract when abdominal pressure increases. Residents are reminded to contract the pelvic muscles in situations when leakage may occur.

Biofeedback

Residents may need repeated guidance over a long period of time. Some nurses recommend using **biofeedback** with Kegel exercises. Biofeedback provides visual and auditory information to give the resident voluntary control. Nurses will teach the residents biofeedback techniques. You will remind residents to use them.

Intake and Output

Record the resident's intake and output during the retraining period. The fluid intake may be increased so the bladder becomes used to holding more urine.

In some facilities, fluids are limited during the evening and night hours. Know and follow your facility policy.

Fluid and Dietary Management During Retraining

Constipation is a common problem in the elderly. The pressure of stool in the rectum increases urinary incontinence. The nurse may have to remove a fecal impaction to relieve pressure. The dietitian will work with the restorative nurse to establish a bowel regimen containing adequate fiber and fluid.

Eliminating caffeine is important for persons with urge incontinence. Coffee, tea, soda, and chocolate contain caffeine. Residents with all types of incontinence may benefit from limiting these items. However, if they continue to ask for these items after an explanation of the effect on incontinence, do not scold them. ⒮ⒶDrinking these beverages and eating chocolate is the residents' right. Report the residents' noncompliance to your supervisor.⒮Ⓐ Restricting fluid is not effective for managing incontinence. Maintaining adequate fluid intake is important. This is particularly true in the elderly, who have a decrease in body water and are at risk for dehydration. Inadequate fluid intake also contributes to constipation. Routine use of stool softeners or laxatives is not recommended. These drugs cause dependence. Residents may become unable to eliminate without them. Emphasis is placed on increasing fluids, high-fiber foods, and fiber supplements. Bulk-forming medications may be used if dietary measures are ineffective.

KEY POINTS IN CHAPTER

- Aging changes to the urinary system include less urine production, decreased muscle tone, reduced bladder capacity, increased frequency of urination, and enlarged prostate gland.
- Incontinence is not a normal aging change.
- An enlarged prostate gland can cause dribbling, urinary retention, and inability to urinate.
- The word diaper is demeaning to adults. Appropriate words to use include adult brief, garment protector, and clothing protector.
- Behavior problems in confused residents may be caused by the inability to communicate the need to use the bathroom.
- Stress incontinence is caused by weak muscles, having multiple children, and aging. The bladder leaks during movement, laughing, coughing, sneezing, and lifting.
- Urge incontinence is frequently caused by infection. Residents have an immediate need to use the bathroom when they feel the urge to urinate.
- Functional incontinence occurs in residents who are physically unable to get to the bathroom due to mobility problems, restraints, or inability to find the bathroom.
- Mixed incontinence is a combination of urge and stress incontinence.

(continues)

KEY POINTS IN CHAPTER *continued*

Overflow incontinence occurs when the bladder is very full. Urine leaks out to relieve the pressure.

Reflex incontinence is loss of urine without awareness. It occurs in residents with paralysis or other neurologic problems.

Independent continence is the ability to maintain continence without assistance.

Dependent continence applies to residents who are physically or mentally impaired, but are kept dry by staff.

Social continence applies to residents who cannot maintain continence independently or through regular toileting by staff. They depend on absorbent products and other measures to contain urine.

Raised toilet seats with arm supports, a safe well-lighted environment, and adaptive devices such as walkers and canes may enable residents to use the bathroom independently.

Incontinence management programs are based on an assessment. They are used for residents who are confused, have behavior problems related to toileting, or cannot communicate the need to eliminate.

Active restorative bowel and bladder programs are based on an assessment. They are individualized to the resident's needs. The programs are adjusted as often as necessary until success is achieved.

Kegel exercises strengthen the lower pelvic muscles. They are done by drawing in or lifting up the muscles surrounding the vagina and anus.

Adequate fluid intake and dietary fiber are important to the success of bowel and bladder management programs.

CLINICAL APPLICATIONS

1. Mrs. Abrams is a mentally confused resident. She sits in the hallway and screams for 30 minutes. Suddenly she is quiet. You notice a large stream of urine under her chair, running down the hallway. This is routine behavior for this resident. She screams, then is quiet. What action should you take? What do you think caused Mrs. Abrams's behavior problem? Should this information be reported to the nurse?

2. Mr. Harris is an ambulatory 75-year-old. He constantly dribbles urine. His clothing must be changed frequently during the shift. What is the most common cause of this problem? What can be done to assist Mr. Harris?

3. Mrs. Hirakawa normally has good bladder control. Over the past week, she has had frequent episodes of incontinence. She says she has little warning of the need to void. When she recognizes the need, it is immediate.

She also complains of back pain above her waist. What type of incontinence is Mrs. Hirakawa experiencing? What is the most common cause of this type of incontinence? What action will you take?

4. The nurse has just started an assessment of a resident's bowel and bladder pattern. The nurse explained the program to the nursing assistants yesterday. Susan, a new CNA, was off yesterday. She sees the paper in the resident's room and asks you what it is for. She says she feels too stupid to ask the nurse. What action will you take? What will you tell Susan?

5. During the bowel and bladder assessment, you notice that the resident has a BM each day within 45 minutes of eating lunch. What does this tell you? Is this information important to the overall assessment? Why or why not? What will you do?

CHAPTER 18

Restorative Care of Residents with Psychosocial and Behavioral Issues

OBJECTIVES

After reading this chapter, you should be able to:

Spell and define key terms.

List some reasons for psychosocial problems in the elderly.

List and define four defense mechanisms.

Describe using the ABC method of behavior management.

Describe how to assist residents with behavior problems that interfere with care.

State the purpose of music therapy.

State the purpose of validation therapy.

State the purpose of reminiscence.

State the purpose of cognitive enhancement.

RESTORATIVE CARE OF RESIDENTS WITH BEHAVIOR PROBLEMS AND PSYCHOSOCIAL NEEDS

Residents in the long-term care facility have suffered many losses. They have many other problems. These range from sadness, stress, and anger to aggressive behavior. Many problems are the result of disease and cognitive loss. Behavior problems occur in both alert and confused residents. Most are caused by the inability to cope with stress or by unmet needs. The unmet needs can be physical or psychosocial. A social worker or licensed psychologist may work with residents to help them cope more effectively. You will work with residents' psychosocial needs during relaxation programs. You will encounter behavior, frustration, and inability to cope during other restorative programs.

Common behavior problems are:

- Physical or verbal aggression
- Wandering
- Yelling or calling out
- Socially inappropriate behaviors, such as undressing

SAProblem behavior may be dangerous to the resident, staff, and other residents on the unit.**SA** Some problems are annoying to the staff, but are harmless.

Fluid is very important. Dehydration contributes to confusion and behavior problems. Working with behavior problems requires using patience, common sense, good communication skills, and a great deal of empathy.

The Meaning of Behavior

All behavior has a meaning. However, the meaning may not be apparent to you. The resident may not even realize that you consider the behavior abnormal. This is particularly true with residents from other cultures. Behavior that is acceptable in one culture may be considered abnormal by persons from other cultures. Behavior patterns develop throughout a person's lifetime. They are affected by heredity, culture, environment, and lifetime experiences.

Normal Coping and Defense Mechanisms

Coping or defense mechanisms are tools residents use to deal with stress. They are also used to help compensate for losses. Residents use these methods

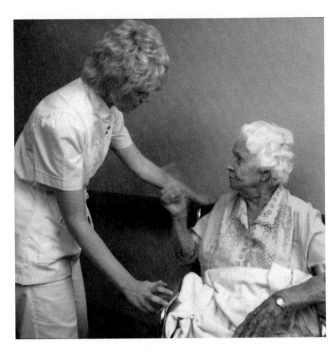

Figure 18–1 Do not take the resident's outburst personally. She is angry with her situation.

Table 18–1	Identify the ABCs
Identify the ABCs	**Definition**
A = Antecedent	The cause or trigger of the behavior
B = Behavior	The behavior itself
C = Consequences	The effect or results of the behavior

throughout their lifetime. Using coping mechanisms helps protect self-esteem. The terms *coping* and *defense* are used interchangeably in this chapter. Common coping/defense mechanisms are:

- **Denial,** or refusing to admit there is a problem
- **Rationalization,** or providing an acceptable but untrue reason for a problem
- **Compensation,** or using strength and overachieving in one area to overcome a weakness in another area
- **Projection,** or blaming someone or something else

Residents are responding to stress when they use coping mechanisms. Do not take angry outbursts or other behavior personally. Residents may say they are angry with you, but this is probably not true **(Figure 18–1).** Usually, the resident is angry about a situation. Observe how the resident responds to you. (SA)Adjust your approach to achieve results. (SA) Practice empathy. Put yourself in the resident's shoes. Try to understand what is happening.

▰▰ THE ABCS OF BEHAVIOR MANAGEMENT

An effective behavior management technique is the ABC plan **(Table 18–1).** It is useful for all residents whether they are alert or cognitively impaired. The theory is that if the **antecedent** or **consequences** of the behavior are eliminated or modified, the behavior will change or stop. The *antecedent* is the

event that causes or triggers a behavior. The *consequences* are the outcome, or what occurs as a result of the behavior.

The Three Steps of Behavior Management

Three steps in the ABC method of behavior management are:

- Step 1—Attempt to learn the cause (trigger for or antecedent) of the behavior. Does the behavior occur in specific environmental conditions? (For example, is the resident hot or cold?) Does it occur at a certain time of day, or during a certain activity? Does the presence or absence of other persons trigger the behavior?
- Step 2—Eliminate the cause of the behavior. Identifying and removing the cause will stop the behavior. This may not happen immediately, but it will over time.
- Step 3—Examine the consequences of the behavior. They may also have to be eliminated or changed before the behavior will be corrected. Modifying the consequences requires practice. For example, a confused resident yells and cries. You discover that if you sit and hold her hand, she stops yelling. Sitting and holding her hand rewards the behavior! To modify the consequences, sit and hold the resident's hand *before* the yelling and crying start **(Figure 18–2).** Pay attention to the resident regularly. Sit and hold her hand for a few minutes several times during your shift. Here, modifying the consequences changes the behavior. If the resident's behavior has been rewarded for a long period of time, you will not see immediate results. The entire team must practice the new approach consistently before results are evident.

Using the ABC Method

Mentally alert residents who use the call signal repeatedly for minor requests are distressing to

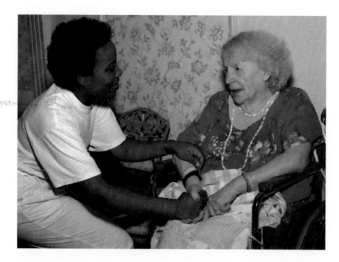

Figure 18–2 Sit and hold the resident's hand before she begins the behavior.

staff. The resident may ask you to turn on the light or refill the water glass. As soon as you leave the room, the resident signals again. Residents with this type of behavior are often lonely and scared. They use the call signal to get attention. Tell the resident what time you will return when you leave. Return at that time. Keeping your word shows the resident that you can be trusted. Stop in the room and check on the resident when you can. As the resident gets more attention, use of the call signal will decrease.

This simple example shows how the ABCs are used effectively. In this case:

A, or antecedent, is the resident's loneliness and fear.

B, or behavior, is using the call signal for minor requests.

C, or consequence, is attention and companionship when you are in the room.

Checking on the resident frequently and keeping promises shows the resident that she can depend on you. This changes the consequences. The resident gets regular companionship and attention. This calms her loneliness and fear. The behavior stops because there is no reason to continue.

In these examples, the consequences were modified to change the behavior. Sometimes the antecedent must be changed. For example, a mentally confused resident is quiet all day. She begins to scream at bedtime after you leave the room. You discover that she stops screaming when you turn on the light. When you turn the light off, she screams again. The resident is afraid of the dark. She stops screaming if you leave a light on in the bathroom. In this case, the consequence is positive. The antecedent caused the problem.

A, or antecedent, is the resident's fear of the dark.

B, or behavior, is screaming when she is alone with the light turned off.

C, or consequence, is the light is turned on, enabling the resident to sleep.

Assisting with Behavior Management Programs

If a resident has a behavior problem, the team will develop a care plan. If you identify a cause for the behavior, or know an approach that works, inform your supervisor. The plan will be based on the resident's strengths and needs. Behavior management is restorative care. The principles of restoration apply. The plan may be modified depending on the resident's response. To be effective, all staff must be consistent in their approaches to the resident.

Implementing the Behavior Management Plan. Become familiar with the care plan. ⓈⒶImplement the approaches listed. Modify your behavior in response to the resident's behavior. Reward residents for positive behavior. *Behavior that is rewarded is usually repeated.*ⓈⒶ The goal is to show the resident a healthy way of directing energy. Verbal praise, positive feedback, and other signs of approval are rewards. Nonverbal rewards, such as a hug, smile, or pat on the back, may also be used. Snacks and privileges are sometimes used as rewards.

Your Role in Assisting Residents with Specific Behavior Problems

There is no universal behavior management program, because each person is unique. Use common sense. Review the behavior information in your nursing assistant textbook. The discussion here is limited to problems that interfere with the resident's participation in restorative programs.

Depression. Depression **(Figure 18–3)** is a feeling of despair or discouragement. It may occur in response to stress and loss. Sometimes the cause is unknown. Depression can interfere with the resident's participation in restorative care. He or she may be unwilling or unable to try. Depression can cause the resident to feel too tired or weak to participate. Take depression seriously. Report your observations to your supervisor. The signs and symptoms of depression vary widely. They may include:

▪ Decreased concentration

▪ Memory loss

▪ Fatigue

▪ Insomnia

▪ Sadness

▪ Crying

General Guidelines for Assisting Residents Who Have Behavior Problems

- Follow the care plan.
- Control your own responses and reactions.
- Remove the cause of the behavior, if known.
- Protect the safety of the resident and others.
- **SA** If the care plan states how to respond to a specific behavior, apply the approaches when the behavior starts. Do not wait until the resident loses control. **SA**
- Use good communication and listening skills.
- Practice empathy.
- Attempt to learn the cause of the behavior. Communicate with other team members.
- Let others know if you discover an approach that works.
- Watch the resident's response to your approaches. Adjust your approach, if necessary.
- Discuss family, friends, or other pleasant information with residents. This provides a source of strength, comfort, and support.
- Meet the resident's physical needs.
- Give residents as much control as possible. Offer choices in care and routines. Encourage them to direct their own care.
- Be patient. Control your reaction to the resident. Make sure your body language does not send the wrong message.
- Be happy. Smile. Make sure your body language sends a positive message. Positive behavior is contagious.

General Guidelines for Assisting Residents with Depression

- Be honest, supportive, and caring.
- Be a good listener. Encourage residents to express feelings. Avoid passing judgment. Do not criticize what the resident feels. Do not interrupt or change the subject.
- Give positive feedback on the resident's strengths and successes.
- Acknowledge the resident's feelings.
- Use touch and hugs, if appropriate.
- Do not make comments like, "Cheer up. Things could be worse."
- Encourage physical activity. Exercise reduces stress.
- Encourage the resident to laugh. Laughter reduces stress.
- Singing reduces stress. You can have fun laughing and singing with the resident!

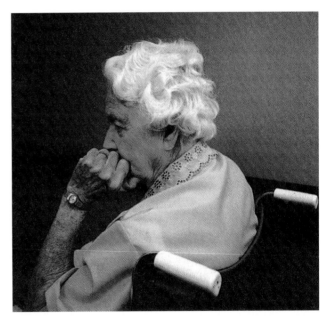

Figure 18–3   Depression is a serious problem in the elderly.

- Loss of appetite
- Overeating
- Apathy
- Despair
- Loss of self-esteem

Cognitive Impairment.   You will work with residents who have cognitive impairment and behavior problems. Restorative approaches are useful in preventing or reducing behavior problems. Behavior problems occur for the same reasons as they do in alert residents. The resident feels stressed or over-

whelmed. You can reduce the resident's stress by modifying your approach. For example, change routines and equipment slightly.

Mentally confused residents who cannot learn new skills will be in maintenance programs. The programs are designed to prevent or slow declines.

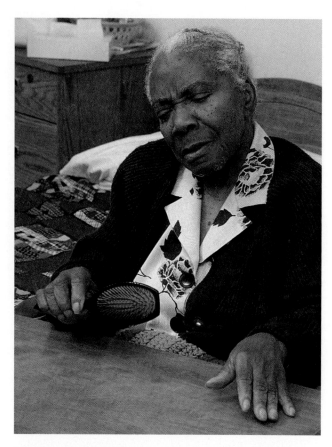

Figure 18–4 Work with residents on simple, familiar tasks. This resident has the motor skill to brush her hair, but she has forgotten what the brush is for. Give verbal cues. If she does not respond, use hand-over-hand technique.

Focus on familiar skills and tasks **(Figure 18–4).** Although the resident cannot learn new tasks, he or she may be able to do familiar ones. Allow enough time for the resident to process your instructions. If he or she does not understand, repeat the instructions. Say things exactly the same way. Break the task down into small, simple steps. Give one direction at a time. Allow the resident time to complete it before giving the next. Telling the resident to complete an entire task is overwhelming. Start with a simple step. When this is done, instruct the resident in the next step. Sincerely compliment him or her for success.

▥ OTHER THERAPEUTIC MODALITIES

You have learned how to use relaxation therapy. This procedure is used to manage stress and pain. Relaxation is also used for residents with stress and behavior problems. Different individuals work with music therapy, validation, reminiscence, and cognitive enhancement in the long-term care facility. Activities or social service may conduct these programs. Like behavior management, the programs

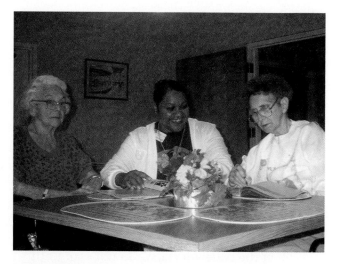

Figure 18–5 The restorative nursing assistant uses pictures in a magazine to help residents reminisce. (Courtesy of East Galbraith Health Care Community, Cincinnati, OH)

are restorative in nature. The restorative nursing department may be responsible for them in your facility **(Figure 18–5).** You must understand the purpose and types of programs used. If you will be working directly with these programs, your supervisor will give you instructions.

Cognitive Enhancement Programs

Cognitive enhancement involves using several techniques. Approaches are taken from memory training, mental stimulation, and reality orientation. The purpose is to help residents become more aware of their environment **(Figure 18–6).** The program also provides a sense of self. Cognitive enhancement provides stimulation gradually. The resident is stimulated throughout the waking hours. He or she is given frequent reminders. For example, color-coding drawers, labeling items, and making lists are used as reminders to the resident. The resident is encouraged to talk about past feelings and events. He or she is asked to write about them, if able. Memory is stimulated with:

▥ games

▥ lists

▥ tags

▥ verbal cues

▥ repetition

▥ pictures

▥ group programs

The resident is asked to repeat the time, date, and activity he or she is doing throughout the day. This is done in a nonthreatening manner. Over time, the resident becomes more oriented.

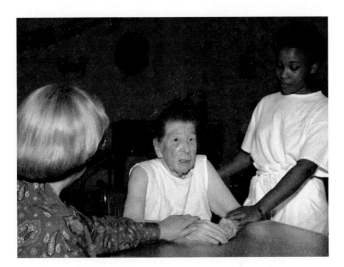

Figure 18–6 Remind the resident of the date, day, and time. Reinforce her self-worth by encouraging her to speak about the past.

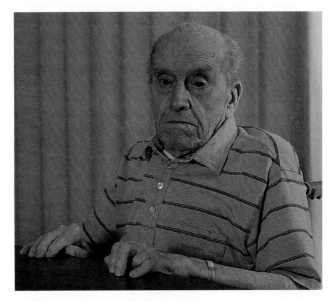

Figure 18–7 This cognitively impaired resident was once a child, then an adult. Use validation to reinforce his feelings of self-esteem and assist him to complete his developmental tasks of old age.

Cognitive enhancement runs through all restorative programs. Reminding the residents of the purpose of an activity is cognitive enhancement. You will remind confused residents several times when you are working with them. Over time, they begin to recognize the environment. They begin to associate it with the activity. The simple measures used in this program have a very positive outcome!

Limit decision making and complex directions that will frustrate the resident. Provide realistic situations in daily routines. Discuss them with the resident. Provide orienting information, if necessary.

Validation Therapy

Validation therapy is a technique developed by Naomi Feil, who is a social worker, an actress, and a researcher. She describes the therapy as a way to communicate with persons over the age of 75. It is also used for residents with Alzheimer's disease and cognitive impairments. The program is based on the belief that developmental tasks from earlier years must be resolved. If they were not resolved, they will emerge in old age. The elderly person may display many emotions in trying to conclude them. Feil's research has shown that using validation reduces the need for restraints. It helps residents regain feelings of dignity and self-control. It also increases staff morale. Feil stresses the following concepts:

- Maintaining the identity and dignity of residents is important.
- People with dementia can feel good about themselves.
- All behavior has a purpose. Some disoriented behavior may be acting out of memories.
- The residents' memories and feelings should be acknowledged.

- Cognitively impaired residents have the right to express their feelings.
- Residents must resolve living in order to prepare for dying.
- The elderly have experienced many losses. Many have lost the ability to cope.
- Living in reality is not the only way to live.
- Disoriented residents are worthwhile. Staff can give them joy by allowing them to express their feelings.
- Each person was once a child, then an adult. Residents deserve to be cared for with dignity in their final years of life **(Figure 18–7)**.

When using validation, allow residents to express their feelings. Reassure them that the feelings are worthwhile. Use a calm, nonthreatening manner. Speak in a loving tone of voice. When the resident describes an emotion, assure him or her that it is okay. A book, videotape, and training program are available for facilities using this technique.

Reality Orientation

Some facilities do not use reality orientation. They believe it worsens agitation in some residents. The subject is controversial. It is presented here for facilities in which the program is used. It is most effective in orienting residents with **delirium.** Memory loss in delirium is caused by an acute illness. It is a temporary condition. After the resident recovers, the confusion clears. Because the condition is temporary, reality orientation may be helpful. Newly admitted residents who are confused by the change

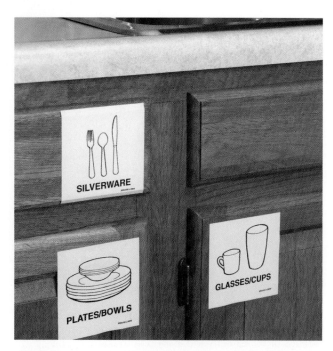

Figure 18–8 Using signs to label areas and personal items helps residents function independently. (Courtesy of Briggs Corporation, Des Moines, IA. (800) 247-2343)

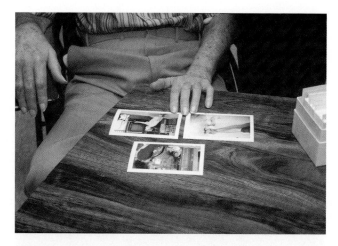

Figure 18–9 Showing residents photographs is a good way of encouraging reminiscence.

in environment may also benefit. A large calendar is placed in the resident's room. Each day is marked off. Large clocks are placed throughout the facility. Signs with large letters label areas, equipment, and personal items **(Figure 18–8).** This enables the resident to find his or her way about the facility.

To be effective, reality orientation must be used by all staff during each resident contact. The goal is to give the resident a sense of identity in time and space. It may decrease anxiety in some residents. When approaching residents, call them by name. Tell them who you are. Do not expect them to remember you.

The principles of reality orientation are to:

- Treat residents as adults
- Treat residents with dignity
- Speak clearly and directly; avoid speaking loudly
- Use repetition; speak slowly if the resident does not understand
- Allow enough time for the resident to process thoughts and respond
- Keep instructions and responses simple and brief
- Maintain structure in routines
- Make sure residents are wearing hearing aids and glasses
- Promote resident independence

- Frequently provide orientation about the day, date, time, season, and weather
- Avoid making residents feel that you are putting them on the spot or criticizing them
- Answer questions honestly, but avoid information that is upsetting
- Avoid reinforcing the resident's confusion
- Avoid teasing the resident about his or her confusion
- Avoid arguing with residents who are delusional

Reminiscing

Reminiscing is the act of remembering the past **(Figure 18–9).** It is a normal activity for all people. One of the developmental tasks of the elderly is a life review. Reminiscence helps residents complete this task. Studies have shown that reminiscence programs can improve cognitive function. A group of women studied had excellent results. Almost everyone enjoys this activity. Reminiscence is a one-to-one activity. The resident discusses his or her past. You will ask questions and make comments. If the resident expresses feelings and emotions, accept them. Reassure the resident that feeling this way is okay. The program can also be done as a group activity. Books **(Figure 18–10),** tapes, and kits are available to facilitate this activity.

Music Therapy

Music therapy dates back to ancient Greece. In that culture, music was part of medical treatment. Think about the effect music has on your own life. Children learn the alphabet by singing the ABCs. We listen to "oldies" and remember events from our past. You can probably remember the words to songs you have not heard in many years.

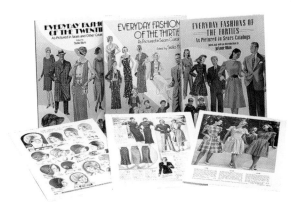

Figure 18–10 Residents enjoy looking at pictures in books. The pictures often stimulate residents to tell interesting stories about the past. (Courtesy of Briggs Corporation, Des Moines, IA. (800) 247-2343)

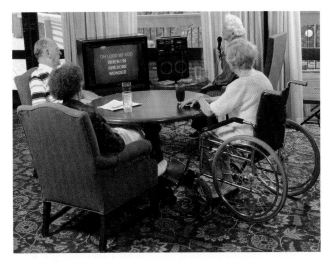

Figure 18–11 A teleprompter can be used so all residents can participate in the activity. Singing is enjoyable and relieves stress. (Courtesy of Briggs Corporation, Des Moines, IA. (800) 247-2343)

Restorative music therapy is used for relieving stress. It may be part of an exercise program. Studies have shown that listening to music has physical benefits:

▨ Increased metabolism
▨ Positive changes in the muscular, circulatory, and respiratory systems

Playing music during exercise makes the activity fun. Music motivates the residents. Singing relieves

stress. Music teleprompters **(Figure 18–11)** are available so that residents can participate if they don't know the words. For relaxation therapy, a personal stereo and headset are used. The activities department may present music activities for other purposes.

KEY POINTS IN CHAPTER

Many behavior problems are caused by illness and cognitive loss.

Behavior problems occur as a result of stress and unmet needs.

Coping and defense mechanisms are tools used to compensate for losses.

The principle of the ABC method of behavior management is that behavior can be changed by changing the antecedent or consequences.

Behavior management is a form of restorative care.

Modify your behavior in response to the resident's behavior.

Reward residents for appropriate behavior. Rewarded behavior is likely to be repeated.

Depression is a feeling of despair or discouragement. It occurs in response to stress and loss.

Reduce stress by modifying your approach. Change routines and equipment slightly.

Cognitive enhancement programs help residents become more aware of their environment.

Validation therapy is used to make residents feel good about themselves.

Reality orientation is used to make residents more aware of time and place.

Music therapy is used for relaxation and exercise.

Reminiscing helps residents with lifetime review and promotes self-esteem.

CLINICAL APPLICATIONS

1. Mrs. Enlow is crying when you enter her room to ambulate her. She tells you that she is going to stop exercising because she will never be able to return home. How can you assist this resident?

2. Miss Jenkins is mentally confused. She doesn't like her roommate, so she wanders in the hallway. Miss Jenkins cries when she can't find her room. When staff see her crying, they give her a hug and take her to her room. Using the ABC method, describe how to modify the resident's behavior. Identify the antecedent and consequences.

3. Dr. Roberto likes to talk about his childhood. He tells some interesting stories. During a story, he describes a person who made him mad in childhood. He says the experience hurt him very deeply. He has never forgiven this person. How will you react to this information in a manner that will help the resident?

4. Mrs. Kraft is a cognitively impaired resident. She is very combative when personal care is given. The social worker has assessed her. She feels that Mrs. Kraft is a candidate for a behavior management program. The restorative nurse feels that the resident is a candidate for a hygiene program. However, the behavior must be eliminated before the resident will cooperate. How will you work with this resident? What approaches will you use?

5. Mr. Hogan's daughter is picking him up at 10:00 AM to take him out for lunch. He is excited and nervous. Breakfast is late this morning. Mr. Hogan yells at you. He tells you that it's your fault. He says he will hold you personally responsible if he doesn't have enough time to get ready before his daughter arrives. What coping mechanism is he using? How can you assist this resident?

Documenting Restorative Care

After reading this chapter, you should be able to:

- Spell and define key terms.
- State the five purposes of documentation.
- Describe the contents of the medical record.
- Explain the differences between narrative and SOAP charting.
- List the guidelines for restorative nursing assistant documentation.
- Define common abbreviations used in restorative and rehabilitative documentation.

■ PURPOSE OF DOCUMENTATION

Documentation is a record of the quality care you have given. You should be proud of the care you give. Accurate, complete documentation is an opportunity to show others that you do a good job. A saying in health care is "if it's not documented it wasn't done." The medical record provides information about the resident. It confirms that care was given. The record shows that the care met acceptable, current standards.

Communication

The medical record is also a means of communication. Many individuals from many departments care for the resident. The physician and others read the medical record. The material there informs others of the resident's problems, needs, solutions, and progress. This helps them plan their care.

Legal Evidence

Documentation is a legal record of the resident's care. As a legal document, it can be used in a court of law. It will be read by lawyers, judges, juries, experts, and others. The notes are admitted as legal evidence. If a medical record is used in a trial, the documentation shows that care was or was not given. This has a major effect on the outcome of the trial. When a note from the chart is used in a lawsuit, the worker who wrote the note may also have to testify at the trial. Testifying is a frightening, stressful experience. Lawsuits move slowly through the courts. They often go to trial several years after care was given. You may not remember exactly

what you did. Your notes must be complete to prove what you did. Thorough notes help you defend your actions.

Reimbursement

Reimbursement is based on documentation. The main purpose of documentation is to provide a record of resident care. However, the medical record is used to evaluate the level and value of the services the facility provides. The information is used to set payment to the facility. Payment is denied if the documentation does not support the care given or that the resident required. The facility and its staff depend on reimbursement for survival. Reimbursement is what pays the bills and meets the payroll. Therefore, documentation is important for many reasons. Documentation requirements change as reimbursement changes.

Surveys

Surveyors review documentation when they visit the facility. Complete, accurate documentation proves that workers have complied with the law. It shows that the residents have received good care. The record should show that the residents' risks and needs were identified, and that care was given to meet them. Missing or absent documentation commonly results in deficiencies. Surveyors may ask questions about information in the chart.

Accountability

Everyone who cares for residents is responsible for documentation. Each worker is responsible for documenting the services he or she provides.

Health care workers cannot document for each other. Each worker is responsible for what he or she has written. Every entry in the chart is evidence that care was given.⑤ As you can see, this evidence is reviewed by many individuals.

CONTENTS OF THE MEDICAL RECORD

Information in the medical record falls into six categories:

- Medical data, or information about the resident's physical condition
- The resident's problems requiring care
- The care and treatment plan to address the problems
- Goals or outcomes of the care or treatment
- Record of care that follows the care/treatment plan
- Effectiveness of the care/treatment plan

The information listed here is found in many different places in the medical record. Most long-term care facilities use a system called **source-oriented medical records (SOMR).** The information in the SOMR is divided into categories. Each discipline has a separate divider in the chart in which their records are stored. The sequence of the record varies from one facility to the next.

Some facilities use the **problem-oriented medical record (POMR).** This type of record is divided into five general categories. All disciplines chart in each category. Facilities that use this system believe it improves communication. They state that it makes finding information easier.

Documentation Format

Many different formats are used for recording information on the medical record. Medications, treatments, and ADLs are recorded on flow sheets. The caregiver initials a box, showing that care was given. Two other common formats are the **narrative** format and **SOAP documentation.** Facilities that use the narrative format describe the resident's care like a story. SOAP is an abbreviation for **S**ubjective, **O**bjective, **A**ssessment, **P**lan. Facilities using this format write an entry for each category. For example:

- *S* stands for subjective. Because symptoms are subjective findings, they are described in this section. The information here is provided by the resident, family member, or caregiver.
- *O* stands for objective. This information is based on observations by the caregiver. The signs of the resident's condition are recorded here. Information about the resident's ability to function goes in this section.

- ⑤*A* stands for assessment. The nurse practice act in most states prohibits unlicensed caregivers from assessing residents. You will assist with assessments by collecting information, such as vital signs. You report your findings to a licensed professional. Because assessment is a professional responsibility, you must be careful about wording the information in this section. You may want to think of the "A" here as an abbreviation for an analysis. You cannot assess, but instead write your analysis of the situation.⑤
- *P* stands for plan. The plan describes the treatment information. You will document your plans for the resident. For example, you will document that you will continue using the same approaches, or that you will notify the restorative nurse of a problem.

A sample SOAP note appears in **Figure 19–1.**

Many nurses prefer to document in narrative format. Some therapists prefer to document in the SOAP format. The SOAP system lends itself well to describing neuromuscular problems. Your supervisor will describe your facility documentation requirements.

Frequency of Documentation

⑤A record is made each time you care for a resident.⑤ At the very least, you will initial a box on a flow sheet. You may be required to write a special note about an unusual situation, significant improvement, or decline. ⑤Always make an entry if the resident refuses treatment.⑤ State the reason, if known. In most facilities, you will write a brief weekly or monthly summary note for each resident. Your note will describe the resident's progress toward the restorative care plan goals. **Figure 19–2** gives examples of summary notes. **Table 19–1** provides suggestions for information to document on specific restorative programs.

S: Res. states he is having LBP today.

O: Charge nurse notified, res. medicated. Amb. res. 1 hour p̄ med. Res. amb. 75 feet to activities room using SBQC et SBA. Balance steady.

A: Res. met goal, med apparently effective. No further c/o pain.

P: Will notify restorative nurse that res. has met goal.

Mary Peterson, RNA, CNA

Figure 19–1 Example of SOAP documentation.

Ambulation Program:

Resident transfers from bed to chair with 1 minimum assist. Walks 50 feet to dining room with transfer belt, wheeled walker, and 1 assist. Walking balance fair. Resident states he sleeps better at night since beginning restorative ambulation program.

Judy King, RNA, CNA

ADL Programs:

Res is dressing UE with min. assist. Is feeding self entire meal p̄ set up et vc. Requires plate guard and built-up utensils, drinks from sippy cup. Res. progressing well.

Stephen Huynh, RNA, CNA

Communication Programs:

Cries when trying to express self. When approached calmly, she attempts to form words. Follows directions. Uses communication board correctly 75% of time. Frequently uses hand gestures to express herself and tries to write a few words. Will continue with program.

Lisa Watson, RNA, CNA

Figure 19–2 Sample summary documentation.

DOCUMENTING IN THE MEDICAL RECORD

You learned basic documentation guidelines in your nursing assistant class. Those will not be repeated here.

(SA) Follow your facility policies and your state's legal guidelines for documentation. Remember that the medical record is a legal document that will be read by others. The information must always be accurate. Never record care you have not given. Avoid making up or overstating information. Information about the resident's care should always be included. (SA)

Abbreviations

Keep your documentation brief and concise. A restorative note should focus on information about the resident's functional ability. Use only acceptable, recognized abbreviations. Abbreviations are easily misunderstood. Some have more than one meaning. Limit the use of abbreviations and make sure they are used correctly. You will use some standard nursing abbreviations in your documentation. You may also learn new abbreviations that describe the resident's functional status. A listing of abbreviations is found in **Table 19–2.** Some of the abbreviations listed here will not be used in your documentation. However, you must understand their

Table 19–1 General Restorative Summary Information	
Restorative Program	**Documentation Information**
Transfers	Sitting balance, amount and type of assistance needed to transfer, how many times a day the resident transfers, changes in vital signs, safety, resident's response.
Ambulation	Number of feet ambulated, assistive devices used, weight bearing, limitations, balance problems, safety concerns, how many times a day the resident transfers, changes in vital signs, resident's response.
ADL programs	Degree of assistance required, where the resident is this week compared to where he or she was last week in relation to goals, assistive devices, how many times a day the resident performs the activity, changes in vital signs, safety, resident's response.
Feeding programs	Degree of assistance required, where the resident is this week compared to where he or she was last week in relation to goals. Also document swallowing ability, special measures used, adaptive devices.
Communication programs	Ability to verbalize and understand, nonverbal behavior, where the resident is this week compared to where he or she was last week in relation to goals.
All programs	Complaints of fatigue, rest requirements; resident's description of pain, specific location of pain, specific nursing measures used to relieve pain; other complaints or concerns.

Table 19-2 Abbreviations Used in Rehabilitation and Restorative Care

Abbreviation	Meaning	Abbreviation	Meaning
↑	increase, or up	amb.	ambulation, ambulate, ambulated
↓	decrease, or down	A/PROM, A&PROM	active and passive range of motion
//	parallel	AROM	active range of motion
>	greater than	assist	assistance
<	less than	B, (B), Ⓑ	bilateral, both
≠	increase	bid	twice a day
Ø (zero with slash through it (/))	none, nothing, decrease	bil.	bilateral
1	first, primary, first degree	BLE	both lower extremities
2	second, secondary, second degree	BPM	beats per minute
3	third, tertiary, third degree	BUE	both upper extremities
1x	one time, one person	C	cane
2°	secondary to	C6	6th cervical vertebra
$\bar{a}$	before	CF	cystic fibrosis
A	assisted	c/o	complains of
AA	actively assisted	COTA	certified occupational therapy assistant
AAROM	active assistive range of motion	CP	compression pump, cerebral palsy, care plan
abd	abduction	CPM	continuous passive motion machine
ACT	active, actively	Cr Tr	crutch training
add	adduction	d/c	discharged, discontinued
ADL	activities of daily living	dep	dependent
AFO	ankle foot orthosis	DJD	degenerative joint disease
AKA	above the knee amputation		
ALS	anterior lateral sclerosis		

(continues)

Table 19–2 Abbreviations Used in Rehabilitation and Restorative Care, *continued*

Abbreviation	Meaning	Abbreviation	Meaning
DOB	date of birth	int.	internal
dx	diagnosis	Int Rot	internal rotation
ES	electrical stimulation	IPPB	intermittent positive pressure breathing
et	and	IR	infrared
Eval	evaluation	KAFO	knee ankle foot orthosis
ex.	exercise	Ⓛ	left
ext.	extension, extremity	L5	5th lumbar vertebra
Ext Rot	external rotation	LA	left arm
flex	flexion	lat.	lateral
F/U	follow up	LB	low back
FWB	full weight bearing	LBP	low back pain
FWW, fw/w	front wheeled walker	LBQC	large based quad cane
Fx	fracture	LL	left leg
G	good	LLC	long leg cast
gluts	gluteal	LLE	left lower extremity
Gt.	gait	LOB	loss of balance
hemi	hemiplegia	LOM	limitation of motion, loss of motion
HNP	herniated nucleus pulposis	LS	lumbar/sacral
HP	hot packs	LTG	long-term goal
Hx	history	LUE	left upper extremity
Ⓘ	independent, independently	max	maximum assistance
ICP	intermittent compression pump	MD	muscular dystrophy
ind	independent	MG	myasthenia gravis

(continues)

Table 19–2 Abbreviations Used in Rehabilitation and Restorative Care, *continued*

Abbreviation	Meaning	Abbreviation	Meaning
MH	moist heat	p̄	after
min.	minimum, minimal assistance	P	poor muscle strength
mmHg	millimeters of mercury	per	by
mm(s)	muscle(s)	PIF	peak inspiratory flow
mod	moderate assistance	POMR	problem-oriented medical record
MS	multiple sclerosis, musculoskeletal	PPV	positive pressure ventilation
ms	muscle	PRE	progressive resistance exercise
Msg	massage	PRN	as needed
MW	microwave	PROM	passive range of motion
N/A	not applicable, not available	PSP	problem, status, plan
NBQC	narrow based quad cane	PSPG	problem, status, plan, goals
NDT	neurodevelopmental treatment	PT	physical therapy, physical therapist (in some states licensure is required; this is LPT)
neg.	negative		
NWB	nonweight bearing		
OA	osteoarthritis	PTA	physical therapy assistant, or physical therapist assistant (in some states licensure is required; this is LPTA)
OOB	out of bed		
ORIF	open reduction, internal fixation		
OT	occupational therapy	PUW	pick-up walker
OTR	occupational therapist, registered	PWB	partial weight bearing
OTR/L	occupational therapist, registered and licensed (in states that require licensure)	QD	daily
		QID	four times a day
		quads	quadriceps

(continues)

Table 19–2 Abbreviations Used in Rehabilitation and Restorative Care, *continued*

Abbreviation	Meaning	Abbreviation	Meaning
Ⓡ	right	sev	severe
RA	rheumatoid arthritis, right arm	sh	shoulder
re:	regarding	SLC	short leg cast
rehab	rehabilitation	SLR	straight leg raise
reps	repetitions	SOB	short of breath
res.	resident	SOMR	source-oriented medical record
ret.	return	ST	speech therapy, speech therapist
RL	right leg		
RLC	residual lung capacity	STG	short-term goal
RLE	right lower extremity	str.	strength
RNA	restorative nursing assistant	STR, STRC	straight cane
		SWD	short-wave diathermy
r/o	rule out	Sx	symptoms
ROM	range of motion	T10	10th thoracic vertebra
rot.	rotation	TDWB	touchdown weight bearing
RT	respiratory therapy, respiratory therapist	TENS	transcutaneous electrical neural stimulation
RUE	right upper extremity		
Rx	treatment	THA	total hip arthroplasty
S	supervision	ther.ex.	therapeutic exercise
SBA	standby assist	THR	total hip replacement
SBQC	small based quad cane	TIW	three times a week
SCI	spinal cord injury	TKA	total knee arthroplasty
sdly	side lying	TKE	terminal knee extension
SEC	single end cane		

(continues)

Table 19–2 Abbreviations Used in Rehabilitation and Restorative Care, *continued*

Abbreviation	Meaning	Abbreviation	Meaning
TKR	total knee replacement	UV	ultraviolet
TMJ	temporomandibular joint	vc	verbal cues
trng.	training	W	walker
TT	tilt table	WB	weight bearing
TTWB	toe-touch weight bearing	WBAT	weight bearing as tolerated
TV	tidal volume	WC, w/c	wheelchair
TWB	touch weight bearing	WFL	within functional limits
Tx	treatment, traction	WNL	within normal limits
TX	traction	wt.	weight
UE	upper extremity	x, X	times
US	ultrasound		

meaning to read restorative and rehabilitation notes. Your facility will have a specific list of abbreviations to use in your charting. ⑤Use only abbreviations that your facility accepts and recognizes.⑤

You may work with the therapy department or read therapy progress notes. Therapists may use terms that you do not understand. **Table 19–3** lists levels of strength. **Table 19–4** lists levels of treatment. **Table 19–5** lists resident responses to treatment. Use these lists as a reference.

Understanding the Information

Your documentation must be clear to anyone who reads the chart. Use your words to paint a picture of the resident's condition. ⑤Your entries must be legible. Illegible information is easily misinterpreted. If your handwriting is not legible, print.⑤

Your punctuation, grammar, and spelling must be correct. An accurate and concise record shows that you are conscientious. It implies that you have given quality care. Errors suggest that you are careless. If you are careless with your documentation, the reader may assume that you are careless with the care you give.

Most facilities have a policy for using colored ink in the medical record. Chart only in the accepted color. Many facilities use only black, because it is clear and copies well. Avoid using erasable or nonpermanent ink.

Timeliness. ⑤Document your care in a timely manner. Never chart before providing care. Document as soon as possible after caring for the resident. Sometimes you cannot document immediately after caring for the resident. Carry a small notebook. Record important information that you can transfer to your notes later. If you forget to document something, then remember later, follow facility policy for late entry documentation. Usually, you will write the date and time the entry is made. You will begin the entry by writing, "Late entry for (date, time)."⑤

Accuracy of the Medical Record. ⑤Avoid providing the opportunity for the record to be altered. For example, notes written in pencil or erasable ink can be changed. Avoid leaving blank lines. These provide space for someone to change the record. If there are blank spaces, draw a line through them. This prevents others from filling them in.

Table 19–3   Levels of Strength

Term	Description
Zero (0)	The resident cannot contract muscles upon command.
Trace (1)	The therapist can palpate muscle contraction, but the contraction does not result in movement of the body part.
Poor (2)	The resident can contract muscles sufficiently to move body parts; however, the strength is less than 50% of normal.
Fair (3)	The resident can contract muscles and complete range of motion with the extremity. He or she cannot sustain the muscle contraction against resistance.
Good (4)	The resident can contract muscles and complete range of motion with the extremity. He or she can sustain the muscle contraction against resistance. He or she can perform repetitive activities. These activities cause the resident to feel tired or fatigued.
Normal (5)	The resident can contract muscles and complete range of motion with the extremity. He or she can sustain the muscle contraction against maximum resistance. He or she can perform repetitive activities without feeling tired or fatigued.

Strength is documented as the amount of force applied during resistance. It is described in pounds or kilograms. The most common scale used in long-term care facilities is from 0 to 5. 0 is the low end of the scale. 5 is normal.

Table 19–4   Level of Treatment

Term	Description
Regression	The resident's condition has deteriorated; he or she has decreased function and increased need for assistance.
Plateau	The resident has not made sufficient progress within a reasonable period of time; there is no apparent reason for lack of progress.
Maintenance	The treatment will prevent decline. It is repetitive in nature. The task can be completed by unlicensed personnel.
Restorative	Care designed to improve the resident's independence with an activity, or to help restore the ability more quickly. Staff must be trained and follow a plan of care to assist the resident. Unlicensed personnel can assist the resident in performing the activity.
Rehabilitative	Care designed to result in significant progress. Treatment must be given by licensed personnel, and is designed to assist the resident to function at the highest level of independence possible, with or without adaptive devices.

Table 19–5   Resident Response

Level of Response	Description
Good	The resident consistently completes a task independently more than 80% of the time.
Fair	The resident completes a task independently more than 50% of the time. With assistance, he or she completes the task more than 75% of the time.
Poor	The resident does not respond, requires maximum assistance, or completes a task less than 50% of the time.

If you make an error, follow your facility policy for correcting it. In most facilities, you will draw a single line through the entry. Write the word "error" next to or above the entry. Sign the changes.⊛

Incidents. If an incident occurs, document the details exactly. Be objective. Chart only the facts. Avoid emotion. Be as thorough as possible. State the resident's condition immediately after the incident. Describe your actions. Include whom you notified of the incident. Describe your follow-up monitoring. An incident report is completed for each unusual event. An *incident report* is a separate record, not part of the chart. Avoid mentioning the incident report in your notes.

Signing the Entry. ⊛Follow your facility policy for signing each entry.⊛ Some facilities require you to sign your complete legal signature. Others use the first initial and last name. Your name is followed by your title and/or certification. Flow sheets will have a key for the initials. Make sure you sign the key each month so your entries can be identified.

Documenting Specific Restorative Information

Your summary notes should include information about the restorative program **(Figure 19–3).** Address the skills the resident is working on. Describe his or her progress, problems, and complaints. Personalize the note to the resident. This helps the reader form a mental image of the resident's progress. The most important thing to chart is the resident's response to the care. Look at the care plan goals for the restorative program. Determine what has been done to work on the goals. Document specific information about the resident's response to the goal. Check with your supervisor if you have questions about content or format of your notes. Consider the information in Table 19–1 when writing restorative notes.

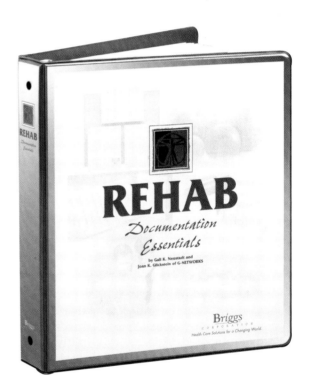

Figure 19–3 Procedure manuals and other guidelines are good sources of information. (Courtesy of Briggs Corporation, Des Moines, IA. (800) 247-2343)

Providing Descriptive Information

Remember that documentation must be clear and easy to read. It should be organized, logical, and suitable to the procedure performed. Documentation should support the effectiveness of the treatment plan and goals. The reader should be able to measure the resident's progress by the notes. Subjective terms, such as "making progress" or "improving," do not describe the resident's condition. Use numbers or other measurable criteria in your notes whenever possible.

KEY POINTS IN CHAPTER

Documentation is a record of quality care.

Documentation supports reimbursement. It is a vehicle for communication. Surveyors use it to evaluate care.

The medical record is a legal document that can be used in court.

Absence of documentation may be interpreted as lack of care.

Entries in the medical record must be accurate, brief, and concise.

Abbreviations in the medical record must be approved for use by the long-term care facility.

Most long-term care facilities use the source-oriented medical record (SOMR).

Care should be documented only after it has been provided.

When documenting care, follow facility policies and state laws.

You will complete a weekly summary of the resident's progress and activities.

CLINICAL APPLICATIONS

1. Mr. Yamaguchi was sick with a cold. He did not participate in his ADL program twice this week. After his illness, he was weak and tired. He could not do as much as he did the previous week. Write a weekly summary note for Mr. Yamaguchi.

2. Mrs. Brady is excited about going to her 50th high school reunion next month. She tells you she wants to use her walker. She does not want to attend using a wheelchair. Last week, Mrs. Brady ambulated 35 feet with a rolling walker and minimal assistance. This week, she walked 50 feet with standby assistance. She said she would advance more by next Friday. Write a weekly summary note for this resident.

3. Mr. Carrerra is in a restorative mobility program. You walked him to the dining room. He slipped and fell when turning to sit in the chair. The resident has a bruise on the left elbow and a skin tear on the left hand. He had no other apparent injuries. He was upset by the incident. You took him back to his room in a wheelchair. He refused to ambulate later in the day. Write a note describing the incident. Write a daily note about this resident.

4. A surveyor asks you the meaning of some abbreviations in your documentation. This makes you very nervous. She asks you why you used the abbreviations. She wants to know if the abbreviations are acceptable according to your facility policy. How will you respond to the surveyor?

5. Mr. Norris is scheduled to ambulate twice a day. Despite your requests, he will only ambulate once a day. He has not made any progress in the past two weeks. Write a SOAP note about this resident.

APPENDICES

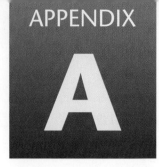

Employment Information

SAMPLE JOB DESCRIPTION FOR RESTORATIVE NURSING ASSISTANT

Definition: A member of the nursing staff specializing in the delivery of restorative care. Works under the direct supervision of the restorative registered nurse.

I. Requirements
  A. Certified Nursing Assistant
  B. Knowledge and training in the principles of restorative nursing, including:
    1. Feeding techniques
    2. Dressing techniques
    3. Bathing techniques
    4. Transfer techniques
    5. Bed mobility
    6. Ambulation
    7. Active and passive range of motion exercises
    8. Heat and cold treatments
    9. Positioning residents in bed and chair
    10. Infection control
  C. Knowledge in applicable safety and precautionary measures related to resident care.
  D. The ability to establish professional rapport with residents and staff.
  E. The ability to effectively demonstrate restorative procedures to nursing assistant staff.

II. Duties
  A. Responsible for assisting the restorative nurse with screening residents for restorative program.
  B. Collecting assessment data such as vital signs, as assigned by restorative nurse.
  C. Assists residents with active restorative programs, as assigned.
  D. Teaches residents how to help themselves.
  E. Explains restorative programs to residents and describes what to expect; demonstrates as necessary.
  F. Uses materials, supplies, and adaptive equipment as necessary.
  G. Teaches nursing assistant staff follow-up care for residents; monitors this care to ensure it is done correctly.
  H. Responsible for feeding retraining program at breakfast and lunch.
  I. Communicates changes in resident goals and approaches to other staff.
  J. Demonstrates techniques and approaches for restorative care to other staff.
  K. Communicates problems, changes in condition, and other information affecting the resident's progress to restorative nurse.
  L. Documents daily on flow sheets; documents weekly observation notes on resident progress.
  M. Attends care conference on assigned residents.
  N. Attends weekly rehabilitation/restorative meetings.

III. Skills, Knowledge, Abilities
  A. Sincerely likes and believes in people.
  B. Is considerate and understanding.
  C. Controls emotions and demonstrates patience in trying situations.
  D. Communicates effectively with staff and residents.
  E. Able to teach others.
  F. Able to follow directions, observe residents' response, and report changes to supervisor.
  G. Able to work independently, with minimal supervision.
  H. Possesses strong communication and documentation skills.

ARISTOCRAT WEST/WEST PARK HEALTH CARE FACILITIES RESTORATIVE NURSING ASSISTANT JOB DESCRIPTION

Responsible to: Restorative Nurse
Responsibilities include, but are not limited to:

1. Participates in and receives nursing report upon reporting to duty.
2. Assists residents with dressing/undressing appropriately as necessary.
3. Answers call lights promptly.
4. Prepares residents for meals, assisting those who need assistance.
5. Performs restorative and rehabilitative procedures as instructed.
6. Completes daily flow sheets.

7. Maintains all resident splints/braces and reports need for repairs to nursing restorative coordinator.
8. Maintains all restorative supplies and equipment, and notifies coordinator in writing of needed repairs.
9. All requests for changes to programs must be in writing and given to the restorative coordinator.
10. Weighs residents as assigned.
11. Assists residents with bowel and bladder functions as outlined in the plan of care; document these functions.
12. Maintains intake and output sheets as needed.
13. Assists residents in preparing for social activities and therapies, in a timely manner.
14. Assists in transporting residents to and from activities, dining rooms, etc., as the need arises.
15. Checks residents routinely to ensure that their personal care needs are met.
16. Reports unusual observations related to resident care, cognitive or functional behaviors.
17. Observes and reports reddened skin, rashes, etc.
18. Observes disoriented and comatose residents; records and reports data to nurses as instructed.
19. Serves between-meal and bedtime snacks if assigned.
20. Attends all mandatory inservices.
21. Releases restraints at least every two hours for range of motion exercises, ambulation, etc.
22. Demonstrates awareness of potential hazards and reports unsafe conditions to supervisor to maintain a safe environment; i.e., reports spills, faulty equipment, maintains a clear path for resident ambulation, etc.
23. Adheres to strict infection control guidelines.
24. Participates in quality assurance programs as assigned.
25. Maintains the confidentiality of all resident care information.
26. Ensures that you treat all residents fairly, with kindness, dignity, and respect.
27. Ensures that all care is provided in privacy.
28. Knocks before entering resident rooms.
29. Reports all grievances and complaints made by residents to the team leader.

Working Conditions and Related Issues

1. Sits, stands, bends, lifts, and moves intermittently during working hours.
2. Is subject to frequent interruptions.
3. Is involved with residents, personnel, visitors, government agencies, etc.
4. Is subject to hostile and emotionally upset residents, family members, personnel, and visitors.
5. Communicates with nursing personnel and other department personnel.
6. Is willing to work beyond normal working hours, on weekends and holidays, and in other positions temporarily, when necessary.
7. Attends and participates in continuing education programs.
8. Is subject to falls, burns from equipment, odors, etc., throughout the work day; takes necessary safety precautions.
9. Is subject to exposure to infectious waste, diseases, conditions, etc., including exposure to the AIDS and hepatitis B viruses; applies the principles of standard precautions.
10. Must be a graduate of an approved nurse aide training program, or be eligible to enter such a program, graduate, and pass a state-approved competency evaluation within 120 days from the date of employment.
11. Must be able to write the English language in a legible and understandable manner.
12. Possesses the ability to make independent decisions when circumstances warrant such action.
13. Possesses the ability to deal tactfully with personnel, residents, family members, visitors, government agencies/personnel, and the general public.
14. Possesses the ability and willingness to work harmoniously with professional and nonprofessional personnel.
15. Must be willing to seek out new methods and principles and be willing to incorporate them into existing nursing practices.
16. Must be able to speak the English language in an understandable manner.
17. Must be able to cope with the mental and emotional stress of the position.
18. Must be able to see and hear, or use prosthetics, that will enable these senses to function adequately to ensure that the requirements of the position are fully met.
19. Must function independently, have flexibility, personal integrity, and the ability to work effectively with residents, personnel, and support agencies.
20. Must be able to relate to and work with the ill, disabled, elderly, emotionally upset, and at times hostile people within the facility.
21. Must be able to lift a minimum of 50 pounds.

Job description provided courtesy of Aristocrat West/West Park Health Care Facilities, Cleveland, Ohio. Used with permission.

Aristocrat West/West Park Health Care
Restorative Flow Sheet

Resident Name: _____ Room # _____ Dr: _____

Resident to receive _____ range of motion to _____ for 15 minutes, 5x week.

Resident to receive _____ range of motion to _____ for 15 minutes, 5x week.

Resident to ambulate _____ feet, with _____

Transfer program _____

Splint/brace to: _____

Adaptive equipment used: _____

May use: _____

Resident ambulates _____ feet in _____ minutes, without resting.

Resident uses parallel bars _____

Month: _____ Year: _____

	1	2	3	4	5	6	7	8	9	10	11	12	13	14	15	16	17	18	19	20	21	22	23	24	25	26	27	28	29	30	31

Month: _____ Year: _____

	1	2	3	4	5	6	7	8	9	10	11	12	13	14	15	16	17	18	19	20	21	22	23	24	25	26	27	28	29	30	31

Month: _____ Year: _____

	1	2	3	4	5	6	7	8	9	10	11	12	13	14	15	16	17	18	19	20	21	22	23	24	25	26	27	28	29	30	31

Initials	Signature	Initials	Signature

(Restorative nursing asssistant documentation form provided courtesy of Aristocrat West/West Park Health Care Facilities, Cleveland, Ohio. Used with permission.)

Monthly Summary for: _____
(month, year)

Overall function has:

improved   declined   remains same

Participates in ADLs:

more   less   same amount

Strength has:

increased   decreased   remains same

Endurance has:

increased   decreased   remains same

Joint range has:

improved   declined   remains same

Ambulation: steady   unsteady

Uses parallel bars: yes   no

Contractures: yes   no

area: _____

Splints: yes   no

needs: _____

Program length:

15 min.   <15 min.   >15 min.

Comments:

Monthly Summary for: _____
(month, year)

Overall function has:

improved   declined   remains same

Participates in ADLs:

more   less   same amount

Strength has:

increased   decreased   remains same

Endurance has:

increased   decreased   remains same

Joint range has:

improved   declined   remains same

Ambulation: steady   unsteady

Uses parallel bars: yes   no

Contractures: yes   no

area: _____

Splints: yes   no

needs: _____

Program length:

15 min.   <15 min.   >15 min.

Comments:

Monthly Summary for: _____
(month, year)

Overall function has:

improved   declined   remains same

Participates in ADLs:

more   less   same amount

Strength has:

increased   decreased   remains same

Endurance has:

increased   decreased   remains same

Joint range has:

improved   declined   remains same

Ambulation: steady   unsteady

Uses parallel bars: yes   no

Contractures: yes   no

area: _____

Splints: yes   no

needs: _____

Program length:

15 min.   <15 min.   >15 min.

Comments:

Monthly Summary for: _____
(month, year)

Overall function has:

improved   declined   remains same

Participates in ADLs:

more   less   same amount

Strength has:

increased   decreased   remains same

Endurance has:

increased   decreased   remains same

Joint range has:

improved   declined   remains same

Ambulation: steady   unsteady

Uses parallel bars: yes   no

Contractures: yes   no

area: _____

Splints: yes   no

needs: _____

Program length:

15 min.   <15 min.   >15 min.

Comments:

(Restorative nursing assistant documentation form provided courtesy of Aristocrat West/West Park Health Care Facilities, Cleveland, Ohio. Used with permission.)

Restorative Nursing Assistant Education and Orientation Record

Employee Name: _____

Dates of orientation: _____ to _____

Topic	Date	Instructor
Ambulation		
Use of walker, cane, and crutches		
Active range of motion		
Passive range of motion		
Transfer activities		
Positioning residents in bed		
Positioning residents in chair		
Using exercise equipment		
Using parallel bars		
Using wheelchairs		
Hot packs		
Whirlpool		
Paraffin bath		
Body mechanics		
Using restraints and restraint alternatives		
Safety		
Using splints and braces		
Handwashing technique		
Standard precautions		
Transmission-based precautions		
Nutrition and hydration		
Resident rights		
Documentation		

The restorative nursing assistant is a certified nursing assistant and reports to the restorative nurse.

_____ CNA/RNA signature _____ Date

_____ Restorative nurse signature _____ Date

Bowel and Bladder Assessment Tool
Aristocrat West/West Park Health Care

Date: _____

Resident: _____ Room #: _____ Bldg: _____ Physician: _____

Choose the number that best corresponds to the resident's status. Total the score for potential bowel and bladder retraining. Proceed if applicable.

Key: **21–18 No need for bowel and bladder program** **17–15 Good candidate for individualized retraining**
14–7 Candidate for scheduled toileting (timed voiding) **6–0 Poor candidate for toileting schedule or retraining**

Assessment	3	2	1	0	Date: score:	Date: score:	Date: score:	Date: score:	Date: score:	Date: score:
Voids correctly in an appropriate place without incontinence	Yes, always	Yes, at least once a day	Yes, but less than once a day	No, never						
Is incontinent of stool	No, never	Yes, 1–3 x/ week	Yes, 4–6x/ week	Yes, daily						
Can walk to bathroom or transfer to toilet/commode. Can manage clothing, wipe, etc.	Alone, with reasonable speed	Alone, but slowly	Needs assistance from 1 aide	Completely immobile/2+ aides						
Mental status	Alert & oriented	Forgetful, but follows commands	Confused, needs physical prompts	Very confused, comatose						
Mentally aware of toileting needs	Yes, always	Usually	Sometimes	Never						
Condition of skin on genital, perineal, or buttocks area	No redness	Some redness	Stage 1–2	Stage 3–4						
Predisposing factors: diabetes, CA of bladder/prostate, frequent UTIs, spinal cord injury, cerebral palsy, MS, CVA, Parkinson's	Absent	Minor	Serious	Debilitating or terminal						

Foley catheter present: _____ Total score: _____

Reviewed by: _____

Comments: _____

(Bowel and bladder assessment tool provided courtesy of Aristocrat West/West Park Health Care Facilities, Cleveland, Ohio. Used with permission.)

Performance Review Checklist

Procedure _____
(Fill in Procedure Number)

Procedure _____
(Fill in Procedure Title)

Name of Nursing Assistant _____ Date of Program _____ to _____

Social Security Number of Nursing Assistant _____

Program Code Number (if any) _____

S=Satisfactory Performance
U=Unsatisfactory Performance

Place a full signature to correspond with each set of initials appearing below:

Initials	Corresponding Signature of Instructor	Title

Procedure Guidelines	S/U	Date	Initials	S/U	Date	Initials

_____   _____
Instructor Signature   Date

_____   _____
Student Signature   Date

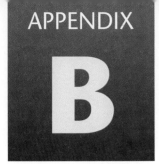

Exercise and Mobility

▆▆▆ SEQUENCE OF JOINT RANGE OF MOTION (SEE FIGURES B–1A THROUGH D)

Neck

▬ Flexion and extension
▬ Rotation

Shoulder

▬ Flexion and extension
▬ Abduction and adduction
▬ Horizontal abduction and adduction
▬ Internal and external rotation
▬ Hyperextension

Elbow

▬ Flexion and extension
▬ Supination and pronation

Wrist

▬ Flexion, extension, hypertension
▬ Ulnar deviation and radial deviation
▬ Circumduction

Fingers

▬ Flexion and extension
▬ Abduction and adduction

Thumb

▬ Flexion and extension
▬ Abduction and adduction
▬ Circumduction
▬ Opposition

Hip

▬ Flexion and extension
▬ Abduction and adduction
▬ Internal and external rotation

Knee

▬ Flexion and extension

Ankle

▬ Dorsiflexion and plantar flexion
▬ Inversion and eversion

Toes

▬ Flexion and extension
▬ Abduction and adduction

Additional exercises to perform if resident can be positioned in the prone position:

Shoulder

▬ Retraction
▬ Hyperextension

Hip

▬ Hyperextension

Knee

▬ Flexion and extension

Ankle

▬ Dorsiflexion and plantar flexion with knees flexed

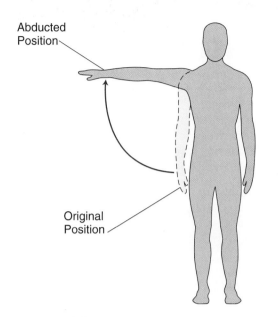

Figure B–1A Abduction.

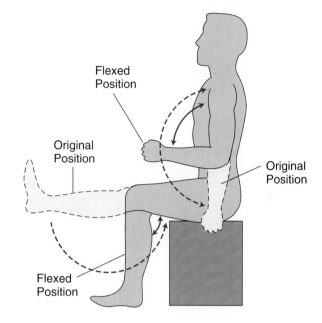

Figure B–1C Flexion.

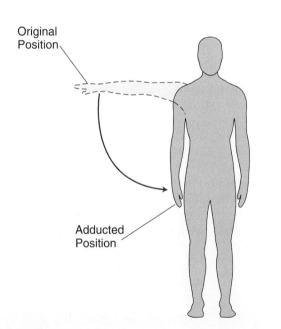

Figure B–1B Adduction.

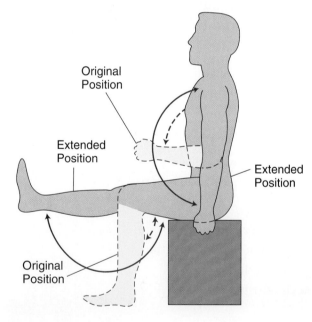

Figure B–1D Extension.

▓▓▓ TEACHING THE RESIDENT WITH HEMIPLEGIA AAROM

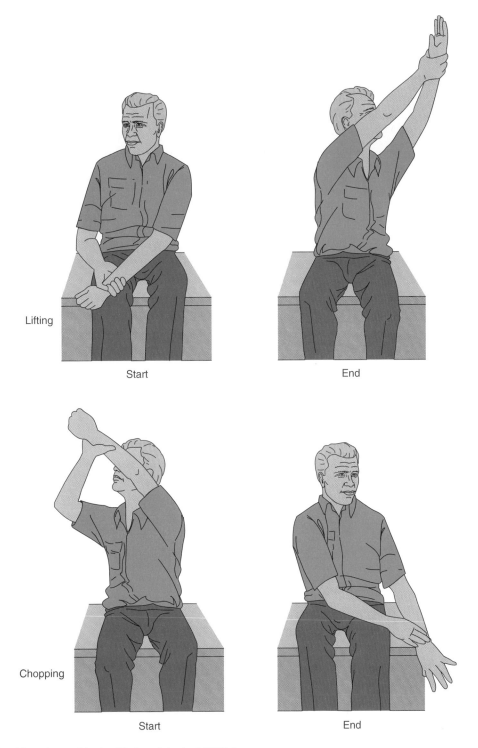

Lifting

Start   End

Chopping

Start   End

Figure B–2 Teaching the resident with hemiplegia AAROM.

NORMAL JOINT RANGE OF MOTION

The nursing assistant may screen residents for joint range of motion. If an abnormality is noted, the restorative nurse will measure the degree of impairment. Figure B-3 is the screening tool used in a long-term care facility for resident screening.

Aristocrat West/West Park Health Care
Range of Motion Screen

RESIDENT: _____ DR: _____

ROOM NO.: _____ BLDG: _____

Date of Screening												
Joint tested	left	left	right	right	left	left	right	right	left	left	right	right
	active	passive	active	passive	active	passive	active	passive	active	passive	active	passive
shoulder flexion												
shoulder abduction												
elbow flexion												
elbow extension												
wrist flexion												
wrist extension												
finger flexion												
finger extension												
hip abduction												
hip adduction												
hip flexion												
hip extension												
knee flexion												
knee extension												
ankle flexion												
ankle extension												
toes flexion												
toes extension												

Figure B–3 Range of motion screening tool. (Courtesy of Aristocrat West/West Park Health Care Facilities, Cleveland, Ohio. Used with permission.)

RANGE OF MOTION ASSESSMENT (continued)

Assess the resident's ROM utilizing the illustrated parameters. Fill in the blanks on the reverse side with the closest percentage of full range shown on the diagrams.

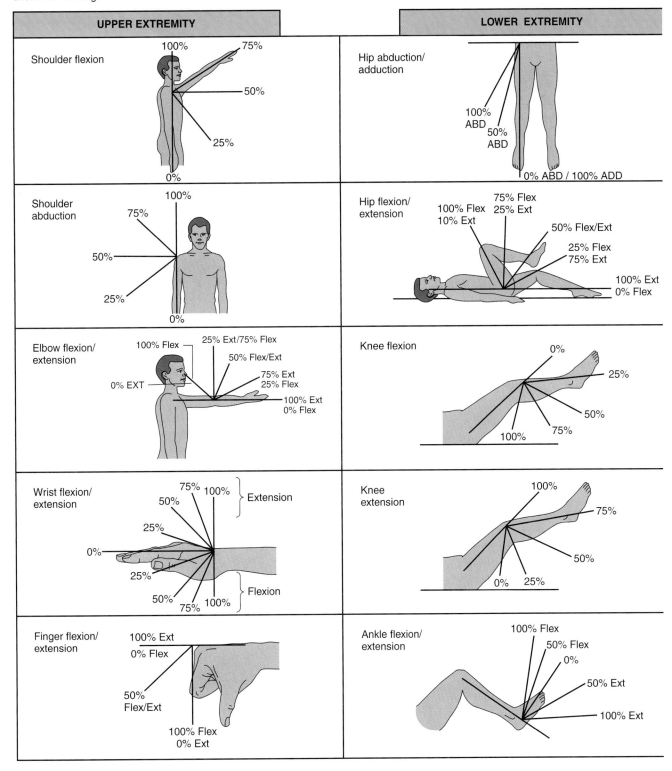

Figure B–3   continued.

SKELETAL SYSTEM

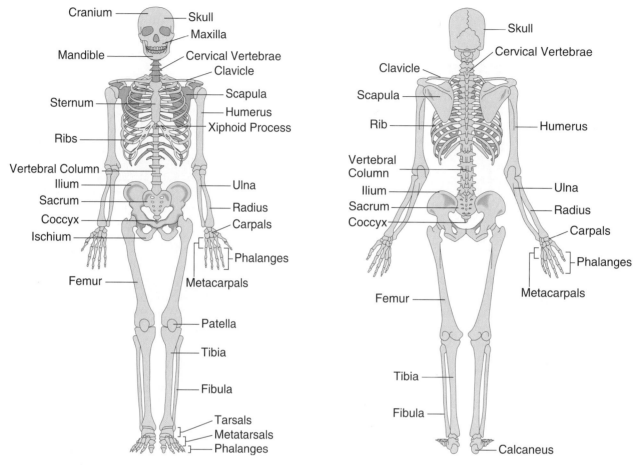

Figure B–4 Skeletal system—anterior (left) and posterior (right) views.

█ MUSCULAR SYSTEM—FRONT OF BODY

█ MUSCULAR SYSTEM—BACK OF BODY

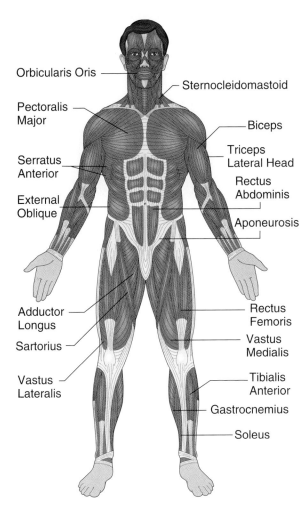

Orbicularis Oris
Sternocleidomastoid
Pectoralis Major
Biceps
Triceps Lateral Head
Serratus Anterior
Rectus Abdominis
External Oblique
Aponeurosis
Adductor Longus
Rectus Femoris
Sartorius
Vastus Medialis
Vastus Lateralis
Tibialis Anterior
Gastrocnemius
Soleus

Figure B–5 Major skeletal muscles of the body—anterior view.

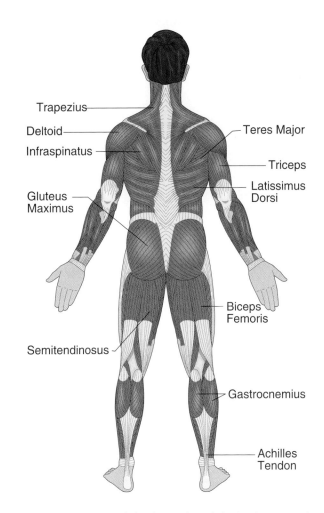

Trapezius
Teres Major
Deltoid
Infraspinatus
Triceps
Latissimus Dorsi
Gluteus Maximus
Biceps Femoris
Semitendinosus
Gastrocnemius
Achilles Tendon

Figure B–6 Major skeletal muscles of the body—posterior view.

▇ PERIPHERAL NERVOUS SYSTEM

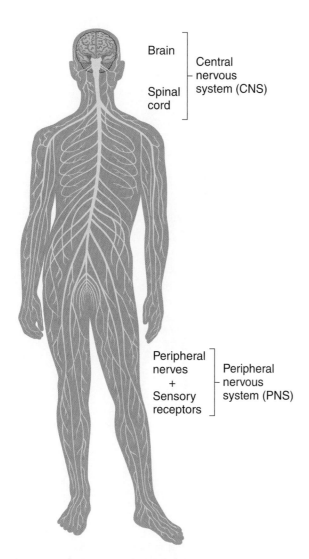

Brain
Spinal cord
Central nervous system (CNS)

Peripheral nerves + Sensory receptors
Peripheral nervous system (PNS)

Figure B–7   The peripheral nervous system connects the central nervous system to the various structures of the body. Messages are relayed from these structures back to the brain through the spinal cord.

▇ FUNCTIONAL AREAS OF THE BRAIN

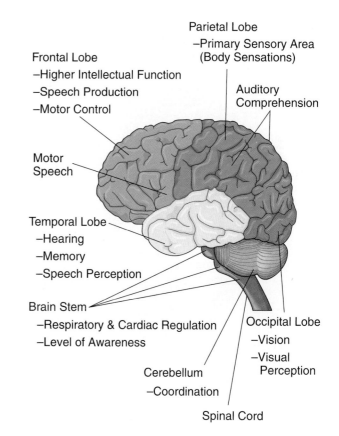

Frontal Lobe
–Higher Intellectual Function
–Speech Production
–Motor Control

Motor Speech

Temporal Lobe
–Hearing
–Memory
–Speech Perception

Brain Stem
–Respiratory & Cardiac Regulation
–Level of Awareness

Cerebellum
–Coordination

Spinal Cord

Parietal Lobe
–Primary Sensory Area (Body Sensations)

Auditory Comprehension

Occipital Lobe
–Vision
–Visual Perception

Figure B–8   Each lobe of the brain is responsible for different function(s).

GAIT PATTERNS

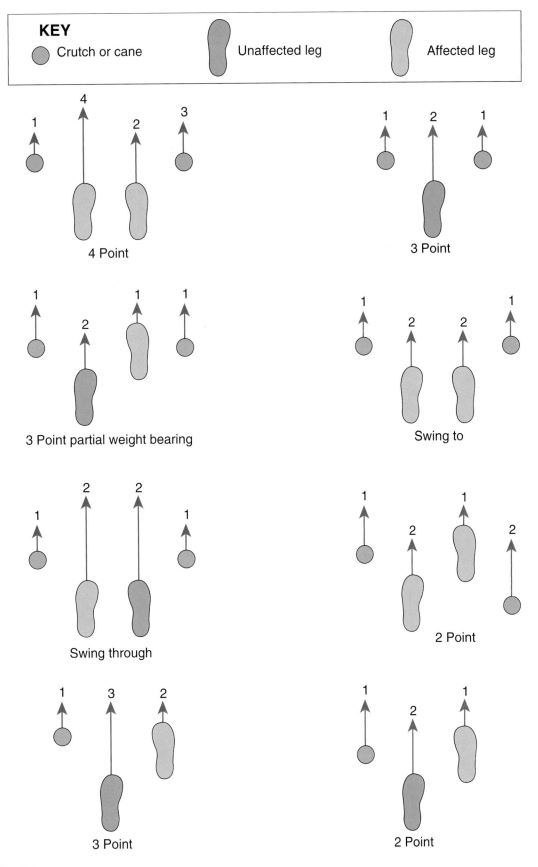

Figure B–9   Gait patterns.

Useful Information

The information in this appendix may be useful reference information for the restorative nursing assistant.

ENVIRONMENTAL FACTORS TO CONSIDER TO REDUCE THE RISK OF ILLNESS AND INJURY

- Adequate lighting without shadows or glare
- Contrasting colors at doorways, stairs, potentially hazardous areas
- Clean, pest-free, odor-free
- Comfortable room temperature (72°–75°)
- Low noise level
- Floor surface even, nonslippery
- Floor free of hazards, obstacles
- Locks on cupboards or closets for chemicals, medications
- Alarms on exit doors
- Emergency call signal system in place
- Nonslip surface in bathroom, tub, and shower
- Hot water temperature regulated to 110° or according to state standards
- Protective covers on electrical outlets, heaters, fans, electrical equipment
- Protected wires
- Simple, uncluttered surroundings
- Familiar objects in room
- Designated locations for storing personal items
- Supervised smoking
- Routine environmental assessment and preventive maintenance

RISK FACTORS FOR FALLS

- History of falls during previous year
- Recent surgery
- Dizziness/other balance problem
- Unsteady gait
- Joint immobility related to arthritis or injury
- Fatigue
- Weakness
- Paresis/paralysis
- Seizure disorder
- Vision impairment
- Hearing impairment
- Mental confusion
- Impaired judgment
- Inability to understand/follow directions
- Unfamiliar surroundings
- Drugs that affect thought processes (sedatives, tranquilizers, antipsychotics)
- Drugs that increase motility of bowel and bladder (diuretics, laxatives, cathartics)
- Other drugs (antihypertensives)
- Use of multiple medications
- Incontinence of urine or stool
- Bandages, cast, etc. on one or both feet
- Footwear with a slippery surface
- Uses walker, cane, crutches, or wheelchair
- Uses restraint or geriatric chair
- Edema
- Postural hypotension
- Neurological disease
- Cardiovascular disease

▰ ADULT NORMAL BODY WEIGHT OVER AGE 51

Women: 60 inches tall = 100 pounds. Add 5 pounds for each additional inch + 10% (add 4 pounds if less than 60 inches tall).

Men: 60 inches tall = 106 pounds. Add 6 pounds for each additional inch + 10% (add 5 pounds if less than 60 inches tall).

	Sedentary	**Moderately Active**
Weight maintenance	30 calories/kg (2.2 pounds)	35 calories/kg (2.2 pounds)
Weight gain	35 calories/kg (2.2 pounds)	40 calories/kg (2.2 pounds)
Weight loss	20–25 calories/kg (2.2 pounds)	30 calories/kg (2.2 pounds)

Weight Range Calculations

Height	Weight Range	Calories Required For Gain	Height	Weight Range	Calories Required For Gain
Women			**Men**		
56"	79–92	1336	58"	86–105	1511
57"	79–97	1400	59"	90–111	1607
58"	81–101	1463	60"	95–117	1686
59"	87–106	1527	61"	101–123	1792
60"	90–110	1590	62"	106–130	1877
61"	95–115	1670	63"	112–136	1973
62"	99–121	1750	64"	117–143	2068
63"	104–126	1830	65"	122–150	2164
64"	108–132	1909	66"	128–156	2259
65"	113–137	1989	67"	133–163	2355
66"	117–143	2068	68"	139–169	2450
67"	122–148	2148	69"	144–176	2545
68"	126–154	2227	70"	149–183	2641
69"	131–159	2306	71"	155–189	2736
70"	135–165	2386	72"	160–196	2832
71"	140–170	2466	73"	166–202	2927
72"	144–176	2545	74"	171–209	3023
73"	144–176	2625	75"	176–216	3118
74"	153–187	2705	76"	182–222	3214
			77"	187–229	3309
			78"	193–235	3405

USDA FOOD GUIDE PYRAMID

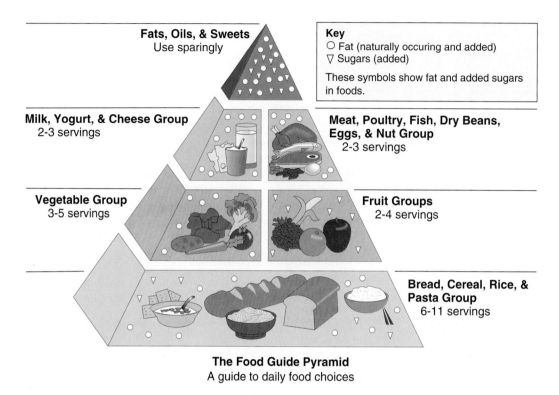

Figure C–1 USDA Food Guide Pyramid. (Courtesy of the U.S. Department of Agriculture)

■■■ PORTION SIZE GUIDE FOR FOOD GUIDE PYRAMID

Food Group	One serving from this group is:	Food Group	One serving from this group is:
Bread ceral, rice, and pasta	1 slice of bread 1 tortilla ½ cup cooked rice, pasta, or cereal 1 ounce ready-to-eat cereal ½ hamburger bun, bagel, or English muffin 3–4 plain crackers 1 pancake (4-inch diameter) ½ large croissant ½ medium doughnut or danish ⅟₁₆ cake (average-size cake) 2 medium cookies ⅟₁₂ of an 8-inch pie	Fruit group	1 piece fruit or melon wedge ¾ cup fruit juice ½ cup chopped, cooked or canned fruit ¼ cup dried fruit
		Milk, yogurt, and cheese group	1 cup milk or yogurt 1½ ounces cheese (natural) 2 ounces cheese (processed) 1½ cups ice cream or ice milk 1 cup frozen yogurt
Vegetable group	½ cup chopped raw or cooked vegetables 1 cup raw, leafy vegetables ¾ cup vegetable juice ½ cup scalloped potatoes ½ cup potato salad 10 french fries	Meat, poultry, dry beans, eggs, and nuts group	2½ to 3 ounces cooked lean beef, pork, lamb, veal, poultry, or fish (a portion the size of a deck of cards) ½ cup cooked beans, 1 egg, or 2 tablespoons peanut butter, or ⅓ cup of nuts equal 1 ounce of meat
		Fates, oils, sweets	Use sparingly

Figure C–2 Portion sizes for the Food Guide Pyramid food groups

■■■ DEGREE MEASUREMENTS

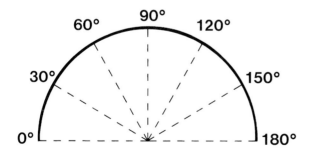

Figure C–3 Degree measurements.

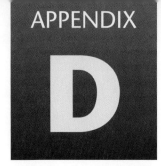

Communication

■ **COMMUNICATION CARDS**

NURSE	DOCTOR	BEDPAN
WATER	FOOD	PILL
BED	WHEELCHAIR	CIGARETTE
PENCIL	PAPER	NEWSPAPER
BATHROBE	TV-RADIO	WATCH
HOT	COLD	FAMILY
OK NO YES	MONEY	PAIN

Figure D–1 Initial communication chart for use with residents with aphasia

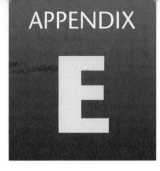

Basic Nursing Assistant Procedure Review

The procedures in this appendix are a review of information learned in your nursing assistant class. As a restorative nursing assistant, you will continue to use these important procedures. They are listed here for reference information.

GUIDELINES FOR GIVING A WHIRLPOOL BATH

Many different types of whirlpool tubs are used in long-term care facilities. Each is operated differently. The manufacturer provides operating instructions. Most tubs use a lift chair to transfer residents to the water. One type of tub has a door that opens in the front, and the resident is transferred in the usual manner.

In general, the water temperature in the whirlpool is lower than that in other types of baths. This is because the whirlpool maintains a constant temperature. The water does not cool off like the water in the bathtub. The warm water is relaxing to the resident, and stimulates circulation. The temperature in most tubs is set at 95° F to 97° F. Do not use the unit if temperatures exceed 105° F.

Little or no soap is used in the whirlpool. The circulating action of the jets cleanses the resident. If soap is used, avoid using more than the recommended amount. Too much soap will cause water and suds to overflow the tub. If soap bubbles overflow the tub, turn the jets off. Rub a bar of soap on the inside walls of the tub to decrease the suds.

PROCEDURE FOR GIVING A WHIRLPOOL BATH

1. Perform your beginning procedure actions. Make sure the tub is clean before beginning the procedure.
2. Gather equipment: 2 or 3 bath towels, washcloth, bath blanket, deodorant, resident's clothing.
3. Take the whirlpool transport chair to the resident's bedside.
4. Assist the resident to undress and put on a robe.
5. Wrap the resident with a bath blanket, so his or her body is not exposed.
6. Transport the resident to the tub room.
7. Fill the tub to within 8 to 10 inches of the top with warm water.

8. Assist the resident to remove the robe. Cover his or her upper torso with a bath towel.
9. Fasten the safety belt to the lift chair.
10. Secure the transport chair to the lift. Make sure it is locked into place before operating the lift. Follow your facility policy. Some facilities require two assistants to be present when the lift is being operated.
11. Operate the controls and elevate the lift so the resident is suspended above the level of the tub.
12. Rotate the chair over the tub. Support and lift the resident's feet and legs over the side of the tub.
13. Operate the controls and lower the resident into the tub.
14. After the resident is seated within the tub, turn on the water jets. Allow the jets to run for the designated period of time.
15. Assist the resident with bathing, as necessary.
16. Turn off the jets. Operate the controls and lift the resident's upper body out of the tub.
17. Assist the resident to dry the upper body. Cover the upper torso with a dry towel.
18. Operate the controls and elevate the seat to the maximum height.
19. Rotate the chair over the side of the tub. Support and lift the resident's feet and legs over the side.
20. Operate the controls and lower the lift chair to the floor.
21. Assist the resident to dry the remainder of the body.
22. Assist the resident to apply deodorant and dress.
23. Return the resident to his or her room.
24. Perform your procedure completion actions.
25. Return to the tub room and disinfect the whirlpool. Clean the room according to facility policy.

PROCEDURE FOR ASSISTING THE RESIDENT WITH A SUSPECTED FRACTURE

1. Stay with the resident and call for help. Reassure the resident.
2. Use standard precautions if contact with blood or moist body fluids (except sweat) is likely.

3. Do not move the resident until the charge nurse has examined the resident and gives approval.

4. Keep the resident as quiet as possible.

5. Immobilize the injured area by supporting it to prevent movement. If the area appears out of shape, bent, or deformed, do not attempt to straighten it.

6. Check the resident's vital signs, and assist her to bed as instructed by the charge nurse.

7. If a fracture is suspected, several staff members must assist the resident to bed. One staff member is assigned to move the injured extremity. Other staff members will move the rest of the resident's body. A sheet or other lifting device may be used to move the resident.

8. Leave the resident in a position of comfort and safety. Leave the call signal and needed personal items within reach.

9. Wash your hands.

10. The charge nurse may direct you to monitor the resident's vital signs frequently until they are stable.

11. You may also be directed to apply a cold treatment to the injured area.

12. Observe for and report:
   - the time of the fall
   - the cause of the fall, if known; avoid guessing and report only what you know to be true
   - measures taken to break the fall
   - measures taken to assist the resident
   - known injuries, such as bleeding, deformities, bruises, or changes in the resident's level of consciousness
   - circulatory problems and abnormal color of the injured extremity
   - appearance of the injured area and steps taken to immobilize it
   - witnesses to the fall
   - vital signs
   - any additional information needed to fill out the incident report

◼◼◼ PROCEDURE FOR APPLICATION OF COLD PACKS TO STRAINS AND BRUISES

1. Notify the charge nurse of the injury.
2. If the resident is on the floor, stay with him and call for help.
3. Do not move the resident until the charge nurse examines him.

4. Wash your hands.

5. Position the resident in a comfortable position.

6. Use standard precautions if contact with blood or moist body fluids (except sweat) is likely.

7. Prepare the cold pack as directed by the charge nurse and according to facility policy:
   - Place a cloth or flannel cover over the cold pack.
   - Apply the cold pack above or on top of the injured area, as directed. If the resident complains that the cold pack increases the pain, remove it and consult the nurse.
   - Secure the cold pack in place, if necessary. You may need to prop it or tie it in place with a gauze bandage.
   - Check the area under the cold pack every 10 minutes and remove it if numbness or discoloration of the skin occurs.
   - Remove the cold pack after 30 minutes.
   - Reapply the cold pack as directed.

8. Wash your hands.

9. Leave the resident in a position of comfort and safety. Leave the call signal and needed personal items within reach.

10. Observe for and report:
   - the time of the injury
   - description of the injured area
   - edema, deformities, or other injuries
   - cause of the injury, if known
   - the type of cold pack applied and time
   - response to the cold pack

◼◼◼ PROCEDURE FOR MOVING THE RESIDENT TO THE SIDE OF THE BED

1. Perform your beginning procedure actions.
2. Cross the resident's arms over the chest.
3. Place your upper hand, palm side up, under the resident's shoulders.
4. Place your lower hand, palm side up, under the mid-back.
5. Lift the upper part of the body toward the near side of the bed.
6. Place your hands under the resident's waist and thighs.
7. Lift the middle section of the body toward the near side of the bed.
8. Place your hands under the thighs and lower legs and lift them toward you.
9. Perform your procedure completion actions.

PROCEDURE FOR TURNING THE RESIDENT ON THE SIDE TOWARD YOU

1. Perform your beginning procedure actions.
2. Move the resident to the side of the bed, if necessary.
3. Cross the resident's arms over the chest.
4. Cross the leg farthest away from you over the near leg.
5. Place your top hand behind the resident's far shoulder. Place your bottom hand on the resident's hip.
6. Roll the resident toward you.
7. Raise the side rail and move to the opposite side of the bed.
8. Lower the side rail.
9. Place your hands under the resident's bottom shoulder and pull back slightly toward the center of the bed. The resident should not be lying directly on the shoulder. Repeat this action for the resident's hips.
10. Roll a pillow or place a positioning device behind the resident's back to maintain the position, if necessary.
11. Raise the side rail and return to the opposite side of the bed.
12. Lower the rail.
13. Bend the knees slightly. The upper leg should be positioned slightly ahead of the lower leg. Place a pillow or folded bath blanket from the knees to the ankles to keep the legs from rubbing together.
14. Place a pillow under the resident's upper arm, if necessary, for support.
15. Check the lower arm to be sure it is not under the resident. If the resident is not able to move the arm, place it in a position of comfort at the side of the body, or bent at the elbow with the hand by the head.
16. Perform your procedure completion actions.

PROCEDURE FOR TURNING THE RESIDENT ON THE SIDE AWAY FROM YOU

1. Perform your beginning procedure actions.
2. Move the resident to the side of the bed, if necessary.
3. Bend the resident's far arm at the elbow, so the hand is near the head. Cross the near arm over the chest.
4. Cross the near leg over the far leg.
5. Place your top hand on the resident's shoulder and your bottom hand on the hip. Turn the resident on the side facing away from you.

6. Roll a pillow or place a positioning device behind the resident's back to maintain the position, if necessary.
7. Raise the side rail and move to the opposite side of the bed.
8. Lower the side rail.
9. Bend the knees slightly. The upper leg should be positioned slightly ahead of the lower leg. Place a pillow or folded bath blanket between the knees, calves, and ankles to keep them from rubbing together.
10. Place a pillow under the resident's upper arm, if necessary, for support.
11. Check the lower arm to be sure it is not under the resident.
12. Perform your procedure completion actions.

PROCEDURE FOR ASSISTING THE RESIDENT TO MOVE TO THE HEAD OF THE BED

1. Perform your beginning procedure actions.
2. Lower the head of the bed.
3. Remove the pillow and place it against the headboard.
4. Instruct the resident to bend the knees and place the feet flat on the bed. The arms should be at the sides with elbows bent.
5. Place your top arm under the shoulders.
6. Place your bottom arm under the hips.
7. On the count of three, instruct the resident to push up with the elbows and feet while you lift.
8. Replace the pillow and straighten the bed linen.
9. Perform your procedure completion actions.

PROCEDURE FOR MOVING THE RESIDENT TO THE HEAD OF THE BED WITH A LIFTING (DRAW) SHEET

1. Ask another nursing assistant to assist you.
2. Perform your beginning procedure actions.
3. Lower the head of the bed.
4. Lower the side rails.
5. Remove the pillow and place it against the headboard.
6. Roll the lift sheet inward until it touches the resident's body.
7. Grasp the lift sheet with your top hand at the level of the resident's shoulder and your bottom hand at the hip.
8. Face the head of the bed. On the count of three, shift your weight from the rear foot to the front foot and lift the resident toward the head of the bed.

9. Replace the pillow.
10. Straighten the lift sheet.
11. Perform your procedure completion actions.

PROCEDURE FOR MOVING THE RESIDENT UP IN BED WITH ONE ASSISTANT

1. Ask another nursing assistant to help you.
2. Perform your beginning procedure actions.
3. Lower the head of the bed.
4. Lower the side rails.
5. Remove the pillow and place it against the headboard.
6. Place your top arm under the resident's shoulders and your bottom arm under the resident's hips. Your assistant should do the same.
7. Grasp arms with your assistant.
8. Face the head of the bed. On the count of three, shift your weight from the rear foot to the front foot and lift the resident toward the head of the bed.
9. Replace the pillow.
10. Perform your procedure completion actions.

PROCEDURE FOR ASSISTING THE RESIDENT TO TRANSFER TO CHAIR OR WHEELCHAIR, ONE PERSON, WITH TRANSFER BELT

1. Perform your beginning procedure actions.
2. Assist the resident to dress and put on nonslip footwear.
3. Apply the transfer belt snugly around the resident's waist and check it with three fingers for tightness.
4. Stand in front of the resident. Keep your feet apart, knees bent, and back straight. Place one hand under each side of the transfer belt, using an underhand grasp.
5. Move the resident so the feet are touching the floor. The resident's knees should be separated to provide a wide base of support.
6. Instruct the resident on the count of three to lean forward and push up from the bed with the hands while you lift up on the belt. Support the resident's knees and feet by placing your knees and feet firmly against them.
7. Assist the resident to pivot until the knees touch the back of the chair and he can reach the armrests with his hands.
8. Bend your knees and assist the resident to lower himself into the chair.
9. Remove the transfer belt.

10. Adjust the wheelchair legs and footrests.
11. Perform your procedure completion actions.
12. Reverse the procedure to return the resident to bed.

PROCEDURE FOR ASSISTING THE RESIDENT TO TRANSFER TO CHAIR OR WHEELCHAIR, TWO PERSONS, WITH TRANSFER BELT

1. Perform your beginning procedure actions.
2. Assist the resident to dress and put on nonslip footwear.
3. Apply the transfer belt snugly around the resident's waist and check it with three fingers for tightness.
4. Stand in front of the resident. Keep your feet apart, knees bent, and back straight. Each nursing assistant places one hand under the front of the belt and one hand under the back of the belt, using an underhand grasp.
5. Move the resident so the feet are touching the floor. The resident's knees should be separated to provide a wide base of support.
6. On the count of three, both nursing assistants will move the resident at the same time. Coordination of movement is important.
7. The nursing assistant on the side closest to the chair stands in a position so that he can pivot and move away, allowing the resident unobstructed access to the chair. This nursing assistant should stand with one leg behind the other, so stepping back quickly is easy.
8. The other nursing assistant uses one knee to support the resident's weak leg. This nursing assistant's other leg is positioned further back.
9. Instruct the resident to lean forward and push off the bed using the palms of the hands on the count of three.
10. The resident's knees should be spread apart. Instruct him to put both feet down with the stronger foot behind the weaker foot.
11. Both nursing assistants bend their knees, squat slightly, and spread their feet to provide a wide base of support.
12. On the count of three, the resident is lifted to a standing position. The nursing assistants pivot slowly and smoothly by moving their feet, legs, and hips to the side left until the resident can feel the back of the wheelchair with the legs.
13. Instruct the resident to place his hands on the armrests of the chair and lean forward slightly.
14. Both nursing assistants bend their knees and lower the resident into the chair.
15. Remove the transfer belt.

16. Adjust the wheelchair legs and footrests.
17. Perform your procedure completion actions.
18. Reverse the procedure to return the resident to bed.

PROCEDURE FOR ASSISTING THE RESIDENT TO TRANSFER FROM BED TO CHAIR OR WHEELCHAIR, ONE ASSISTANT

Note: For the safety of both the nursing assistant and the resident, use this procedure only if use of the transfer belt is contraindicated.

1. Perform your beginning procedure actions.
2. Assist the resident to dress and put on nonslip footwear.
3. Bring the resident to the edge of the bed so the feet touch the floor. The resident's knees should be separated to provide a wide base of support.
4. Place your hands under the resident's arms and around the back of the shoulders.
5. Brace the resident's knees and feet with your knees and feet.
6. On the count of three, pull the resident to a standing position. Avoid pulling upward under the arms.
7. Pivot the resident until the knees touch the back of the chair and she can reach the armrests with her hands.
8. Bend your knees and assist the resident to lower herself into the chair.
9. Adjust the wheelchair legs and footrests.
10. Perform your procedure completion actions.
11. Reverse the procedure to return the resident to bed.

PROCEDURE FOR TRANSFERRING THE RESIDENT USING A MECHANICAL LIFT

1. Perform your beginning procedure actions.
2. Place the chair at right angles to the foot of the bed, facing the head.
3. Lower the side rail on the side nearest you.
4. Roll the resident on the side.
5. Position the sling under the resident's body so it supports the shoulders, buttocks, and thighs. Straighten the sling.
6. Roll the resident onto the sling and properly position it on the other side.
7. Position the lift over the bed. Spread the legs of the lift to the widest open position, to maintain a broad base of support.
8. Attach the suspension straps or chains to the sling. The "S" hook should face *away* from the resident to prevent injury.

9. Position the resident's arms comfortably inside the sling.
10. Attach the straps or chains to the lift frame.
11. Reassure the resident, lock the hydraulic mechanism, and slowly raise the boom of the lift until the resident is suspended over the bed.
12. Slowly guide the lift away from the bed.
13. Position the lift above the chair.
14. The nursing assistant helping you holds the sling back and helps lower the resident slowly into the chair, keeping the hips back while you slowly release the hydraulic mechanism and lower the lift.
15. When lowering the lift, monitor the location of the resident's feet and arms to prevent injury.
16. Unhook the straps or chains and remove the lift. The lift seat remains under the resident.
17. Position the footrests to support the feet.
18. Perform your procedure completion actions.
19. Reverse the procedure to return the resident to bed. When raising the resident from the chair, monitor the position of the "S" hooks, which sometimes catch under the arms of the chair.

PROCEDURE FOR APPLYING ANTI-EMBOLISM STOCKINGS

1. Perform your beginning procedure actions.
2. Obtain hosiery in the correct size.
3. Expose one leg.
4. Hold the stocking with both hands at the top and roll or gather toward the toe end.
5. Apply the stocking over the toes and over the leg by rolling it upward.
6. Check the fit to be sure the stocking is even and there are no wrinkles. Pull up slightly on the toes to ensure that the stocking is not too tight.
7. Expose the other leg.
8. Repeat the procedure.
9. Perform your procedure completion actions.

PROCEDURE FOR ASSISTING THE RESIDENT WITH DRESSING AND UNDRESSING

1. Perform your beginning procedure actions.
2. Gather needed supplies: bath blanket, clothing, deodorant, disposable gloves.
3. If the resident has a weak or paralyzed arm, work from the strong side.
4. Cover the resident with the bath blanket and remove the upper linens without exposing the resident.

5. For pants:
   a. Put one foot at a time into underwear. Slide them up over the feet and ankles.
   b. Gather the leg of the pants on the weak side. Slide the pant leg over the foot and ankle. Repeat with the strong leg.
   c. Slide the pants and underwear up the resident's legs.
   d. Ask the resident to raise the hips and buttocks while you pull underwear and pants into position.
   e. If the resident is unable to assist, roll onto the strong side. Pull the underwear and pants up on the weak side. Turn the resident to the weak side and finish pulling the clothing up. Fasten at the waist, if necessary.
6. Apply deodorant before putting on a shirt or sweater.
7. To put on garments that go over the arms or head:
   a. Stretch the neck as widely as possible and pull it over the resident's head.
   b. Put your hand into the sleeve of the garment on the resident's weaker side. Grasp the resident's weak hand. Slide the sleeve off your wrist and pull resident's hand and wrist through the sleeve.
   c. Pull the sleeve up and adjust it at the shoulder.

   d. Lift the resident's arms and shoulders. Adjust the garment in the back.
   e. Ask the resident to put the strong arm into the other sleeve. If unable, repeat step 7b.
   f. Lift the resident's arms and shoulders, or roll the resident to the side. Pull down and adjust the garment in back.
8. To put on a shirt or blouse that opens in front:
   a. Put your hand into the sleeve of the garment on the resident's weaker side. Roll the sleeve over your wrist. Grasp the resident's weak hand. Slide the sleeve off your wrist and over the resident's hand and wrist.
   b. Pull the garment up the arm and adjust it at the shoulder.
   c. Lift the resident's head and shoulders and pull the garment around the back. If you cannot lift the resident, roll him toward you and tuck the garment under him. Turn the resident away from you and pull the garment out. Then return the resident to the supine position.
   d. Ask the resident to put the strong arm into the other sleeve. If unable, repeat step 8a.
   e. Pull the garment up the arm and adjust it at the shoulder.
   f. Fasten the garment in the front.
9. Reverse the procedure for undressing the resident.

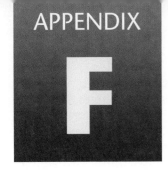

Professional Organizations and Continuing Education Resources

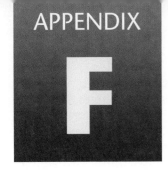 NATIONAL GROUPS AND PUBLICATIONS

Career Nurse Assistants Programs, Inc.
3577 Easton Rd.
Norton, OH 44203-5661
(216) 825-9342

The Career Nurse Assistants Programs, Inc. (CNAP) is a tax-exempt, nonprofit, volunteer organization provided for, by, and with nurse assistants and nurse assistant related groups, organizations, publishers, and researchers.

CNAP is the founder and sponsor of the annual nationwide observance of Nurse Assistants' Week and Career Nurse Assistants' Day. Other initiatives include the National Classroom, the National Twenty-Year Club, and National Most Service Years Award for nurse assistants. Since 1993, CNAP has also sponsored the Annual Forum on Nurse Assisting held in conjunction with the National Citizens' Coalition for Nursing Home Reform. The *Network News* is published four times a year to foster connections among members and other participating groups. The very popular booklet series, "Tips by Nurse Assistants for Nurse Assistants," are published on a regular basis on a variety of topics.

CNAP has taken the lead to develop programs in support of nurse assistants and provides guidelines and materials to others desiring to replicate this work in another state or area. Today, CNAP plays an important role to provide a voice for the direct care worker nationwide, foster connections among nurse assistant related groups, organizations, publishers, and researchers, and involve the community in recognizing and validating the nurse assistant in nursing homes and other long-term care settings. For its work to improve the professionalism of nurse assistants, CNAP was named the recipient of the American College of Health Care Administrators' Annual Public Service Award in 1997.

Journal of Nurse Assistants
P.O. Box 23365
Chagrin Falls, OH 44023
(216) 247-5668
Fax (216) 247-8925

The *Journal of Nurse Assistants* promotes positive self-image, stresses proper patient care, and enhances standards of professionalism. A mission of this journal is to encourage nurse assistants to form peer support groups. An individual subscription is available for $25.00 for 4 issues. The group rate for 10 or more to the same address is $15.00 per subscription.

National Association of Geriatric Nursing Assistants
403 W. 5th St.
Joplin, MO 64801
(800) 784-6049 or (417) 623-6049
Fax (417) 623-2230

This is a professional trade association for long-term care facilities and their CNAs. Educational and motivational video programs, newsletters, and low-cost insurance are available to members. Membership entitles a member facility to four video seminars per year, bimonthly newsletters, lapel pins, a certificate of membership, membership identification cards, and bumper stickers. The organization helps facilities improve morale, enhance personal and professional growth, and teach nursing assistants that they have a key role in retaining new employees. The group helps facilities with recruitment, provides public relations tools, reduces turnover through REM programs (recognition, education, motivation), and provides group uniform purchasing below retail prices. Member facilities pay fees depending on the number of employees. The organization is developing a similar program to be used for home health assistants.

The National Nurse Assistants Association
6091 South Perkins Rd.
Bedford, OH 44146
(216) 439-7867

If possible, please write instead of calling. Send a self-addressed, stamped envelope for information requests.

The goal of this organization is to encourage groups of nursing assistants to form support groups and work together for the good of all nursing assistants, whatever the employment setting. The organization advises members of specific nursing assistant-related legislation and provides educational information so that nursing assistants can take responsibility for their own growth and development. The group advocates that nursing assistants learn how to become responsible and articulate members of the health care team. The association recommends that members learn problem-solving techniques to enhance their capabilities in any organization. A speaker's bureau is available to discuss how to improve communication, peer support, and self-identity. The fee is $24.00 annually for support groups.

Nursing Assistant Monthly

Frontline Publishing Corp.
12 Arrow St.
Cambridge, MA 02138
(800) 348-0605
Fax (617) 661-1530

The result of more than 10 years of research into the lives of nursing assistants by Dr. Karl Pillemer of Cornell University, *Nursing Assistant Monthly* is a multifaceted training and communications program, now in use in 43 states. The program is designed to address the critical interpersonal and psychosocial aspects of caregiving.

Each month's training package includes a fully developed lesson plan for the in-service coordinator, a guide to additional resources, and a quiz to measure learning and provide documentation that fulfills OBRA requirements for ongoing training of CNAs. The text for each month's topic is delivered to each CNA in an attractive newsletter that serves as a professional journal, building pride, confidence, and self-esteem. The facility pays for cost of membership for this program.

Shari's CNA Page

http://members.tripod.com/~CNA_MUNCHKIN/
Shari.htm

For nursing assistants with access to the Internet, this site is an excellent source of support, educational, and other miscellaneous information. It offers online resources and support specifically for nursing assistants.

▇▇ REGIONAL AND STATE GROUPS AND PUBLICATIONS

Colorado Association of Certified Nurse Aides

Mailing addresses and telephones:
Pat Cloyd
5601 Federal Blvd., #8B
Denver, CO 80221
(303) 477-4386
or
Erma Gallardo
8670 Pratt Place
Westminster, CO 80030
(303) 429-4488

The Association of Nurse Aides is a group working to help solve work-related challenges. Members work in hospitals, rehabilitation centers, care centers, board and care homes, nursing homes, and private homes. The objectives of the group are to improve skills, exchange ideas, improve care, be recognized as professional health care providers, and establish a support network for each other. The group offers professional speakers at monthly meetings, continuing education hours, additional training opportunities, and updated information from the Colorado State Board of Nursing related to changes in maintaining state certification. Criteria for membership are current CNA certification in the state of Colorado, and $15.00 per year annual dues.

Florida Association of Nurse Assistants, Inc.

M. T. Carleton-Bucher, LPN, Director
6039 Cypress Gardens Blvd., #266
Winter Haven, FL 33884
(914) 324-5136

This organization provides an opportunity for nursing assistants, home health aides, and resident caregivers to come together in mutual support of one another and continue to advance in knowledge, for their personal development as well as the enhancement of patient/resident care. They promote the development of individual facility/agency support groups. These groups are encouraged to meet regularly to discuss solutions to problems, identify ways to keep current, and support one another through the development of good listening skills. Meetings are held in various locations throughout Polk County, Florida. The organization is exploring the feasibility of becoming an official organization in the state of Florida, with each county forming its own chapter within an established framework. Membership is open to any CNA, nurse assistant, HHA, or resident caregiver.

Certified Nursing Assistant Association of Georgia, Inc.

235 Bay St.
Fairburn, GA 30213
(404) 969-9779

The motto of this group is "We serve because we care." The group represents nursing assistants, home health aides, therapy aides, psychiatric technicians, Alzheimer's technicians, and other related caregivers. The goal of the organization is to broaden the horizons of all CNAs and elevate the status of the nursing assistant profession. The vision is to develop a team of dedicated, enthusiastic paraprofessionals, encouraging creativity, and innovation to accomplish their mission.

This organization was founded in response to quality-of-life and quality-of-care issues associated with direct care. They seek pen pals as a support team, and offer services to improve CNA morale and assist with training and motivational programs designed to benefit the patient/resident/client. Other services include a quarterly newsletter, in-services, conferences, and workshops. Individual membership is $20.00 per year. Facility membership is also available.

Iowa Caregivers Association
1117 Pleasant St., #221
Des Moines, IA 50309
(515) 241-8697
Fax (515) 241-5038

This is a nonprofit, statewide professional association for certified nurse assistants (CNAs) and home care aides (HCAs). The goals of the organization are to promote CNAs and HCAs as professionals and to provide the tools of education, support, recognition, and advocacy to make that possible. ICA sponsors the governor-proclaimed Iowa Caregivers Month each June, along with a ribbon campaign to increase awareness of the important role of direct caregivers.

ICA member advantages include a system of outside support, annual and regional conferences, support groups, quarterly newsletters, business discounts, and opportunities to serve on the ICA board and committees.

ICA is a model that easily can be duplicated in any state. Speakers are available for conventions.

PROFESSIONAL NURSING ORGANIZATIONS RELATED TO RESTORATIVE NURSING

These organizations may be useful to the restorative nursing assistant as a source of educational information about specific diseases and conditions.

American Association of Diabetes Educators
444 N. Michigan Ave., Suite 1240
Chicago, IL 60611-3901
(312) 644-2233
Fax (312) 644-4411
Web site: http://www.aadenet.org

American Association of Spinal Cord Injury Nurses
75-20 Astoria Blvd.
Jackson Heights, NY 11370-1177
(718) 803-3782
Fax (718) 803-0414
Spinal cord hotline: 1-800-526-3456
E-mail: scihotline@aol.com
Web site: http://members.aol.com/scihotline

American Society of Pain Management Nurses
7794 Grow Dr.
Pensacola, FL 32514
(850) 473-0233
(850) 484-8762
1-888-342-7766
E-mail: aspmn@aol.com

Association of Nurses in AIDS Care
11250 Roger Bacon Dr., Suite 8
Reston, VA 20190-5202
(703) 925-0081
Fax (703) 435-4390
E-mail: aidsnurses@aol.com
Web site: http://www.anacnet.org/aids/

Association of Rehabilitation Nurses
4700 W. Lake Ave.
Glenview, IL 60025-1485
(847) 375-4710
Fax (847) 375-4777
E-mail: info@rehabnurse.org
Web site: http://www.rehabnurse.org

National Association of Directors of Nursing in Long Term Care
10999 Reed-Hartman Hwy, Suite 233
Cincinnati, OH 45242-8301
1-800-222-0539
Fax (513) 791-3699

National Association of Orthopaedic Nurses, Inc.
E. Holly Ave., Box 56
Pittman, NJ 08071-0056
(609) 256-2310
Fax (609) 589-7463
E-mail: naon@mail.ajj.com
Web site: http://www.inurse.com/~naon

National Gerontological Nursing Association
7250 Parkway Dr., Suite 510
Hanover, MD 21076
1-800-723-0560
Fax (410) 712-4424
E-mail: susan.sibiski@mosby.com

National Pressure Ulcer Advisory Panel (NPUAP)
2834 Bourbon Red Dr.
St. Louis, MO 93131
(314) 909-6815
Fax (314) 909-6814
E-mail: thomasjn@worldnet.att.net
Web site: http://www.npuap.org/

Oncology Nursing Society
501 Holiday Dr.
Pittsburgh, PA 15220-2749
(412) 921-7373
Fax (412) 921-6565
E-mail: members@ons.org
Web site: http://www.ons.org

Respiratory Nursing Society
7794 Grow Dr.
Pensacola, FL 32514
(850) 474-8869
1-888-330-4767
Fax (850) 484-8762
E-mail: rnsatpns@aol.com

Wound, Ostomy and Continence Nurses Society
1550 S. Coast Hwy, #201
Laguna Beach, CA 92651
1-888-224-9626
Fax (949) 376-3456
Web site: http://www.wocn.org

▆▆ OTHER RESOURCES LISTED IN THE TEXT

Materials Referenced in Text

For forms, adaptive devices, restorative nursing products, and the Americans with Disabilities Act featured in your text:

Americans with Disabilities Act Summary Information
http://www.ada-infonet.org/ovrvew.htm

Briggs Corporation
P.O. Box 1698
Des Moines, IA 50306-1698
1-800-247-2343
Web site: http://www.briggscorp.com

Medline Industries, Inc.
One Medline Pl.
Mundelein, IL 60060
1-800-MEDLINE

National Pressure Ulcer Advisory Panel
12834 Bourbon Red Drive
St. Louis, MO 63131
(314) 909-6814
Fax (314) 909-6815
E-mail: thomasjn@worldnet.att.net

Restorative Medical, Inc.
139 Sunny View
Brandenburg, KY 40108
1-800-793-5544
Fax (502) 422-5453

Sammons-Preston Corporation
P.O. Box 5071
Bollingbrook, IL 60440-5071
1-800-323-5547
Fax 1-800-547-4333
Skil-Care Corporation
167 Saw Mill River Rd.
Yonkers, NY 10701
1-800-431-2972
Fax (914) 963-2567

Validation Training Institute
Naomi Feil, Executive Director
21987 Byron Rd.
Cleveland, OH 44122
(216) 561-0357 or (216) 881-0040
Fax (216) 751-6434
E-mail: naomifeil@aol.com
Web site: http://www.pangea.ca/~naomi/

Federal Agencies

Agency for Health Care Policy and Research (AHCPR) (guidelines for urinary incontinence, pressure ulcers, and other information)
Division of Communications
2101 E. Jefferson St.
Rockville, MD 20852
(301) 594-1364
Web site: http://www.ahcpr.gov

Centers for Disease Control and Prevention (CDC) (information on standard precautions and transmission-based precautions)
2000 Building 1
1600 Clifton Rd., NE
Atlanta, GA 30333
(404) 639-3311
Web site: http://www.cdc.gov

Health Care Financing Administration (HCFA) (information on federal standards for long-term care)
Security Office Park Bldg, Room 1A11
7008 Security Blvd.
Baltimore, MD 21207
(410) 597-5110
Web site: http://www.hcfa.gov

Occupational Safety and Health Administration (OSHA) (information on ergonomics, back safety, and employee injuries)
Department of Labor
200 Constitution Ave. NW
N-36-47
Washington, DC 20010
(202) 523-8148
Web site: http://www.osha.go

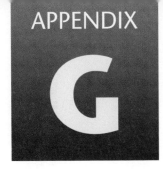

APPENDIX G

Federal Law

▰▰ QUALITY OF CARE (OBRA 483.25)

§483.25 Quality of care.

Each resident must receive and the facility must provide the necessary care and services to attain or maintain the highest practicable physical, mental, and psychosocial well-being, in accordance with the comprehensive assessment and plan of care.

(a) *Activities of daily living.* Based on the comprehensive assessment of a resident, the facility must ensure that—

(1) A resident's abilities in activities of daily living do not diminish unless circumstances of the individual's clinical condition demonstrate that diminution was unavoidable. This includes the resident's ability to—

(i) Bathe, dress, and groom;

(ii) Transfer and ambulate;

(iii) Toilet;

(iv) Eat; and

(v) Use speech, language, or other functional communication systems.

(2) A resident is given the appropriate treatment and services to maintain or improve his or her abilities specified in paragraph (a)(1) of this section; and

(3) A resident who is unable to carry out activities of daily living receives the necessary services to maintain good nutrition, grooming, and personal and oral hygiene.

(b) *Vision and hearing.* To ensure that residents receive proper treatment and assistive devices to maintain vision and hearing abilities, the facility must, if necessary, assist the resident—

(1) In making appointments, and

(2) By arranging for transportation to and from the office of a practitioner specializing in the treatment of vision or hearing impairment or the office of a professional specializing in the provision of vision or hearing assistive devices.

(c) *Pressure sores.* Based on the comprehensive assessment of a resident the facility must ensure that—

(1) A resident who enters the facility without pressure sores does not develop pressure sores unless the individual's clinical condition demonstrates that they were unavoidable; and

(2) A resident having pressure sores receives necessary treatment and services to promote healing, prevent infection and prevent new sores from developing.

(d) *Urinary Incontinence.* Based on the resident's comprehensive assessment, the facility must ensure that—

(1) A resident who enters the facility without an indwelling catheter is not catheterized unless the resident's clinical condition demonstrates that catheterization was necessary; and

(2) A resident who is incontinent of bladder receives appropriate treatment and services to prevent urinary tract infections and to restore as much normal bladder function as possible.

(e) *Range of motion.* Based on the comprehensive assessment of a resident, the facility must ensure that—

(1) A resident who enters the facility without a limited range of motion does not experience reduction in range of motion unless the resident's clinical condition demonstrates that a reduction in range of motion is unavoidable; and

(2) A resident with a limited range of motion receives appropriate treatment and services to increase range of motion and/or to prevent further decrease in range of motion.

(f) *Mental and psychosocial functioning.* Based on the comprehensive assessment of a resident, the facility must ensure that—

(1) A resident who displays mental or psychosocial adjustment difficulty, receives appropriate treatment and services to correct the assessed problem, and

(2) A resident whose assessment did not reveal a mental or psychosocial adjustment difficulty does not display a pattern of decreased social interaction and/or increased withdrawn, angry, or depressive behaviors, unless the resident's clinical condition demonstrates that such a pattern was unavoidable;

(g) *Naso-gastric tubes.* Based on the comprehensive assessment of a resident, the facility must ensure that—

(1) A resident who has been able to eat enough alone or with assistance is not fed by naso-gastric tube unless the resident's clinical condition demonstrates that use of a naso-gastric tube was unavoidable; and

(2) A resident who is fed by a gastrostomy tube receives the appropriate treatment and services to prevent aspiration, pneumonia, diarrhea, vomiting, dehydration, metabolic abnormalities, and nasalpharyngeal ulcers and to restore, if possible, normal eating skills.

(h) *Accidents.* The facility must ensure that—

(1) The resident environment remains as free of accident hazards as is possible; and

(2) Each resident receives adequate supervision and assistance devices to prevent accidents.

(i) *Nutrition.* Based on a resident's comprehensive assessment, the facility must ensure that a resident—

(1) Maintains acceptable parameters of nutritional status, such as body weight and protein levels, unless the resident's clinical condition demonstrates that this is not possible; and

(2) Receives a therapeutic diet when there is a nutritional problem.

(j) *Hydration.* The facility must provide each resident with sufficient fluid intake to maintain proper hydration and health.

(k) *Special needs.* The facility must ensure that residents receive proper treatment and care for the following special services:

(1) Injections;

(2) Parenteral and enteral fluids;

(3) Colostomy, ureterostomy, or ileostomy care;

(4) Tracheostomy care;

(5) Tracheal suctioning;

(6) Respiratory care;

(7) Foot care; and

(8) Prostheses.

(l) *Unnecessary drugs*—(1) *General.* Each resident's drug regimen must be free from unnecessary drugs. An unnecessary drug is any drug when used:

(i) In excessive dose (including duplicate drug therapy); or

(ii) For excessive duration; or

(iii) Without adequate monitoring; or

(iv) Without adequate indications for its use; or

(v) In the presence of adverse consequences which indicate the dose should be reduced or discontinued; or

(vi) Any combinations of the reasons above.

(2) *Antipsychotic drugs.* Based on a comprehensive assessment of a resident, the facility must ensure that—

(i) Residents who have not used antipsychotic drugs are not given these drugs unless antipsychotic drug therapy is necessary to treat a specific condition as diagnosed and documented in the clinical record; and

(ii) Residents who use antipsychotic drugs receive gradual dose reductions, and behavioral interventions, unless clinically contraindicated, in an effort to discontinue these drugs.

(m) *Medication errors*—The facility must ensure that—

(1) It is free of medication error rates of five percent or greater; and

(2) Residents are free of any significant medication errors.

Interpretive Guidelines for Restorative Care

TAG NUMBER

*F309

REGULATIONS

§483.25 Quality of Care.

Each resident must receive and the facility must provide the necessary care and services to attain or maintain the highest practicable physical, mental, and psychosocial well-being, in accordance with the comprehensive assessment and plan of care.

*(Use F309 for quality of care deficiencies not covered by §483.25(a)-(m).)

GUIDANCE FOR SURVEYORS

Interpretive Guidelines: §483.25

"Highest practicable" is defined as the highest level of functioning and well-being possible, limited only by the individual's presenting functional status and potential for improvement or reduced rate of functional decline. Highest practicable is determined through the comprehensive resident assessment and competently and thoroughly addressing the physical, mental or psychosocial needs of the individual.

The facility must ensure that the resident obtains optimal improvement or does not deteriorate within the limits of a resident's right to refuse treatment, and within he limits of recognized pathology and the normal aging process.

In any instance in which there has been a lack of improvement or a decline, the survey team must determine if the occurrence was unavoidable or avoidable. A determination of unavoidable decline or failure to reach highest practicable well-being may be made only if all of the following are present:

An accurate and complete assessment (see §483.20);
A care plan which is implemented consistently and based on information from the assessment;
Evaluation of the results of the interventions and revising the interventions as necessary.

Determine if the facility is providing the necessary care and services based on the findings of the RAI. If services and care are being provided, determine if the facility is evaluating the outcome to the resident and changing the interventions if needed. This should be done in accordance with the resident's customary daily routine. Use Tag F309 to cite quality of care deficiencies that are not explicit in the quality of care regulations.

Intent: §483.25(a)

The intent of this regulation is that the facility must ensure that a resident's abilities in ADLs do not deteriorate unless the deterioration was unavoidable.

(a) Activities of daily living. Based on the comprehensive assessment of a resident, the facility must ensure that—

TAG NUMBER

F310

REGULATIONS

(1) A resident's abilities in activities of daily living do not diminish unless circumstances of the individual's clinical condition demonstrate that diminution was unavoidable. This includes the resident's ability to—

(i) Bathe, dress, and groom;

(ii) Transfer and ambulate;

(iii) Toilet;

(iv) Eat; and

(v) Use speech, language, or other functional communication systems.

GUIDANCE FOR SURVEYORS

Interpretive Guidelines: §483.25(a)

The mere presence of a clinical diagnosis, in itself, justifies a decline in a resident's ability to perform ADLs. Conditions which may demonstrate unavoidable diminution in ADLs include:

The natural progression of the resident's disease;

Deterioration of the resident's physical condition associated with the onset of a physical or mental disability while receiving care to restore or maintain functional abilities; and

The resident's or his/her surrogate's or representative's refusal of care and treatment to restore or maintain functional abilities after aggressive efforts by the facility to counsel and/or offer alternatives to the resident, surrogate, or representative. Refusal of such care and treatment should be documented in the clinical record.

Determine which interventions were identified on the care plan and/or could be in place to minimize or decrease complications. Note also that depression is a potential cause of excess disability and, where appropriate, therapeutic interventions should be initialed.

Appropriate treatment and services includes all care provided to residents by employees, contractors, or volunteers of the facility to maximize the individual's functional abilities. This includes pain relief and control, especially when it is causing a decline or a decrease in the quality of life of the resident.

If the survey team identifies a pattern of deterioration in ADLs, i.e., a number of residents have deteriorated in more than one ADL or a number of residents have deteriorated in only one ADL (one in bathing, one in eating, one in toileting) and it is determined there is deficient practice, cite at F310.

For evaluating a resident's ADLs and determining whether a resident's abilities have declined, improved or stayed the same for up to the last twelve months, use the following definitions as specified in the State's RAI:

Independent—No help or staff oversight; or staff help/oversight provided only 1 or 2 times during prior 7 days.

TAG NUMBER

F310 cont.

REGULATIONS

GUIDANCE FOR SURVEYORS

Supervision—Oversight, encouragement or cueing provided three or more times during the last seven days, or supervision plus physical assistance provided only one or two times during the last seven days.

Limited Assistance—Resident highly involved in activity, received physical help in guided maneuvering of limbs, and/or other non-weight bearing assistance on at least 3 or more occasions; or more help provided only 1 or 2 times over 7-day period.

Extensive Assistance—While resident performed part of activity, over prior 7-day period, help of following type(s) was provided 3 or more times;

- Weight-bearing support; or
- Full staff performance during part (but not all) of week.

Total Dependence—Full staff performance of activity over entire 7-day period.

BATHING, DRESSING, GROOMING

Interpretive Guidelines: §483.25(a)(1)(i)

This corresponds to MDS section E; version 2.0, section G, when specified for use by the State.

"Bathing" means how resident takes full-body bath, sponge bath, and transfers in/out of tub/shower. Exclude washing of back and hair.

"Dressing" means how resident puts on, fastens, and takes off all items of street clothing, including donning/removing prosthesis.

"Grooming" means the resident maintains personal hygiene, including preparatory activities, combing hair, brushing teeth, shaving, applying make-up, washing/drying face, hands and perineum. Exclude baths and showers.

Procedures: §483.25(a)(1)(i) BATHING, DRESSING, GROOMING

For each sample resident selected for the comprehensive review or the focused review, as appropriate, determine:

1. Whether the resident's ability to bathe, dress and/or groom has changed since admission, or over the past 12 months.
2. Whether the resident's ability to bathe, dress and groom has improved, declined or stayed the same;

TAG NUMBER	REGULATIONS	GUIDANCE FOR SURVEYORS
F310 cont.		

GUIDANCE FOR SURVEYORS

3. Whether any deterioration or lack of improvement was avoidable or unavoidable by:

4. Identifying if resident triggers RAPs for ADL functional/rehabilitation potential.

   a. What risk factors for decline of bathing, dressing, and/or grooming abilities did the facility identify?

   b. What care did the resident receive to address unique needs to maintain his/her bathing, dressing, and/or grooming abilities (e.g., resident needs a button hook to button his shirt; staff teaches the resident how to use it; staff provides resident with dementia with cues that allow him/her to dress him or herself)?

   c. Were individual objectives of the plan of care periodically evaluated, and if the objectives were not met, were alternative approaches developed to encourage maintenance of bathing, dressing, and/or grooming abilities (e.g., resident now unable to button dress, even with encouragement; will ask family if we may use velcro in place of buttons so resident can continue to dress herself)?

TRANSFER AND AMBULATION

Interpretive Guidelines: §483.25(a)(1)(ii)
This corresponds to MDS section E; MDS 2.0 section G when specified for use by the State.

"Transfer" means how resident moves between surfaces—to/from: bed, chair, wheelchair, standing position. (Exclude to/from bath/toilet.)

"Ambulation" means how resident moves between locations in his/her room and adjacent corridor on same floor. If in wheelchair, self-sufficiency once in chair.

Procedures: §483.25(a)(1)(ii) TRANSFER AND AMBULATION
Determine for each resident selected for a comprehensive review, or a focused review as appropriate, whether the resident's ability to transfer and ambulate has declined, improved or stayed the same and whether any deterioration or decline in function was avoidable or unavoidable.

TAG NUMBER

F310 cont.

REGULATIONS

GUIDANCE FOR SURVEYORS

TOILETING

Interpretive Guidelines: §483.25(a)(1)(iii)
This corresponds to MDS section E; MDS 2.0 sections G and H when specified for use by the State.

"Toilet use" means how the resident uses the toilet room (or commode, bedpan, urinal); transfers on/off the toilet, cleanses self, changes pad, manages ostomy or catheters, adjusts clothes.

Procedures: §483.25(a)(1)(iii) TOILETING
Determine for each resident selected for a comprehensive review, or focused review as appropriate, whether the resident's ability to use the toilet has improved, declined or stayed the same and whether any deterioration or decline in improvement was avoidable or unavoidable.

EATING

Interpretive Guidelines: §483.25(a)(1)(iv)
This corresponds to MDS sections E, L1 and MI; MDS 2.0 sections G and K when specified for use by the State.

"Eating" means how resident ingests and drinks (regardless of self-feeding skill).

Procedures: §483.25(a)(1)(iv) EATING
Determine for each resident selected for a comprehensive review, or focused review, as appropriate, whether the resident's ability to eat or eating skills has improved, declined, or stayed the same and whether any deterioration or lack of improvement was avoidable or unavoidable.

If the resident's eating abilities have declined, is there any evidence that the decline was unavoidable?
1. What risk factors for decline of eating skills did the facility identify?
   a. A decrease in the ability to chew and swallow food
   b. Deficit in neurological and muscular status necessary for moving food onto a utensil and into the mouth
   c. Oral health status affecting eating ability
   d. Depression or confused mental state

TAG NUMBER

F310 cont.

REGULATIONS

GUIDANCE FOR SURVEYORS

2. What care did the resident receive to address risk factors and unique needs to maintain eating abilities?
   a. Assistive devices to improve resident's grasp or coordination
   b. Seating arrangements to improve sociability
   c. Seating in a calm, quiet setting for residents with dementia
3. Is there sufficient staff time and assistance provided to maintain eating abilities (e.g., allowing residents enough time to eat independently or with limited assistance)?
4. Identify if resident triggers RAPs for ADL functional/ rehabilitation potential, feeding tubes, and dehydration/fluid maintenance, and the RAPs were used to assess causal reasons for decline, potential for decline or lack of improvement.
5. Were individual objectives of the plan of care periodically evaluated, and if the objectives were not met, were alternative approaches developed to encourage maintaining eating abilities?

USE OF SPEECH, LANGUAGE, OR OTHER FUNCTIONAL COMMUNICATION SYSTEMS
Interpretive Guidelines: §483.25(a)(1)(v)
This corresponds to MDS, section C; MDS 2.0 sections B and C when specified for use by the State.

"Speech, language or other functional communication systems" is defined as the ability to effectively communicate requests, needs, opinions, and urgent problems; to express emotion, to listen to others and to participate in social conversation whether in speech, writing, gesture or a combination of these (e.g., a communication board or electronic augmentative communication device).

Procedures: §483.25(a)(1)(v) USE OF SPEECH, LANGUAGE OR OTHER FUNCTIONAL COMMUNICATION SYSTEMS
Determine for each resident selected for a comprehensive review, or focused review, as appropriate, if resident's ability to communicate has declined, improved or stayed the same and whether any deterioration or lack of improvement was avoidable or unavoidable.

TAG NUMBER

F310 cont.

F311

REGULATIONS

(2) A resident is given the appropriate treatment and services to maintain or improve his or her abilities specified in paragraph (a)(1) of this section

GUIDANCE FOR SURVEYORS

Identify if resident triggers RAPs for communication, psychosocial well-being, mood state, and visual function, and if the RAPs were used to assess causal factors for decline, potential for decline or lack of improvement.

Intent: §483.25(a)(2)
The intent of this regulation is to stress that the facility is responsible for providing maintenance and restorative programs that will not only maintain, but improve, as indicated by the resident's comprehensive assessment to achieve and maintain the highest practicable outcome.

Procedures: §483.25(a)(2)
Use the survey procedure and probes at §483.25(a)(1)(i) through (v) to assist in making this determination.

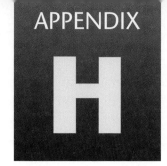
The Americans with Disabilities Act

INTRODUCTION

The Americans with Disabilities Act (ADA) was passed in 1990. This comprehensive legislation was designed to eliminate discrimination against individuals with disabilities. Health care facilities cannot discriminate against individuals with disabilities. The act is lengthy, and is not duplicated here. This summary information is reproduced from: http://www.ada-infonet.org/ovrvew.htm/ with permission of Mr. Duncan C. Kinder.

SUMMARY OF THE ADA

The ADA prohibits discrimination on the basis of disability in employment, State and local government, public accommodations, commercial facilities, transportation, and telecommunications. It also applies to the United States Congress.

To be protected by the ADA, one must have a disability or have a relationship or association with an individual with a disability. An individual with a disability is defined by the ADA as a person who has a physical or mental impairment that substantially limits one or more major life activities, a person who has a history or record of such an impairment, or a person who is perceived by others as having such an impairment. The ADA does not specifically name all of the impairments that are covered.

OVERVIEW OF THE AMERICANS WITH DISABILITIES ACT

Over 43 million Americans with physical or mental impairments that substantially limit daily activities are protected under the ADA. These activities include working, walking, talking, seeing, hearing, or caring for oneself. People who have a record of such an impairment and those regarded as having an impairment are also protected.

The ADA has the following five titles:

Title I—Employment (all Title II employers and private employers with 15 or more employees)

Title II—Public Services (state and local government including public school districts and public transportation)

Title III—Public Accommodations and Services Operated by Private Entities

Title IV—Telecommunications

Title V—Miscellaneous Provisions

The following is a brief summary of some of the major requirements contained in the ADA statute.

To determine all of the requirements that a covered entity must satisfy, it is necessary to refer to the regulations, guidelines, and/or technical assistance materials that have been developed by the Department of Justice (DOJ), the Equal Employment Opportunity Commission (EEOC), the Department of Transportation (DOT), the Federal Communications Commission (FCC), and the Architectural and Transportation Barriers Compliance Board (the Access Board). In addition, the Internal Revenue Service (IRS) has developed regulations on the tax relief available for certain costs of complying with the ADA, such as small business tax credits.

Title I—Employment

Title I of the ADA prohibits discrimination in employment against people with disabilities. It requires employers to make reasonable accommodations to the known physical or mental limitations of a qualified applicant or employee, unless such accommodation would impose an undue hardship on the employer. Reasonable accommodations include such actions as making worksites accessible, modifying existing equipment, providing new devices, modifying work schedules, restructuring jobs, and providing readers or interpreters.

Title I also prohibits the use of employment tests and other selection criteria that screen out, or tend to screen out, individuals with disabilities, unless such tests or criteria are shown to be job-related and consistent with business necessity. It also bans the use of pre-employment medical examinations or inquiries to determine if an applicant has a disability. It does, however, permit the use of a medical examination after a job offer has been made if the results are kept confidential; all persons offered employment in the same job category are required to take them; and the results are not used to discriminate.

Employers are permitted, at any time, to inquire about the ability of a job applicant or employee to perform job-related functions. The EEOC is the enforcement agency for Title I.

Title II—Public Services

Title II of the ADA requires that the services and programs of local and State governments, as well as other non-Federal government agencies, shall operate their programs so that when viewed in their entirety are readily accessible to and usable by individuals with disabilities.

Title II entities:

- do not need to remove physical barriers, such as stairs, in all existing buildings, as long as they make their programs accessible to individuals who are unable to use an inaccessible existing facility.
- must provide appropriate auxiliary aids to ensure that communications with individuals with hearing, vision, or speech impairments are as effective as communications with others, unless an undue burden or fundamental alteration would result.
- may impose safety requirements that are necessary for the safe operation of a Title II program if they are based on actual risks and not on mere speculation, stereotypes, or generalizations about individuals with disabilities.

In addition, Title II seeks to ensure that people with disabilities have access to existing public transportation services. All new buses must be accessible. Transit authorities must provide supplementary paratransit services or other special transportation services for individuals with disabilities who cannot use fixed-route bus services, unless this would present an undue burden.

Title III—Public Accommodations

Public accommodations include the broad range of privately-owned entities that affect commerce, including sales, rental, and service establishments; private educational institutions; recreational facilities; and social service centers. In providing goods and services, a public accommodation may not use eligibility requirements that exclude or segregate individuals with disabilities, unless the requirements are "necessary" for the operation of the public accommodation. As an example, restricting people with Down's Syndrome to a certain area of a restaurant would violate Title III. It also requires public accommodations to make reasonable modifications to policies, practices, and procedures, unless those modifications would fundamentally alter the nature of the services provided by the public accommodation.

Title III also requires that public accommodations provide auxiliary aids necessary to enable persons who have visual, hearing, or sensory impairments to participate in the program, but only if their provision will not result in an undue burden on the business. Thus, for example, a restaurant would not be required to provide menus in braille for blind patrons if it requires its wait persons to read the menu. The auxiliary aid requirement is flexible. A public accommodation may choose among various alternatives as long as the result is effective communication.

With respect to existing facilities of public accommodations, physical barriers must be removed when it is "readily achievable" to do so (i.e., when it can be accomplished easily and without much expense). Tax write-offs are available to minimize the costs associated with the removal of barriers in existing buildings or in providing auxiliary aids, including interpreters for the deaf. Modifications that would be readily achievable in most cases include the ramping of a few steps. However, all construction of new building facilities and alterations of existing facilities in public accommodations, as well as in commercial facilities such as office buildings, must comply with the ADA Accessibility Guidelines (ADAAG) so they are accessible to people with disabilities. New privately owned buildings are not required to install elevators if they are less than three stories high or have less than 3,000 square feet per story, unless the building is a shopping center, mall, or a professional office of a health care provider.

Title III also addresses transportation provided by private entities.

Title IV—Telecommunications

Title IV of the ADA amends the Communications Act of 1934 to require that telephone companies provide telecommunication relay services. The relay services must provide speech-impaired or hearing-impaired individuals who use TTYs or other non-voice terminal devices opportunities for communication that are equivalent to those provided to other customers.

Title V—Miscellaneous Provisions

This title addresses such issues as the ADA's relationship to other laws including the Rehabilitation Act of 1973, requirements relating to the provision of insurance, regulations by the Access Board, prohibition of State immunity, inclusion of Congress as a covered entity, implementation of each title, promotion of alternative means of dispute resolution, and provision of technical assistance.

Additional Information

For additional information and answers to your questions, call
1-800-949-4232.

ADA Information Line

The U.S. Department of Justice provides information about the Americans with Disabilities Act (ADA) through a toll-free ADA Information Line. This service permits businesses, State and local governments, or others to call and ask questions about general or specific ADA requirements including questions about the ADA Standards for Accessible Design.

ADA specialists are available Monday through Friday from 10:00 AM until 6:00 PM (eastern time) except on Thursday when the hours are 1:00 PM until 6:00 PM.

Spanish language service is also available. For general ADA information, answers to specific technical questions, free ADA materials, or information about filing a complaint, call:

800 - 514 - 0301 (voice)
800 - 514 - 0383 (TDD)

http://www.usdoj.gov/crt/ada/adahom1.htm

Glossary

Note: The number in parentheses following the term is the chapter in which the term is first introduced.

abduction (11)—moving an extremity away from the body.

abduction pillow (6)—a special pillow to keep the legs apart in residents who have had hip replacement surgery.

abrasion (8)—superficial scrape in the top layer of skin.

active assisted range of motion (AAROM) exercises (11)—exercises that are either started or completed by the resident.

active range of motion (AROM) exercises (11)—exercises done by residents each day during movement, ADLs, certain activities, and in exercise groups.

adaptive devices (9)—equipment used to assist residents in performing everyday tasks.

adduction (11)—moving an extremity *toward* the body.

airborne precautions (4)—isolation precautions used for residents whose disease is spread by the airborne method of transmission.

all-inclusive (1)—covers all care the individual receives.

antecedent (18)—an event that causes or triggers a behavior.

aphasia (7)—loss of the ability to speak or understand what is spoken.

apraxia (15)—the inability to plan a motor activity.

aquathermia pad (6)—localized heat treatment in which water circulates through the coils inside a plastic pad.

arthritis (6)—a condition of the joints that can cause mild discomfort to severe deformities and disability; it is common in the elderly.

aspiration (14)—a serious condition in which food is inhaled into the lungs, causing complications.

assessment (2)—an evaluation of the resident's condition; the first step of the nursing process.

assisted transfers (12)—transfers in which the nursing assistant moves the resident; the resident actively assists in the transfer.

associate reactions (15)—muscle spasms caused by an increase in muscle tone; may be the result of insecurity, excitement, fear, or overactivity.

ataxic gait (13)—a way of walking that appears uncoordinated; the resident keeps the legs farther apart than normal for support.

atrophy (11)—muscle weakness and wasting from lack of use.

autoimmune disorder (7)—a condition in which the individual makes antibodies that work against his or her own body.

avulsion fracture (6)—a fracture in which a bone fragment is pulled off at the point of ligament or tendon attachment.

axilla (11)—the armpit or underarm.

axillary crutches (13)—crutches made of wood or aluminum; provide moderate stability.

biofeedback (17)—a process of providing visual and auditory information to give the resident voluntary control.

bridging (9)—a technique used to elevate an area off the surface of the bed, completely relieving pressure.

cerebrovascular accident (CVA) (7)—a stroke or brain attack; caused by a sudden interruption of blood flow to the brain.

chorea (7)—rapid, jerking, involuntary movements.

circumduction (11)—a circular movement of a joint, such as the thumb or wrist.

clavicle strap (6)—an appliance used to immobilize and treat a fractured clavicle (collarbone).

closed (simple) fracture (6)—a fracture in which the skin is intact and not broken.

comminuted fracture (6)—a fracture in which the bone is shattered and splintered into more than three fragments.

compensation (18)—using strength and overachieving in one area to overcome a weakness in another area.

complete fracture (6)—break across the entire cross-section of the bone.

compound fracture. *See* open fracture.

compression fracture (6)—a fracture of the vertebrae of the spine, in which the bone collapses inward.

congenital disorders (7)—conditions present at birth.

consequence (18)—the outcome of a behavior.

consistency (1)—sameness; means that all staff members approach and care for the resident in the same manner.

constrict (6)—to make smaller.

contact precautions (4)—type of isolation used to contain pathogens that are spread by direct or indirect contact; the microbes are usually found in infections of the skin, wounds, mucous membranes, urine, and fecal material.

continuity of care (1)—goal achieved when all staff members approach and care for the resident in the same manner.

cumulative trauma disorders (10)—bodily injuries to nerves, tissues, tendons, and joints that occur from repeated stress and strain over a period of months to years.

cryotherapy (6)—cold treatments.

debride (4)—a method of cleaning wounds to remove eschar, or dead tissue.

decline (1)—deterioration in condition that is not permitted, according to OBRA '87, unless it is medically unavoidable.

dehydration (14)—a serious condition in which liquid intake is not adequate to maintain minimum body functions; untreated, it can lead to many complications, including death.

delirium (18)—mental confusion caused by an acute medical illness.

demonstration (5)—showing the resident what you want him or her to do.

denial (18)—refusing to admit there is a problem.

dependent continence (17)—term used to describe residents who are physically or mentally impaired, but are kept dry by staff.

dependent transfers (12)—transfers in which the nursing assistant does the work; resident participation is minimal.

depressed fracture (6)—a fracture of the skull or face, in which the bone is depressed and forced inward.

dermis (8)—the thick, inner layer of skin.

diaphragmatic breathing (16)—a method of slowing the respiratory rate and increasing the ability to take a deep breath.

diathermy (6)—heat treatments.

dietary personnel (2)—the team members who provide proper nutrition and ensure that residents' dietary needs are addressed.

dietitian (2)—the team member who plans the menus and develops special diets to address residents' medical problems and needs.

digits (9)—fingers and toes.

dilate (6)—enlarge; make larger.

displaced (6)—improperly aligned.

disuse atrophy (13)—muscular wasting from lack of use.

dorsal flexion (dorsiflexion) (11)—pulling the foot upward toward the head (toward the shin).

droplet precautions (4)—type of isolation precautions used for some residents whose infection is spread by droplets in the air; the droplets remain within three feet of the resident.

duration (10)—the length of time a person is continually exposed to a risk factor.

dynamic splints (9)—flexible splints that are recommended for most immobility contractures. They enable the resident to move the joint in flexion and extension.

dynamometer (13)—instrument used to measure hand and grip strength.

dysphagia (14)—difficulty swallowing food and liquids.

ecchymosis (6)—bruising.

emotional lability (7)—crying or laughing uncontrollably for no apparent reason.

empathy (1)—understanding how the resident feels.

enabler (9)—a device that empowers residents and assists them to function at their highest level.

epidermis (8)—the outer layer of skin.

ergonomic hazards (10)—workplace conditions that create biomechanical stress on the worker.

ergonomics (10)—a method of fitting or matching the job to the worker.

eschar (8)—black, leathery, devitalized tissue.

evaluation (2)—the fourth step in the nursing process; involves critically reviewing care plan goals and approaches to see if they are working.

eversion (11)—turning a joint outward.

exacerbations (6)—times in which a condition seems to worsen; an aggravation of symptoms or an increase in the severity of a chronic condition.

expressive aphasia (7)—the inability to form or express thoughts.

extension (11)—straightening a joint.

external fixation devices (6)—metal appliances that are sometimes used to treat fractures and other orthopedic conditions.

external rotation (6)—a condition in which a fractured leg is shortened with the toes pointing outward. Also (11), turning a joint outward, away from the median line.

fine motor exercises (6)—exercises to develop skill using small muscles.

flaccid paralysis (7)—loss of muscle tone and absence of tendon reflexes.

flexion (11)—bending a joint.

fluid restrictions (14)—limiting the total amount of fluid the resident can have in a 24-hour period.

Fowler's position (8)—semi-sitting position, in which the head of the bed is elevated.

fracture (6)—a break in a bone.

friction (8)—damage to the skin that occurs when the skin rubs against another surface.

functional distance (12)—the distance a resident must ambulate to reach a specific location or activity.

functional incontinence (17)—incontinence related to the inability to reach the bathroom in time; may be caused by mobility problems, restraints, disorientation, or inability to find the bathroom.

gait (13)—the way a person walks.

gait training (13)—a method of teaching a resident to walk; also involves teaching the resident to get in and out of a chair, walk on uneven or irregular surfaces, go up and down stairs and curbs, and use assistive ambulation devices.

generalized application (6)—treatment that delivers heat or cold to the entire body.

global aphasia (7)—loss of all speech and language ability.

goniometer (11)—an instrument used for measuring a resident's range of motion.

gout (6)—a severely disabling metabolic disease caused by increased uric acid, which deposits in the joints, causing pain.

greenstick fracture (6)—a fracture in which one side of the bone is broken and the other side is bent.

gross motor exercises (11)—exercises for large muscle groups; done with residents who have a limited response to the environment.

guarding (12)—positioning and using your body in a manner that keeps the resident safe.

habit training (17)—a toileting program used for residents who are mentally confused and urinate at fairly predictable times.

hand-over-hand technique (5)—placing your hand over the resident's hand and guiding him or her to perform the desired action.

health maintenance organization (HMO) (1)—group of health care providers funded by Medicare, Medicaid, or private money.

hemianopsia (7)—loss of half the visual field.

hemiplegia (7)—paralysis on one side of the body.

holistic (2)—emphasizing the organic or functional relation between parts and the whole.

holistic care (2)—a method of caring for residents in which caregivers consider the whole person.

hydrocollator (6)—a rectangular tank containing very hot water used to warm hot packs.

hydromassage (6)—the massaging effect of circulating hot water in the whirlpool.

hydrotherapy (6)—hot water therapy.

hyperextension (11)—gentle, excessive extension of a joint, slightly past the point of resistance.

impacted fracture (6)—a fracture in which the fragment from one bone is wedged into another bone.

implementation (2)—the third step in the nursing process; involves putting the care plan into action.

incentive spirometry (16)—a form of goal-directed therapy in which the goal is deep breathing.

incomplete fracture (6)—a fracture involving part of the cross-section of bone.

incontinence management program (catch program) (17)—method that involves toileting the resident on a regular schedule to prevent incontinence; residents that benefit from this program have no potential for retraining and cannot communicate the need to use the bathroom.

independent continence (17)—the ability to maintain continence without assistance.

instantaneous injuries (10)—injuries that occur suddenly and without warning, such as accidents.

instrumental activities of daily living (IADLs) (15)—higher-level tasks that are required for living in the community, such as paying bills, planning a menu, making a shopping list, or driving a car.

internal rotation (11)—turning a joint inward toward the median line.

inversion (11)—turning a joint inward.

ischemic area (8)—an area that has been deprived of blood flow and oxygen.

isometrics (11)—the science of physical exercise without movement.

isometric exercises (11)—exercises that help maintain strength when a joint is immobilized; these exercises use the body's own resistance.

Kegel exercises (17)—pelvic floor exercises used to strengthen muscles and prevent incontinence.

lateral position (8)—side-lying position; the resident can be positioned on either side.

licensed and certified therapy assistants (2)—individuals with several years of education in their specialty; assistants can do many of the things licensed therapists do, but cannot perform evaluations.

licensed nurses (RN, LPN/LVN) (2)—members of the interdisciplinary team who communicate the residents' needs and progress to the physician; responsible for seeing that the medical plan of care and orders for restorative services are followed.

lifting technique (12)—method used when three or more staff members must physically lift a resident who is lying down from one surface to another.

localized application (6)—treatment that delivers heat or cold to a specific area.

Lofstrand crutches (forearm or Canadian crutches) (13)—crutches with a cuff that fits around the forearm, so the resident can release the hand grip without dropping the crutch.

mechanical debridement (4)—a method of removing dead tissue from wounds; the procedure is done by licensed personnel using sterile instruments.

medial (11)—pertains to or is situated toward the midline of the body.

median (11)—situated in the median plane or in the midline of the body.

Medicaid (1)—health care program funded by both the state and federal governments; pays for health care for individuals with low income.

medical model (5)—a method of caring for residents in which the emphasis is on treating the illness or medical condition.

Medicare (1)—federally funded health care program for individuals who are elderly or disabled.

Medicare Part A (1)—the part of the Medicare program that pays the hospital or long-term care facility a set rate for room, board, and all care and supplies.

Medicare Part B (1)—the part of Medicare that pays for some diagnostic tests, splints, braces, prosthetics, and therapy evaluations and services.

Minimum Data Set 2.0 (MDS 2.0) (2)—assessment component of the RAI; information about the resident is gathered using this document.

mixed incontinence (17)—a combination of urge and stress incontinence.

mobility (1)—the ability to move about.

modified barium swallow (14)—a special x-ray study that shows the resident's potential for aspiration.

moribund (8)—near death; dying.

narrative (19)—information given in story format.

nebulizer (4)—a hand-held unit used for administering medications by inhalation.

necrosis (8)—tissue death; necrotic tissue is black and leathery in appearance.

negative-pressure environment (4)—the atmosphere in an airborne precautions room, in which the ventilation is reversed so that room air is drawn upward into the vents.

neurogenic bladder (7)—a condition in which the resident is unaware of the sensation of urine in the bladder; in this condition, the bladder does not empty completely.

neuropathy (8)—a painful condition of the nervous system that affects the lower legs and predisposes residents to ulcerations.

NIOSH-approved respirator (4)—type of mask approved by the National Institute for Occupational Safety and Health; worn in an airborne precautions room; the masks have tiny pores that most pathogens cannot fit through.

nonrapid eye movement (NREM) sleep (3)—consists of approximately 80% of the sleep cycle; NREM sleep has four phases, progressing from light to very deep.

nursing assistants (2)—team members who reinforce the teaching that the therapist, restorative nurse, and restorative nursing assistant have done.

nursing process (2)—process used when caring for residents; involves assessment, planning, implementation, and evaluation.

oblique fracture (6)—a fracture that runs at an angle across the bone.

OBRA '87 (1)—abbreviation for the Omnibus Budget Reconciliation Act of 1987, which caused significant changes in the long-term care industry.

occupational therapist (2)—team member who evaluates and treats residents for self-care, work, and ADLs.

open (compound) fracture (6)—a fracture in which the skin over the fracture is broken.

open reduction internal fixation (ORIF) (6)—a method of treating a fracture in which the fracture is stabilized with a metal plate, screws, nails, or pins.

opposition (11)—touching each of the fingers against the thumb.

orthopneic position (16)—same as high Fowler's position; used for residents with respiratory conditions.

orthotic devices (5)—appliances that improve function and prevent deformities.

osteoarthritis (6)—a chronic condition that causes deterioration of the joints.

osteoporosis (6)—a metabolic disorder of the bones in which bone mass is lost; causes bones to become porous, spongy, and easily broken.

overflow incontinence (17)—urine release that occurs when the bladder is very full and the resident cannot hold the urine.

palmar flexion (11)—bending the hand down toward the palm.

paralysis (7)—loss of sensation and voluntary movement below the level of a spinal cord injury.

paraplegia (7)—paralysis of the lower half of the body, including both legs.

paresis (11)—weakness; slight paralysis.

passive range-of-motion (PROM) exercises (11)—exercises performed by the restorative assistant for residents with conditions such as paralysis, contractures, orthopedic and neurologic disorders, or severe cognitive impairment, or when independent movement is impossible.

pathologic fracture (6)—a fracture in a diseased bone that occurs as a result of osteoporosis, a tumor, or cancer.

percussion (16)—a treatment performed by a licensed practitioner for obstructive airway disorders; done by covering the resident's back with a towel, cupping the hands, and clapping against the chest wall to loosen secretions.

phantom pain (6)—pain from severed nerves in an extremity that has been removed.

physical restraints (9)—any manual method or physical or mechanical device, material, or equipment attached or adjacent to the body that the resident cannot remove easily and that restricts the resident's freedom of movement or normal access to his or her own body.

physical therapist (2)—team member concerned with preventing physical disability; uses physical methods to evaluate and treat pain, disease, and injury.

physician (2)—team member who directs the resident's medical care.

pivot technique (12)—a method of moving residents who can bear weight on at least one leg.

planning (2)—second step in the nursing process; describes problems, goals, and approaches to use when caring for the resident.

plantar flexion (9)—a position in which the foot is extended with the toes facing downward; bending the foot downward, away from the body.

postural support (9)—a device used as an enabler that maintains body position and alignment.

preferred provider organization (PPO) (1)—organization that provides reimbursement for health care.

pressure ulcer (8)—an ischemic ulceration and/or necrosis of tissues overlying a bony prominence that has been subjected to pressure, friction, or shear.

problem-oriented medical record (POMR) (19)—a method of maintaining the medical record in which information is divided into five general categories.

progressive mobility (12)—exercises that increase the resident's activity level gradually.

projection (18)—blaming someone or something else for a problem.

prompted voiding (17)—a toileting program for cognitively impaired residents who cannot participate in more complex incontinence retraining programs; each time staff enters the room, they ask the resident if he or she is wet or dry; the resident is assisted and encouraged to use the toilet.

pronation (11)—moving a joint to face downward.

prone position (8)—lying on the abdomen, with the head turned to one side.

prostate gland (17)—a gland surrounding the urethra just below the bladder in the male; this gland often enlarges in elderly residents, causing urinary retention and other complications.

prosthetic devices (5)—replacements for body parts.

pursed-lip breathing (16)—one type of breathing exercises for residents with obstructive airway disease; exercises help relieve shortness of breath by slowing down rapid respirations and allowing more complete exhalation.

quad cane (13)—a cane with four feet; provides extra stability.

quadriplegia (7)—paralysis affecting the arms and legs.

radial deviation (11)—turning the forearm toward the radius.

rapid eye movement (REM) sleep (3)—the portion of the sleep cycle in which there is rapid eye movement. Dreams occur during this part of sleep. Mental function is restored during REM sleep.

rationalization (18)—providing an acceptable but untrue reason for a problem.

reasonable accommodation (5)—changing things in the facility or environment to meet a resident's needs.

receptive aphasia (7)—inability to understand the spoken word.

reflex incontinence (17)—loss of urine in residents with paralysis and neurologic disorders; the resident is unaware of the urge to void.

rehabilitation (1)—services delivered by licensed therapists to assist the resident to attain and maintain his or her highest potential.

rehabilitation programs (5)—programs designed by licensed therapists to help residents regain lost skills or to teach new skills.

rehabilitation team (2)—licensed therapists, licensed and certified therapy assistants, and specially trained restorative nursing assistants; team members evaluate and treat residents, design rehabilitation and restorative programs, teach and train facility staff and family members, and provide consultation when needed.

reminiscence (18)—remembering the past.

remissions (6)—times in which a disease appears stable or retreats.

repetitive motions (10)—movements repeated frequently for prolonged periods; these movements increase fatigue and cause muscle and tendon strain over time.

Resident Assessment Instrument (RAI) (2)—written tool developed by the government to assess residents; consists of the MDS, triggers, and RAPs.

resident assessment protocols (RAPs) (2)—lists of information and guidelines that help link the comprehensive assessment (MDS) with care plan goals.

resistive range-of-motion exercises (11)—exercises prescribed by the licensed therapist to increase strength; residents perform these exercises by working against manual or mechanical resistance.

respiratory therapist (2)—team member who works with residents having problems with oxygenation; performs breathing treatments and exercises.

restorative environment (5)—an environment in which residents can be as independent as possible.

restorative nurse (2)—RN who has special training in rehabilitation and restoration; oversees the restorative care program and acts as a liaison with therapies.

restorative nursing assistant (RNA) (1)—team member who works directly with residents to meet their needs for restorative care.

restorative nursing care (1)—services given by nursing personnel based on a belief in the dignity and worth of each resident as a unique individual; designed to assist residents to attain and maintain the highest level of function possible in their individual situations.

retraction (11)—drawing back, away from the body.

rheumatoid arthritis (6)—a systemic, inflammatory condition that attacks muscles, tendons, ligaments, and blood vessels in the joints, causing severe deformities.

risk factors (1)—conditions with the potential to cause the resident's health to worsen.

rotation (11)—moving a joint in, out, and around.

safe lifting zone (10)—the area between your knees and your shoulders.

scheduled toileting (17)—term used to describe a toileting program for residents who recognize the urge to use the toilet, but do not have the physical or mental ability to get there without help.

self-actualization (3)—a sense of accomplishment and success.

self-esteem (3)—the mental image a person has of himself or herself.

self-care deficit (5)—a state in which a resident cannot perform or complete an activity.

self-limiting (2)—conditions that will resolve themselves without intervention.

semiprone position (8)—variation of the prone position; minimizes pressure ulcer development.

semisupine position (tilt position) (8)—variation of the supine position; minimizes pressure ulcer development; the resident is tilted at an angle, slightly to the side.

senile purpura (8)—bruising in the elderly; caused by fragile blood vessels.

set up (5)—to prepare equipment and supplies for an activity.

shearing (8)—stretching the skin in one direction while the underlying bone moves in the opposite direction.

simple fracture. *See* closed fracture.

skeletal traction (6)—treatment for a fracture that involves surgically placing a wire, pin, or tongs into or through the fractured bone.

skilled therapy (5)—treatment by a licensed therapist that is designed to restore recently lost function.

skilled unit (1)—the area of the hospital or long-term care facility in which residents receiving Medicare Part A services reside.

skin traction (6)—treatment for a fracture that uses a halter or foam belt, boot, or other device attached to a weight on the injured extremity.

sliding technique (12)—method of moving residents from one surface to another when the resident cannot bear weight.

sling and swathe (6)—an appliance used to immobilize and treat a fractured humerus.

SOAP documentation (19)—SOAP is an abbreviation for **S**ubjective, **O**bjective, **A**ssessment, **P**lan. Facilities using this documentation format write an entry for each category.

social continence (17)—term used to describe residents who cannot maintain continence independently or through regular toileting by staff and who depend on absorbent products and other measures to contain urine.

social worker (2)—team member who helps residents make the adjustment from living in the community to life in the facility.

source-oriented medical record (SOMR) (19)—a method of managing medical records in which information in the record is divided into categories by discipline.

spastic paralysis (7)—absence of voluntary movement; extremities move in an involuntary pattern, similar to muscle spasms.

spasticity (7)—muscle spasms; involuntary movements.

spatial-perceptual deficit (7)—inability to differentiate right from left or up from down.

speech therapist (2)—team member who uses special techniques and skills to help residents with communication and swallowing disorders.

spiral fracture (6)—a fracture that twists around the bone.

staff development director (SDC) (2)—team member who orients and teaches the facility's restorative philosophy to all personnel. He or she teaches new staff members the skills and techniques necessary to provide basic restorative care.

standard precautions (4)—infection control guidelines introduced in 1996; used in the care of all residents.

standby assistance (12)—supervising the resident.

static splints (9)—stiff splints; these increase the risk of injury in residents with increased spasticity.

stress incontinence (17)—a condition in which the bladder leaks urine when the pelvic muscles are strained (when the resident moves, laughs, coughs, sneezes, or lifts).

subcutaneous tissue (8)—the fatty layer beneath the dermis; the deepest layer of skin.

subluxation (7)—dislocation.

supination (11)—moving a joint so it faces upward.

supine position (8)—lying on the back, face up.

sympathy (1)—feeling sorry for the resident.

task analysis (5)—an analysis of the steps in a task that the resident can complete independently.

therapeutic exercises (11)—exercises that are specifically planned for individual residents to maintain or improve joint function.

thermotherapy (6)—heat treatments.

traction (6)—a treatment for fractures in which the bone ends are pulled into place with ropes and weights.

transition (12)—movement between two surfaces.

transmission-based precautions (4)—the second tier of the 1996 CDC recommendations; designed to replace the isolation categories previously used.

transverse fracture (6)—a break completely across a bone.

trapeze (6)—equipment applied to the bed (overhanging bar) to assist the resident with movement.

triggers (2)—conditions identified by the MDS 2.0 as needing further assessment; most require a care plan intervention; conditions trigger because the resident has an actual condition with the potential for declines, the resident has a risk factor, or the resident is a candidate for a restorative program. If a condition triggers, personnel must review a RAP.

tunneling (8)—deep areas or "tunnels" extending far back from a wound crater into the subcutaneous tissue.

ulnar deviation (11)—turning the forearm toward the ulna.

ultrasonic treatments (4)—treatments that use high-frequency sound waves; performed by licensed therapists to reduce inflammation.

ultrasound (6)—high-frequency sound.

undermining (8)—a lip, rim, or edge surrounding a wound bed; similar to tunneling.

unilateral neglect (7)—condition in which the resident ignores the affected side of the body.

urge incontinence (17)—having to use the bathroom immediately after taking a drink, or hearing running water; if the resident does not reach the toilet immediately, the bladder will empty completely and involuntarily.

urinary retention (17)—the inability to empty the bladder completely.

validation therapy (18)—a technique developed by Naomi Feil to maintain the identity and dignity of residents, and make persons with dementia feel good about themselves.

vascular (6)—an area containing many blood vessels, which bleeds readily.

verbal cues (5)—brief, clear, and concise directions or hints that prompt the resident to do something.

Index